RECENT ADVANCES IN

# Sexually Transmitted Diseases and AIDS

RECENT ADVANCES IN

# Sexually Transmitted Diseases and AIDS

Edited by

## John R.W. Harris MB BCh BAO MRCP

Senior Consultant Physician, St Mary's Hospital, London, UK

## Susie M. Forster MRCP

Senior Lecturer, St Mary's Hospital Medical School, London, UK

NUMBER FOUR

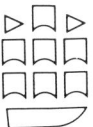

CHURCHILL LIVINGSTONE
EDINBURGH LONDON MELBOURNE NEW YORK AND TOKYO 1991

CHURCHILL LIVINGSTONE
Medical Division of Longman Group UK Limited

Distributed in the United States of America by Churchill
Livingstone Inc., 1560 Broadway, New York, NY 10036, and
by associated companies, branches and representatives
throughout the world

First published 1991

ISBN 0-443-04123-7
ISSN 0143-6805

Produced by Longman Singapore Publishers Pte Ltd

Printed in Singapore

# Preface

The main means of transmission of HIV across the world is by sexual contact and the emergence of this infection has produced a well overdue resurgence of interest in sexually transmitted diseases in general. The title of this issue has changed from that of its predecessors in the series, reflecting the belief of the editors that the management of HIV infection and AIDS cannot be separated from that of all sexually transmitted diseases, and an interest in one must presuppose an interest in the others. In this and future issues we hope to achieve a balance between representing the enormous volume of work in the field of HIV with the equally important advances being made in the field of all sexually transmitted disease. We would like to thank all our contributors, the patient staff of Churchill Livingstone, and in particular Miss Jackie Harris for her excellent secretarial assistance.

J. R. W. H.
S. M. F.

London, 1991

# Contributors

**Jane E. Armes** BMedSci BM BS
Department of Pathology, University of Melbourne, Victoria, Australia

**Susan Barter** MB BS MRCP DMRD FRCR
Consultant Radiologist, Royal Masonic Hospital, London

**Raymond P. Brettle** BSc MB ChB FRCP
Consultant, Infectious Diseases Unit, The City Hospital, Edinburgh; Part-time Senior Lecturer, Department of Medicine, University of Edinburgh

**Sophie Day** PhD
Research Associate, Department of Anthropology,
London School of Economics; Honorary Research Fellow,
Academic Department of Public Health, St Mary's Hospital Medical
School, London

**Anthon De Schryver** MD DPH
Associate Professional Officer, Programme of Sexually Transmitted
Diseases,World Health Organization, Geneva

**A Doble** MB FRCS
Formerly Research Registrar, Department of Urology, St Mary's Hospital
Medical School, London; Currently Registrar in Urology, Battle Hospital,
Reading

**Charles S.F. Easmon** MD PhD MRCPath
Fleming Professor of Medical Microbiology, St Mary's Hospital Medical
School, London

**Peter J. Flegg** MRCP DTM&H
Research Fellow, Infectious Diseases Unit, The City Hospital, Edinburgh

**George E. Griffin** BSc PhD FRCP
Wellcome Trust Senior Lecturer, Department of Molecular & Cellular
Sciences, Head of Infectious Diseases Section, St George's Hospital
Medical School, London

**Catherine A. Ison** PhD MSc FIMLS
Research Fellow, Department of Bacteriology, St Mary's Hospital Medical School, London

**Linda R. MacCallum** MB ChB
Clinical Medical Officer, Infectious Diseases Unit, The City Hospital, Edinburgh

**André Meheus** MD DPH Phd
Programme Manager Programme of Sexually Transmitted Diseases, World Health Organisation, Geneva

**Rory Shaw** BSc MD MRCP
Senior Lecturer and Honorary Consultant, Department of Respiratory Medicine, St Mary's Hospital Medical School, London

**David Taylor-Robinson** MD FRCPath
Head, Division of Sexually Transmitted Diseases, Clinical Research Centre, Harrow; Professor of Genitourinary Microbiology and Medicine, St Mary's Hospital Medical School, London

**Helen Ward** MB ChB
Research Fellow in Epidemiology, Academic Department of Public Health, St Mary's Hospital Medical School, London

**Jon Weber**
Senior Lecturer, Department of Medicine, Royal Postgraduate Medical School, Hammersmith Hospital, London

# Contents

# *Pneumocystis carinii* pneumonia diagnosis, treatment and prophylaxis

*R.J. Shaw*

## INTRODUCTION

*Pneumocystis carinii* pneumonia (PCP) is a common sequeli of compromised host immunity. In AIDS, it is a frequent cause of pneumonitis, occurring in over 60% of cases (Centers for Disease Control 1986, Wharton et al 1986, Haverkos et al 1984, Federal Drug Administration 1985). The organism is a protozoa similar to *Toxoplasma gondii*, and has trophozoite and cystic forms.

## *P. CARINII* LIFE CYCLE

Studies in animal tissue suggest that free-floating trophozoites attach to host cells, where the walls appear to thicken and internal convolutions develop. The cysts then detach from the host cell and are seen to contain up to eight intra-cystic sporozoites. The cysts rupture to release these as trophozoites (Pifer et al 1977).

## PATHOLOGY

With only rare exceptions *P. carinii* infection is confined to the lung. On hematoxylin and eosin staining, the alveoli are seen to contain a foamy eosinophilic material which contains few inflammatory cells, but which with a silver stain is observed to contain the cysts of *P. carinii* (Weber et al 1977). With increasing severity, an increase in the number of alveolar macrophages occurs. In the interstitium between the alveoli, there is a mild to moderate infiltration by lymphocytes. In a proportion of cases, there is also evidence of some fibrosis within the interstitium (LeGlovan & Heidelberger 1973). These observations derive from PCP in patients immunocompromised for reasons other than HIV infection, but it is thought that the pathology in PCP is similar irrespective of whether it is associated with HIV or non-HIV immunocompromise (Sterling et al 1984).

## DIAGNOSIS

The clinical features of PCP may be subtle, and a high index of suspicion is required. A number of non-invasive tests are available to help identify patients

1

with minor symptoms who merit further investigation by more invasive means to confirm the diagnosis. Arguments to treat patients with a presumptive clinical diagnosis of PCP and thus avoid further investigation have not been generally accepted. Such a policy poses difficulty if a patient deteriorates despite treatment, when they may be too ill for further investigation to identify other pathogens. It is also difficult for discussions of prognosis to take place in the face of uncertainty as to whether a patient has a definite complication of AIDS or merely a bacterial pneumonia and positive HIV serology.

## Symptoms

PCP may occur in a previously healthy individual, or new respiratory symptoms may be superimposed on those due to other HIV-related conditions. The symptoms of PCP are dyspnoea (68%), dry cough (81%) and fevers (81%) (Kovacs et al 1984). When compared to other immunodeficiency states, there is a longer prodrome in AIDS, with fever for an average of 7 weeks and cough and dyspnoea for 3 to 5 weeks (Engelberg et al 1984, Kovacs et al 1984, Sterling et al 1984). Other pulmonary symptoms such as chest pain (14–23% of cases) and sputum production (23–30%) may be present. Systemic symptoms are common, including weight loss (32–100%), night sweats (12–66%), chills (12–26%), fatigue or malaise (12–100%) (Barron et al 1985, Engelberg et al 1984, Kales et al 1987, Kovacs et al 1984, Sterling et al 1984, Tuazon et al 1985). However, 6–7% of cases may be completely asymptomatic (Barron et al 1985, Engelberg et al 1984).

## Physical examination

Three quarters of the patients with PCP have a temperature above 38°C and the majority an increase in respiratory rate (Kales et al 1987, Kovacs et al 1984, Tuazon et al 1985). Examination of the chest is usually unremarkable, with inspiratory crackles present in less than one third of the patients. Thus the absence of adventitial breath sounds is not helpful in excluding the presence of PCP. Signs suggestive of consolidation or pleural effusion are more often due to pathology other than PCP.

## Chest X-ray

The single most useful investigation in suspected PCP is the chest X-ray. There are a wide variety of changes which reflect the severity of the infection. In up to 15% of cases the chest X-ray is normal. At the next level of severity there is a perihilar haze (see Fig. 1.1) which, as the disease progresses, coalesces to give homogeneous airspace shadowing extending bilaterally from the hilum, but often sparing the apices and costophrenic angles (Stover et al

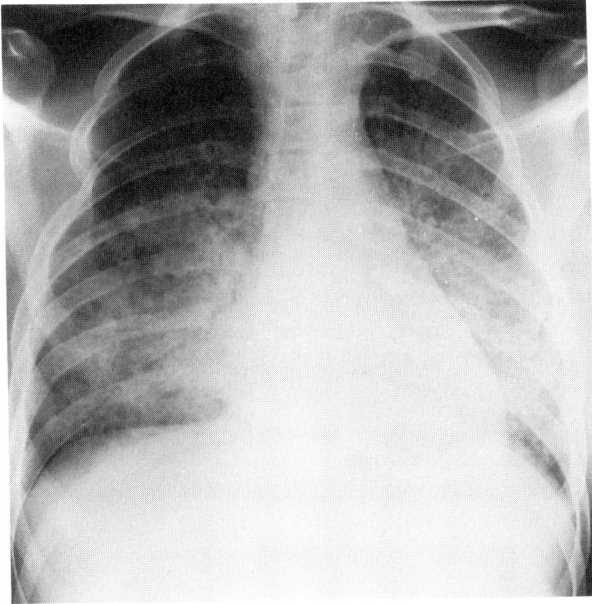

**Fig. 1.1**   Chest X-ray of *P. carinii* pneumonia, showing perihilar infiltrate

1985). In the final stages there is dense bilateral homogeneous consolidation with air bronchograms.

A review of the chest X-ray finding in 104 cases of PCP in AIDS, identified a high incidence of atypical features (DeLorenzo et al 1987). An interstitial pattern, defined as granular, nodular, reticular, or reticulonodular appearances were observed in 75%. An alveolar pattern with airspace filling, air-bronchograms or a confluent acinar infiltrate was seen in 12.5%, and a combination in 12.5% of cases. The distribution of the infiltrations involved both peripheral and central lung fields in 84%, peripheral only in 14%, and central only in 2%. Five patients of the 104 had a unilateral infiltrate. In addition to these findings, 4 patients had bilateral hilar enlargement, 7 patients had thin walled cysts and 4 honeycomb lesions. In this series of 104 patients, 6 developed spontaneous pneumothoraces, and 3 pneumomediastinum during the illness. Fifteen more developed pneumothoraces after diagnostic procedures or mechanical ventilation. This series did not report pleural effusions, but others have observed small bilateral effusions in severe PCP (Stover et al 1985). There are also rare reports of cavitating or non-cavitating opacities in the lung during PCP (Suster et al 1986, Barrio et al 1986).

Having outlined the possible chest X-ray abnormalities in PCP, it is important to state that lobar shadowing, pulmonary nodules, pleural effusions and mediastinal or hilar lymphadenopathy while reported in PCP, are more commonly associated with other pathology, e.g. infection with pyogenic organisms, mycobacteria or fungi, or involvement by Kaposi's sarcoma, lymphoma or primary lung carcinoma.

## Radioisotope imaging

Gallium 67 localises in areas of inflammation. Initial hope that this would provide a method to screen those with suspected PCP was disappointed by the lack of specificity of the test. Scans have been reported to be abnormal in over 90% of cases of PCP. However, up to 50% of cases without PCP also may have an abnormal scan (Murray et al 1984). The specificity can be improved when the uptake in the lung is only considered abnormal when it exceeds that by the liver (Coleman et al 1984). A Gallium scan can be useful in a patient in whom other non-invasive tests are equivocal, as a negative test has a high predictive value (Barron et al 1985).

Technetium-99 DTPA clearance from the lung is a measure of lung permeability. This is increased in PCP, but smoking and other lung diseases have a marked effect on this test and it has yet to find a place in routine clinical practice.

## Blood tests

AIDS patients with PCP have positive HIV serology and reduced CD4 T-cells in their peripheral blood. Marked lymphopenia suggests a high degree of compromised host immunity, and biases one in favour of urgent investigation of a patient with respiratory symptoms.

Serum lactate dehydrogenase (LDH) concentrations are increased in over 90% of cases of PCP (Silverman & Rubinstein 1985, Zaman & White 1988). This is due to an increase in LDH-3/LDH-4 isoenzyme derived from lung parenchyma. Unfortunately the test does not discriminate from other lung infections unless isoenzymes are measured, but high levels (greater than 450 i.u.) strongly suggest a diagnosis of PCP. Some studies have found higher LDH concentrations in patients who died from PCP versus those who survived (Kales et al 1987, Zaman & White 1988).

## Lung function tests

Reductions in transfer factor (DLCO), vital capacity (VC), and total lung capacity have been described in PCP (Curtis et al 1986). The single breath diffusing capacity for carbon monoxide/transfer test (DLCO) is the most sensitive test, with values close to those predicted for age, sex and height, in only 10% of cases of PCP. However, it lacks specificity, and reductions are observed with other causes of lung involvement, as well as in AIDS patients without pulmonary complications (Shaw et al 1988). It is particularly difficult to interpret in intravenous drug abusers who may have a decreased DLCO irrespective of HIV disease (Overland et al 1980). In general, a DLCO of less than 60% predicted, or a value that has declined in the same patient by more than 10% is an indication for further investigation.

## Blood gases

Hypoxaemia with or without hypocarbia is common and reflects the severity of the pneumonia. A fall in $PO_2$ or widening of the alveolar-arterial (A-a) oxygen tension gradient, following exercise, is a useful non-specific indicator of pulmonary complications in HIV infected patients (Stover et al 1985).

## Sputum induction

Although most patients with PCP do not spontaneously cough up sputum, this can be induced following a 5–20 minute inhalation of a 3–5% hypertonic saline solution. This induced sputum provides material for cytological examination and is the least invasive method of acquiring samples from the lung. Giemsa staining of the sample is essential, as this permits identification of the trophozoites of *P. carinii*, which are more readily seen than the cysts. Centres using this test have been able to identify PCP in up to 80% of the ultimately confirmed cases (Bigby et al 1986, Pitchenik et al 1986).

## Bronchoalveolar lavage

In an increasing number of centres, fibreoptic bronchoscopy and bronchoalveolar lavage are used to obtain samples when induced sputum fails to yield a diagnosis. To collect the sample, the tip of the bronchoscope is wedged in one of the segments of the right middle lobe or lingula, and 60 ml aliquots of normal saline are instilled and aspirated to a total volume of 180–240 ml. The fluid can be examined cytologically by centrifugation to precipitate the cells followed by staining with methanamine silver to show the cysts of *P. carinii*. The fluid can also be cultured to grow bacteria, fungi or viruses. Up to 90% of cases of PCP can be diagnosed by bronchoalveolar lavage (Ognibene et al 1984, Orenstein et al 1986, Stover et al 1984, Broaddus et al 1985, Warren et al 1985).

## Biopsy

Transbronchial biopsy performed at the time of the fibreoptic bronchoscopy is the least traumatic method of acquiring tissue. In the context of diffuse chest X-ray abnormalities seen in suspected PCP, it can safely be performed without fluoroscopy (Milligan et al 1988). It is associated with a 10% incidence of pneumothorax, half of which require aspiration, and a low incidence of lung haemorrhage, which rarely causes respiratory embarrassment. To minimise bleeding, abnormal clotting due to hepatitis or thrombocytopenia should be corrected prior to the procedure, and biopsy should be avoided when extensive endobronchial Kaposi's sarcoma is seen. Hypoxia is a relative contra-indication and arterial $PO_2$ or oxygen saturation should be measured, with supplemental oxygen administered during the procedure.

'Touch preparations' are obtained by scraping a fresh biopsy across a microscope slide, which is fixed and stained with a silver stain to show the black cysts of *P. carinii*. Histological examination of a transbronchial biopsy from a patient with PCP reveals the alveoli to be full of amorphous eosinophilic material and black staining cysts, which are approximately the same size as an erythrocyte.

### Diagnostic algorithm

An appropriate sequence of diagnostic studies in patients with, or suspected of having, AIDS who may have respiratory symptoms, is outlined in Figure 1.2. Respiratory symptoms plus an X-ray compatible with PCP should prompt

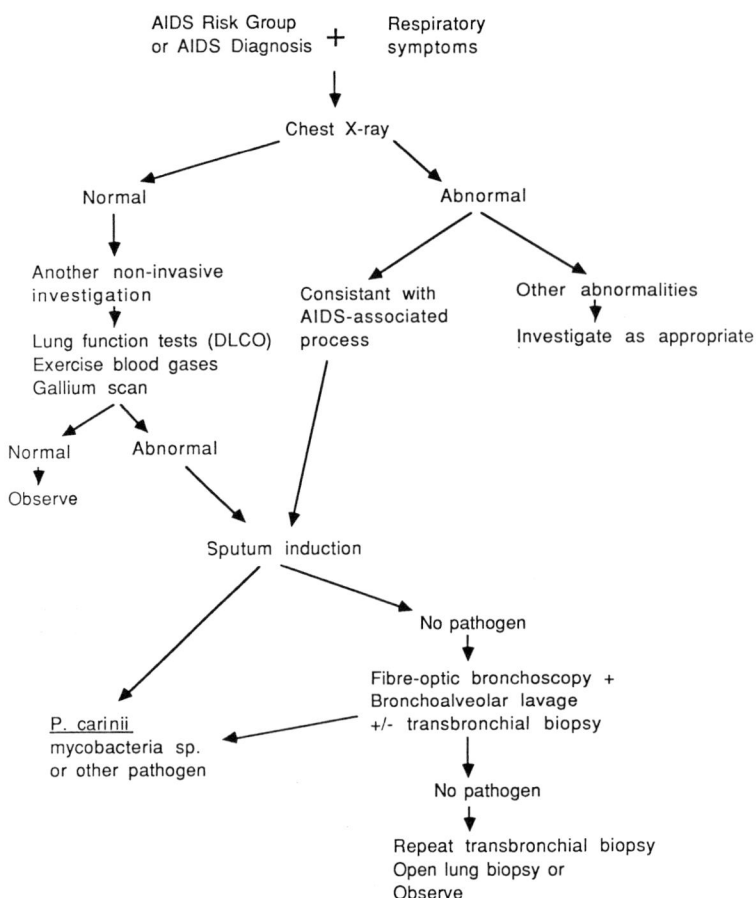

**Fig. 1.2**  Algorithm of the investigations in HIV seropositive patients with dyspnoea or cough. (Modified from Hopewell & Luce 1986.)

immediate further investigation with sputum induction, bronchoalveolar lavage or transbronchial biopsy, until a pathogen is identified. In patients with a normal chest X-ray, an abnormal DLCO on lung function testing, or an abnormal gallium scan, will identify those who should be further investigated. Patients with only mild symptoms and normal non-invasive investigation results can be observed.

## Differential diagnosis

Although PCP is by far the most common pulmonary complication of HIV infection many other complications of HIV infection may occur in the lung (Table 1.1). These can be divided into opportunistic infections compatible with a degree of immunocompromise only seen in AIDS, and thus pathognomonic of AIDS, while others are caused by organisms found in subjects with normal immunity, but take advantage of the decreased host immunity in HIV infection, e.g. *M. tuberculosis* and pyogenic bacteria. There are also non-infectious causes of pulmonary involvement in HIV infection e.g. Kaposi's sarcoma and non-Hodgkins lymphoma.

## Concurrent pulmonary infections

Ten to 20% of cases of PCP are accompanied by another pulmonary complication, which may alter the clinical picture and therapeutic requirements (Cohen et al 1984, Stover et al 1985, Rodriguez et al 1986, Kales et al 1987). Concurrent infection may occur commonly with *M. tuberculosis, M. avium-intracellulare,* cryptococcus, toxoplasma, cytomegalovirus, and rarely

**Table 1.1**  Differential diagnosis of pulmonary complications of HIV infection. (Modified from Murray et al 1987.)

| |
|---|
| *Opportunistic infections diagnostic of AIDS* |
| *Pneumocystis carinii* pneumonia (PCP) |
| Pulmonary toxoplasmosis |
| Extraintestinal (e.g. pulmonary) strongyloidiasis |
| Bronchopulmonary candidiasis |
| Pulmonary cryptococcosis |
| Disseminated histoplasmosis |
| Disseminated *Mycobacterium avium* complex or *M. kansasii* |
| Cytomegalovirus pneumonia |
| *Herpes simplex* pneumonia |
| |
| *HIV-related pulmonary infections* |
| Tuberculosis |
| Nocardiosis |
| |
| *Presumed HIV-related pulmonary disorders* |
| Pyogenic bacterial pneumonia |
| Lymphocytic interstitial pneumonitis (LIP) |
| Non-specific interstitial pneumonitis (NIP) |
| |
| *AIDS-related pulmonary neoplasia* |
| Kaposi's sarcoma |
| Non-Hodgkins lymphoma |

nocardia. In addition, pulmonary Kaposi's sarcoma or lymphocytic interstitial pneumonitis may be present.

## TREATMENT

The two main drugs for the treatment of PCP are co-trimoxazole and pentamidine. Numerous comparisons of the efficacy of these two alternatives have found both to have similar survival rates (greater than 75%), both to have a high incidence of side effects and that there is no advantage in combining co-trimoxazole and pentamidine. There exist certain circumstances where one or other drug is preferred. Co-trimoxazole has antibacterial action and should be used if there is also a bacterial infection. In renal failure, co-trimoxazole should be given in reduced doses. Pentamidine is used if there is a prior history of allergic reactions to sulpha-containing drugs.

### Co-trimoxazole (trimethoprim-sulphamethoxazole)

Following its success in treating PCP in patients immunocompromised for reasons other than HIV infection, co-trimoxazole (trimethoprim-sulphamethoxazole), has become the first line agent in treating PCP in AIDS patients. Its antimicrobial action results from inhibition of microbial tetrahydrofolate production. Sulphamethoxazole inhibits conversion of p-aminobenzoate to dihydrofolate, and trimethoprim prevents the reduction of dihydrofolate to tetrahydrofolate. Co-trimoxazole may be given orally or intravenously (trimethoprim 20 mg/kg/day and sulphamethoxazole 100 mg/kg/day) (e.g. for a 65 kg man give 16 tablets containing 400 mg sulphamethoxazole and trimethoprim 80 mg per day) for 14–21 days. Intravenous administration is preferred for severe disease, but can be converted to oral therapy after 1–2 weeks. HIV infected patients are more prone to side effects than those with compromised immunity from other causes and adverse reactions may occur in up to 65% of patients (Kovacs et al 1984). There are many adverse reactions and they need to be compared with those from pentamidine, which is the major therapeutic alternative (see Table 1.2). The most common side effects are fever and an erythematous maculopapular rash, which are felt to be due to immunologically mediated hypersensitivity, due to the rapid onset and prompt recurrence following re-exposure (Jaffe et al 1983). Leucopenia is also common. This may be immunologically mediated, or due to the antifolate activity of trimethoprim, although it does not respond to administration of folic acid (Jaffe et al 1983, Kovacs et al 1984).

The adverse reactions may be severe, and require dose reduction, completing the therapy with trimethoprim alone, or changing to pentamidine. In most studies the most common causes for a change in therapy were rash, haematological side effects or hepatitis. The incidence of these varied with extremes at 18 and 52% of cases (Kovacs et al 1984, Gordin et al 1984).

**Table 1.2** Comparison of the adverse effects of co-trimoxazole (trimethoprim plus sluphamethoxazole) and pentamidine. (From Sattler et al 1988.)

|  | Co-trimoxazole % of 36 patients | Pentamidine % of 33 patients | P value |
|---|---|---|---|
| *Clinical toxicity* |  |  |  |
| Fever | 78 | 82 |  |
| Hypotension | 0 | 27 | P<0.002 |
| Nausea and vomiting | 25 | 24 |  |
| Rash | 44 | 15 | P<0.001 |
| *Laboratory toxicity* |  |  |  |
| Anaemia | 39 | 24 | P<0.05 |
| Leucopenia | 72 | 47 |  |
| Thrombocytopenia | 3 | 18 |  |
| Increased serum creatinine | 14 | 64 | P<0.0001 |
| Increased alanine aminotransferase | 22 | 15 |  |
| Increased alkaline phosphatase | 11 | 18 |  |
| Hypoglycaemia | 0 | 21 | P<0.05 |
| Hypocalcaemia | 0 | 3 |  |

**Pentamidine**

Although first used for trypanosomiasis in the 1930s, the exact mechanism of action of pentamidine is unknown. Pentamidine isethionate (4 mg/kg) or pentamidine methone-sulphonate (2.3 mg/kg) was initially given by intramuscular injection. A prominent side effect of this route of administration was the development of cold abcesses. More recently it has been administered as a single daily intravenous infusion in 250 ml of 5% dextrose in water (Navin & Fontaine 1984). Pentamidine has a long half life, with 15–20% of the daily dose excreted in the urine over 24 hours. It is also commonly accompanied by adverse effects (see Table 1.2). These occur in up to 55% of cases (Wharton et al 1986). The most frequent major adverse effects are nephrotoxicity (25–66%), hepatic dysfunction (30–66%) and neutropenia (6–41%). These tend to resolve on discontinuation of the drug. Hypoglycaemia occurred in 27% of patients in one study commencing approximately 11 days after the start of pentamidine, and persisting for an average of 10 days (Stahl-Bayliss et al 1986). In four of the patients hypoglycaemia developed after pentamidine had been discontinued. It is therefore recommended that if a patient receiving pentamidine experiences mental changes, an urgent blood glucose estimation should be performed. A proportion of patients who experience hypoglycaemia will develop overt diabetes mellitus. It has been hypothesised that pentamidine has a streptazocin-like effect, with resultant islet cell destruction.

To reduce the incidence of side effects, there has been recent interest in site-specific delivery of pentamidine via the inhaled route. Numerous trials are in progress, with encouraging results in one study using up to 8 mg/kg/day of pentamidine administered daily for 2 to 3 weeks via an acorn nebuliser to patients with mild PCP (Godfrey-Fausett et al 1988). An unresolved issue is the optimal device to nebulise particles such that they deposit in the alveoli. One study comparing different nebulisers recommended either a system 22 Mizer (Medicaid) or a Respigard II (Marquest) (O'Doherty et al 1988). Inhaled pentamidine has the advantage that it provides adequate alveolar concentrations of the drug, low serum concentrations and a low incidence of adverse effects. It is thus likely to play an increasing role in treatment and prophylaxis of PCP.

## Alternative agents

Dapsone has an action similar to other sulphonamides. It has been used alone (100 mg once daily for 3 weeks) when a high relapse rate was observed (Mills et al 1986), or in combination with trimethoprim, when it was effective but accompanied by a high incidence of side effects namely nausea, vomiting, hepatitis, anaemia and rash (Leoung et al 1986).

Difluoromethylornithine (DFMO) prevents the biosynthesis of polyamines necessary for cell growth. Few studies on DFMO use are available. In one group of 10 patients who had failed on conventional therapy, intravenous administration (400 mg/kg/day) for 1–2 weeks was followed by oral administration (300 mg/kg/day) for several weeks, and four patients survived (Gilman et al 1985). Its use was accompanied by many side-effects including anaemia (40%), thrombocytopenia (20%), leucopenia (10%), gastrointestinal disturbances (e.g. diarrhoea, nausea, vomiting) (70%) and hepatic dysfunction (20%). DFMO has been advocated for use as an alternative agent or in those who have failed on conventional therapy, but randomised trials are awaited.

Trimetrexate is an analogue of methotrexate, which is 1500 times more potent as an inhibitor of protozoan dihydrofolate reductase than trimethoprim. Concurrent administration of Leucovorin (5-formyl tetrahydrofolate), prevents myelosuppression or intestinal epithelial toxicity. Allegra and colleagues in an uncontrolled pilot study found that of 16 patients in whom conventional therapy was not tolerated or had failed, 69% responded to trimetrexate-Leucovorin administered as salvage therapy (Allegra et al 1987). In another 16 with a prior history of toxicity or failure with conventional therapy, 63% had a positive initial response. There was however a 60% relapse rate within 3 months. This was prevented in another 17 patients who received trimetrexate-Leucovorin plus sulphadiazine as initial therapy for either a first or second episode of PCP. This group had a 71% response rate and only a 6% relapse rate. Toxicity from trimetrexate-Leucovorin is mild and only one of the total of 49 patients in the above study required discontinuation of therapy following the development of a maculopapular rash.

## Corticosteroids

Concern that short courses of corticosteroids might exacerbate immunosuppression have given way to the view that in severe PCP concurrent administration of corticosteroids might act as an adjunct to antimicrobial therapy by decreasing the associated lung inflammation. Many studies are currently addressing this question. Initial reports suggest that, in life threatening PCP, a short course of high dose corticosteroids (e.g. methylprednisolone 240 mg for 3 days, 120 mg for 3 days, 60 mg for 3 days), may improve mortality and shorten the duration of hypoxia and fever (Mottin et al 1987).

## Supportive measures

Hypoxic patients require increased inspired $PO_2$ up to 100%. A CPAP mask may aid $O_2$ delivery. Antipyretics e.g. paracetamol, should be used, as $O_2$ requirement increases with metabolic rate and temperature.

## Artificial ventilation

In nearly all studies, the mortality from PCP in those patients who require mechanical ventilation is over 85%. This has prompted the view that, following careful discussion with the patient and relatives, it may be compassionate not to offer mechanical ventilation, or do so only for a finite period (Luce et al 1988).

## CHEMOPROPHYLAXIS

PCP has a high relapse rate of 10–40% (Engelberg et al 1984, Haverkos et al 1984). The mechanism of recurrence is not known. Although *P. carinii* cysts persist in the lung after completion of therapy, respiratory problems within the first 3 months of an episode of PCP are not usually due to recurrences. These occur 4 to 6 months after the first episode (Barrio et al 1987, Fitzgerald et al 1987, Levine & White 1988). This high relapse rate has prompted studies into a number of chemoprophylactic regimes.

Co-trimoxazole at reduced dosage is effective in patients immunocompromised for reasons other than HIV infection, in preventing a recurrence of PCP, when it is associated with few side effects (Hughes et al 1977). AIDS patients experience a high incidence of side effects with co-trimoxazole, compared to patients not infected with HIV, and thus there is little information available from studies on the use of co-trimoxazole as chemoprophylaxis in AIDS.

Fansidar (pyrimethamine 25 mg and sulfadoxine 500 mg) may be given orally once a week as it has a long half-life. Its efficacy in AIDS associated PCP has yet to be confirmed, but is recognised in PCP not associated with AIDS (Post et al 1971). It is generally well tolerated even in a proportion of patients who have previously demonstrated co-trimoxazole hypersensitivity (Gottlieb et al 1984), but Stevens-Johnson syndrome has been reported in four AIDS patients given this drug (Navin et al 1985).

Taking advantage of aerosolised delivery and the long half-life, pentamidine delivered to the lungs via the inhaled route provides high sustained local drug levels in the lungs, with few side effects. Aerosolised pentamidine is an attractive chemoprophylactic agent, and human studies are underway.

Azidothymidine (AZT) acts against the HIV virus by inhibiting reverse trancriptase. It was first shown to help protect patients from recurrent PCP, in 282 patients with AIDS, manifest by an episode of PCP or severe AIDS related complex (Fischl et al 1987). AZT was associated with a mortality of 1 in the treatment group compared to 19 in the placebo group. AZT also causes an improvement in host immunity (Yarchoan et al 1986, Fischl et al 1987). The recommended dose is 200 mg 4 hourly. AZT is associated with profound bone marrow depression (Richman et al 1987) to the extent that patients may become transfusion dependent and a full blood count should be performed at 2 weekly intervals. Other side effects include nausea, myalgia and insomnia.

## CHILDREN

PCP is the most frequent opportunistic infection in paediatric AIDS (Oleske et al 1983, Rogers et al 1987, Rubinstein et al 1983, Rubinstein 1986). Unlike adult cases, the disease usually has an acute onset with fever, respiratory distress and hypoxia. The investigations, treatment and prognosis are similar to adult cases. In the differential diagnosis, lymphocytic interstitial pneumonitis is seen more commonly than in adults and may be differentiated on clinical and laboratory grounds (Table 1.3).

## PROGNOSIS

In the past the prognosis has been poor with between 30 and 55% of episodes of PCP resulting in death (Public Health Service 1986, Haverkos 1984, Federal Drug Administration 1985, Murray et al 1984, Kovacs et al 1984,

**Table 1.3** Comparison of clinical and laboratory features of lymphocytic interstitial pneumonitis (LIP) and *P. carinii* pneumonia (PCP) for differential diagnosis in paediatric AIDS (From Rubinstein et al 1988.)

|  | LIP | PCP |
|---|---|---|
| *Symptoms* | | |
| Acute onset | − | + |
| Insidious onset | + | Seldom |
| Fever | − | + |
| Tachypnoea | Late | Early, acute |
| Hypoxia | Late | Early, severe |
| Diminished breath sounds | − | + |
| Wheezes | Rare | + |
| Digital clubbing | + | − |
| Nodules on chest X-ray | + | − |
| Salivary gland enlargement | + | − |
| Generalised lymphadenopathy | + + | − |
| | | |
| *Laboratory tests* | | |
| Isomorphic serum lactate dehydrogenase elevation | + | + + |
| Elevated serum IgG | + + | + |
| Increased T8 lymphocytes in bronchoalveolar lavage fluid | + | − |
| Tissue contains: HIV genome | + | − |
| Epstein-Barr virus genome | + | − |

Wachter et al 1986). In a study of 43 patients with PCP, severe abnormalities on initial chest X-ray and alveolar-arterial (A-a) oxygen gradient of greater than 30 mm Hg were associated with a high early mortality (Brenner et al 1987). Decreased long term survival after PCP correlated with the severity of interstitial oedema on the initial transbronchial biopsy, a high A-a oxygen gradient, and the persistence of *P. carinii* cysts after 3 weeks of therapy. The outcome has improved in recent years with better diagnostic and treatment regimes.

REFERENCES

Allegra C J, Chabner B A, Tuzon C U et al 1987 Trimetrexate for the treatment of *Pneumocystis carinii* pneumonia in patients with the acquired immunodeficiency syndrome. New England Journal of Medicine 317: 978.

Barrio J L, Harcup C, Baier H J et al 1987 Value of repeat fibreoptic bronchoscopies and significance of non-diagnostic bronchoscopic results in patients with the acquired immunodeficiency syndrome. American Review of Respiratory Disease 135: 422

Barrio J L, Suarez M, Rodriguez J L, Saldana M J, Pitchenik A E 1986 *Pneumocystis carinii* pneumonia presenting as cavitating solitary pulmonary nodules in patients with the acquired immunodeficiency syndrome. American Review of Respiratory Disease 134: 1094

Barron T F, Birnbaum N S, Shane L B et al 1985 *Pneumocystis carinii* pneumonia studied by gallium-67 scanning. Radiology 154: 791

Bigby T D, Margolskee D, Curtis J L 1986 The usefulness of induced sputum in the diagnosis of *Pneumocystis carinii* pneumonia in patients with the acquired immunodeficiency syndrome. American Review of Respiratory Disease 133: 515

Brenner M, Ognibene F P, Lack E E et al 1987 Prognostic factors and life expectancy of patients with acquired immunodeficiency syndrome and *Pneumocystis carinii* pneumonia. American Review of Respiratory Disease 136: 1199

Broaddus C, Dake M D, Stulbarg M S et al 1985 Bronchoalveolar lavage and transbronchial biopsy for the diagnosis of pulmonary infections in the acquired immunodeficiency syndrome. Annals of Internal Medicine 102: 747

Centers for Disease Control 1986 Update: acquired immunodeficiency syndrome (AIDS)—United States. MMWR 35: 17

Cohen B A, Pmeranz S, Rabinowitz J G et al 1984 Pulmonary complications of AIDS: Radiologic features. American Journal of Radiology 143: 115

Coleman D L, Hattner R S, Luce J M et al 1984 Correlation between gallium lung scans and fiberoptic bronchoscopy in patients with suspected *Pneumocystis carinii* pneumonia and the acquired immune deficiency syndrome. American Review of Respiratory Disease 130: 1166

Curtis J, Goodman P, Hopewell P C 1986 Non-invasive tests in the diagnostic evaluation for *Pneumocystis carinii* pneumonia in patients with or suspected of having AIDS. American Review of Respiratory Disease 133: A132

DeLorenzo L J, Huang C T, Maguire G P, Stone D J 1987 Roentgenographic patterns of *Pneumocystis carinii* pneumonia in 104 patients with AIDS. Chest 91: 323

Engelberg L A, Lerner C W, Tapper M L 1984 Clinical features of *Pneumocystis* pneumonia in the acquired immune deficiency syndrome. American Review of Respiratory Disease 130: 689

Federal Drug Administration 1985 Drug bulletin: progress on AIDS 15: 26

Fischl M A, Richman D D, Grieco M H et al 1987 The efficacy of azidothymidine (AZT) in the treatment of patients with AIDS and AIDS-related complexes. New England Journal of Medicine 317: 185

Fitzgerald W, Bevelaqua F A, Garay S M et al 1987 The role of open lung biopsy in patients with the acquired immunodeficiency syndrome. Chest 91: 659

Gilman A G, Goodman L S, Rall T W et al 1985 The pharmacological basis of therapeutics, 7th edn. MacMillan. New York

Godfrey-Fausett P, Miller R F, Semple S J G 1988 Nebulized pentamidine Lancet 2: 645

Gordin F M, Simon G L, Wofsy C B et al 1984 Adverse reactions to trimethoprim-sulfamethoxazole in patients with the acquired immunodeficiency syndrome. Annals of Internal Medicine 100: 495

Gottlieb M S, Knight S, Mitsuyasu R et al 1984 Prophylaxis of pneumocystis infection in AIDS patients with pyrimethamine-sulfadoxine. Lancet 2: 398

Haverkos H W 1984 Assessment of therapy for *Pneumocystis carinii* pneumonia. American Journal of Medicine 76: 501

Hopewell P, Luce J M 1986 Pulmonary manifestations of the acquired immunodeficiency syndrome. Recent Advances in Respiratory Medicine 4: 45

Hughes W T, Kuhn S, Chandhary S et al 1977 Successful chemoprophylaxis for *Pneumocystis carinii* pneumonia. New England Journal of Medicine 297: 1419

Jaffe H S, Abrams D I, Ammann A J et al 1983 Complications of co-trimaxazole in treatment of AIDS-associated *Pneumocystis carinii* pneumonia in homosexual men. Lancet 2: 11098

Kales C P, Murren J R, Torres R A et al 1987 Early predictors of in-hospital mortality for *Pneumocystis carinii* pneumonia in the acquired immunodeficiency syndrome. Archives of Internal Medicine 147: 1413

Kovacs J A, Hiemenz J W, Macher A M 1984 *Pneumocystis carinii* pneumonia: A comparison between patients with the acquired immunodeficiency syndrome and patients with other immunodeficiencies. Annals of Internal Medicine 100: 663

LeGolvan D P, Heidelberger K P 1973 Disseminated, granulomatous *Pneumocystis carinii* pneumonia. Archives of Pathology 95: 344

Leoung G S, Mills J, Hopewell P C et al 1986 Dapsone-trimethoprim for *Pneumocystis carinii* pneumonia in the acquired immunodeficiency syndrome. Annals of Internal Medicine 105: 45

Levine S J, White D A 1988 *Pneumocystis carinii*. Clinics in Chest Medicine 9: 395

Luce J M, Wachter R M, Hopewell P C 1988 Intensive care of patients with the acquired immunodeficiency syndrome: time for a reassessment? (editorial) American Review of Respiratory Disease 137: 1261

Milligan S A, Luce J M, Golden J et al 1988 Transbronchial biopsy without fluoroscopy in patients with diffuse roentgenographic infiltrates and acquired immunodeficiency syndrome. American Review of Respiratory Disease 137: 486

Mills J, Leoung G, Medina I et al 1986 Dapsone is ineffective therapy for *Pneumocystis carinii* pneumonia in patients with AIDS. Clinical Research 34: 101A

Mottin D, Denis M, Dombret H et al 1987 Role of steroids in treatment of *Pneumocystis carinii* pneumonia in AIDS. Lancet ii: 519

Murray J F, Felton C P, Garay S M et al 1984 Pulmonary complications of the acquired immunodeficiency syndrome: Report of a National Heart, Lung and Blood Institute workshop. New England Journal of Medicine 310: 1682

Murray J F, Garay S M, Hopewell P C et al 1987 Pulmonary complications of the acquired immunodeficiency syndrome: an update: Report of the Second National Heart, Lung and Blood Institute Workshop. American Review of Respiratory Disease 135: 504

Navin T R, Fontaine R E 1984 Intravenous versus intramuscular administration of pentamidine. New England Journal of Medicine 311: 1701

Navin T R, Miller K D, Satriale R F 1985 Adverse reactions associated with pyrimethamine-sulfadoxine (letter) Lancet i: 1332

O'Doherty M J, Thomas S, Page C et al 1988 Differences in relative efficiency of nebulisers for pentamidine administration. Lancet ii: 1283

Ognibene F P, Shelhamer J, Gill V et al 1984 The diagnosis of *Pneumocystis carinii* pneumonia in patients with the acquired immunodeficieny syndrome using subsegmental bronchoalveolar lavage. American Review of Respiratory Disease 129: 929

Oleske J, Minnefor A, Cooper R et al 1983 Immune deficiency syndrome in children. Journal of the American Medical Association 249: 2345

Orenstein M, Webber C A, Cash M et al 1986 Value of bronchoalveolar lavage in the diagnosis of pulmonary infection in acquired immune deficiency syndrome. Thorax 41: 345

Overland E S, Nolan A J, Hopewell P C 1980 Alteration of pulmonary function in intravenous drug abusers: prevalence, severity and characterization of gas exchange abnormalities. American Journal of Medicine 68: 231

Pifer L L, Hughes W T, Murphy M J Jr 1977 Propagation of *Pneumocystis carinii* in vitro. Pediatric Research 11: 305

Pitchenik A E, Ganjei P, Torres A et al 1986 Sputum examination for the diagnosis of

*Pneumocystis carinii* pneumonia in the acquired immunodeficiency syndrome. American Review of Respiratory Disease 133: 226

Post C, Fakouhi T, Dutz W et al 1971 Prophylaxis of epidemic infantile pneumocytosis with a 20:1 sulfadoxine plus pyrimethamine combination. Current Therapeutic Research 13: 273.

Public Health Service 1986 Coolfont report: a PHS plan for prevention and control of AIDS and the AIDS virus. Public Health Report 101: 341

Richman D D, Fischl M A, Grieco M M et al 1987 The toxicity of azidothymidine (AZT) in the treatment of patients with AIDS and AIDS-related complex. New England Journal of Medicine 317: 192

Rodriguez J L, Barrio J L, Pitchenik A E 1986 Pulmonary nocardiosis in the acquired immunodeficiency syndrom: diagnosis with bronchoalveolar lavage and treatment with non-sulphur containing drugs. Chest 90: 912

Rogers M F, Thomas P A, Starcher E T et al 1987 AIDS in children: report of the Centers for Disease Control, national surveillance, 1982–1985. Pediatrics 79: 1008

Rubinstein A 1986 Pediatric AIDS. Current Problems in Pediatrics 16: 7

Rubinstein A, Sicklick M, Gupta A et al 1983 Acquired immunodeficiency with reversed T4/T8 ratios in infants born to promiscuous and drug-addicted mothers. Journal of the American Medical Assoication 249: 2350

Rubinstein A, Morecki R, Goldman H 1988 Pulmonary disease in infants and children. Clinics in Chest Medicine 93: 507

Sattler F R, Cowan R, Nielsen D M, Ruskin J 1988 Timethoprim-sulfamethoxazole compared with pentamidine for treatment of *Pneumocystis carinii* pneumonia in the acquired immunodeficiency syndrome. A prospective, noncrossover study. Annals of Internal Medicine 109: 280

Shaw R J, Roussak C, Forster S M, Harris J R W, Pinching A J, Mitchell D M 1988 Lung function abnormalities in patients infected with the human immunodeficiency virus with and without overt pneumonitis. Thorax 43: 436

Silverman B A, Rubinstein A 1985 Serum lactate dehydrogenase levels in adults and children with acquired immune deficiency syndrome (AIDS) and AIDS-related complex: possible indicator of B-cell lymphoproliferation and disease activity. American Journal of Medicine 78: 728

Stahl-Bayliss C M, Kalman C M, Laskin O L 1986 Pentamidine-induced hypoglycemia in patients with the acquired immune deficiency syndrome. Clinical Pharmacology and Therapeutics 39: 271

Sterling R P, Bardley B B, Khalil K G, Kerman R H, Conklin R H 1984 Comparisons of biopsy-proven *Pneumocystis carinii* pneumonia in acquired immune deficiency syndrome patients and renal allograft recipients. Annals of Thoracic Surgery 38: 494

Stover D E, White D A, Romano P A et al 1984 Diagnosis of pulmonary disease in acquired immune deficiency syndrome (AIDS): role of bronchoscopy and bronchoalveolar lavage. American Review of Respiratory Disease 130: 659

Stover D E, White D A, Romano P A, Gellene R A, Robeson W A 1985 Spectrum of pulmonary diseases associated with the acquired immune deficiency syndrome. American Journal of Medicine 78: 429

Suster B, Akerman M, Orenstein M, Wax M R 1986 Pulmonary manifestations of AIDS: review of 106 episodes. Radiology 161: 87

Tuazon C U, Delaney M D, Simon G L et al 1985 Utility of gallium-67 scintigraphy and bronchial washings in the diagnosis and treatment of *Pneumocystis carinii* pneumonia in patients with the acquired immune deficiency syndrome. Amercian Review of Respiratory Disease 132: 1087

Wachter R M, Luce J M, Turner J et al 1986 Intensive care of patients with the acquired immunodeficiency syndrome. American Review of Respiratory Disease 134: 891

Warren J B, Shaw R J, Weber J N et al 1985 Role of fiberoptic bronchology in management of pneumonia in acquired immune deficiency syndrome. British Medical Journal 291: 1012

Weber W R, Askin F B, Dehner L P 1977 Lung biopsy in *Pneumocystis carinii* pneumonia: a histopathologic study of typical and atypical features. American Journal of Clinical Pathology 67: 11

Wharton M J, Lewis D C, Constance B, et al 1986 Trimethoprim-sulfamethoxazole or pentamidine for *Pneumocystis carinii* penumonia in the acquired immunodeficiency syndrome; a prospective randomized trial. Annals of Internal Medicine 105: 37

Yarchoan R, Klecker R W, Weinhold K J et al 1986 Administration of

3'-azido-3'-deoxythymidine, an inhibitor of HTLV-III/LAV replication, to patients with AIDS or AIDS related complex. Lancet i: 575

Zaman M K, White D A 1988 Serum lactate dehydrogenase levels and *Pneumocystis carinii* pneumonia: diagnostic and prognostic significance. American Review of Respiratory Disease 137: 3402

# Gastrointestinal manifestations of human immunodeficiency virus disease

*George E. Griffin*

## INTRODUCTION

The gastrointestinal tract is a major target organ for human immunodeficiency virus (HIV) infection (Jaffe et al 1983, Malebranche et al 1983, Quinn 1985). Weight loss, diarrhoea and malnutrition are the major clinical presentations of the acquired immunodeficiency syndrome (AIDS) in Africa (Serwadda et al 1985, Colebunders et al 1987). In addition children with AIDS may suffer from major gastrointestinal problems (McLoughlin et al 1987). The gastrointestinal problems encountered in this condition may cause profound chronic morbidity (diarrhoea, abdominal pain, weight loss and malnutrition) or mortality (intestinal obstruction and perforation). It is therefore important to accurately diagnose the aetiology of these clinical manifestations if rational treatment is to be attempted. It is estimated that between 45–60% of intestinal infections are amenable to treatment (Smith & Janoff 1988).

The relationship between diarrhoeal disease and proctitis and homosexual practice (gay bowel syndrome) has been known for several years and the polymicrobial nature of enteric infections in these conditions has been well documented (Quinn et al 1983). However the nature of abdominal symptoms and diarrhoea has made it apparent that gastrointestinal disease related to HIV is chronic, often intractable, and generally severe in nature.

The purpose of this chapter is to document clinical presentations of gastrointestinal involvement in HIV disease, their aetiology, diagnosis and management. In addition current knowledge relating to the intestinal immune response in HIV disease and the possible direct involvement of HIV per se in inducing enteropathy will be discussed.

## CLINICAL GASTROINTESTINAL MANIFESTATIONS OF HIV DISEASE

### Abdominal pain

Abdominal pain is not an uncommon complaint in HIV infection; some 12.3% of a series of 235 North American patients suffering from AIDS were investigated for this problem and it was found that surgical exploration was rarely necessary for diagnosis but had to be used for intestinal perforation or obstruction (Barone et al 1988). The causes of abdominal pain include all of those normally encountered in HIV antibody negative patients but special attention must be made to the presence of opportunistic infection or disseminated malignancy related specifically to HIV disease. For example cramping mid-abdominal pain is often a feature of cryptosporidiosis and of many of the other enteric infections encountered in HIV infection. A problem may arise when multiple intestinal pathologies are present, for example when infection coexists with lymphoma and surgery may be required to relieve obstruction (Steinberg et al 1985). Kaposi's sarcoma (KS) may be found throughout the gastrointestinal tract in about 50% of patients with cutaneous KS (Friedman-Kein et al 1982). However visceral involvement may be detected in the absence of cutaneous disease and gastrointestinal symptoms (Lemlich et al 1987). Kaposi's sarcoma may lead to life threatening events such as intestinal obstruction (often second part of duodenum, Fig. 2.1), perforation or haemorrhage (Potter et al 1984). The pathophysiological significance of KS detected on endoscopic 'blind' upper intestinal tract biopsy in the aetiology of abdominal pain is unknown.

### Anorectal pain

Anorectal disease is common in homosexual men with AIDS related complex (ARC) or AIDS (Wexner et al 1986) and surgery for these conditions is complicated by poor healing and considerable mortality. The aetiology of anorectal disease in AIDS patients is multifactorial in terms of enteropathogens, trauma and malignant disease (Barone et al 1988) and needs careful microbiological and anatomical investigation before treatment (Quinn 1986). In general terms AIDS patients requiring major anorectal surgery have poor prognosis with significantly increased morbidity (poor wound healing, infection) and mortality.

### Dysphagia and odynophagia

Many of the causes of odynophagia and dysphagia are treatable and thus accurate diagnosis based on history, examination and microbiological data is very important. Distinction should be made between these two clinical entities: odynophagia refers to painful swallowing whereas dysphagia relates to perceived difficulty in propelling ingested food from the mouth to the stomach (Rauffman 1988). Both symptoms related to candidiasis were complained of by about 75% of patients during the clinical course of their HIV disease (Farman et al 1986). Disease of the oropharynx and oesophagus are present with equal frequency in all groups at risk for AIDS while other features, e.g. anorectal disease, which specifically relate to homosexual men (Rauffman et al 1986) are seen less frequently in other risk groups.

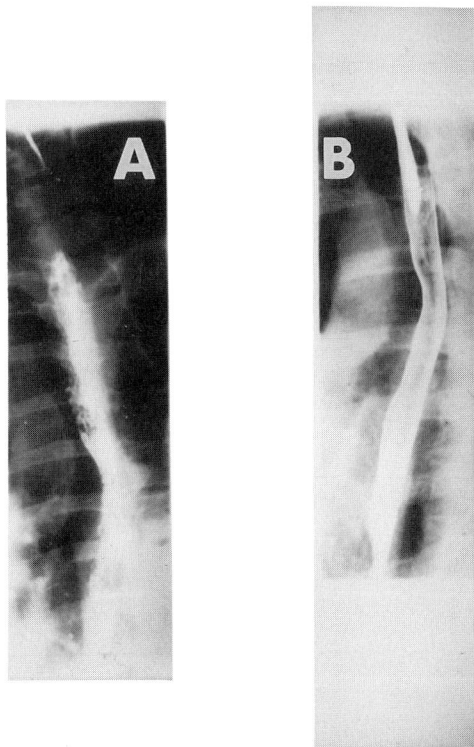

**Fig. 2.1** Barium contrast swallow study of an HIV antibody positive male presenting with odynophagia and dysphagia. Severe oral candidiasis was present on physical examination and had failed to respond to topical antifungal treatment. **A.** Multiple mucosal lesions typical of severe oesophageal candidiasis. **B.** 10 days after treatment with oral Fluconazole the contrast study showed complete resolution of the oesophageal candidiasis and the patient's symptoms had resolved within 5 days of starting treatment. Clinical relapse occurred 2 weeks after stopping treatment but thereafter prophylaxis with Fluconazole controlled the infection for a further 9 months when the patient died.

### Candidiasis

The most common cause of dysphagia and odynophagia in AIDS is candidiasis. Oral candidiasis was shown to be a very common presenting feature of AIDS, (Revision of CDC Surveillance case definition for Acquired Immunodeficiency Syndrome; MMWR, 36, 1987) and that within 3 months of this presentation further major complications of AIDS e.g. KS or pneumocystis pneumonia would ensue (Klein et al 1984). Oesophageal candidiasis may be present in the absence of oral candidiasis and the association of odynophagia or dysphagia is such a strong marker of candidiasis that many physicians now embark upon a therapeutic trial of antifungal agents (vide infra) without resorting to diagnostic investigations (Rauffman 1988).

The management of candidiasis affecting the upper gastrointestinal tract is usually successful but after induction of remission it is important to maintain prophylactic treatment (Fig. 2.2). Topical treatment of oral candidiasis, e.g. Nystatin, clotrimazole, may be initially successful but systemic antifungal agents are required to treat oesophageal candidiasis. Imidazoles (ketoconazole or its derivative fluconazole) are the mainstay of treatment for oesophageal candidiasis. Failures have been reported and may be related to decreased acid secretion (Lake-Bakaar et al 1988), reducing absorption of ketoconazole, or fungal resistance to the drug (Tavitian et al 1986). In general terms the use of fluconazole is preferred to ketoconazole since it appears to be as effective and is thought to have a lower incidence of hepatotoxicity. Patients who successfully respond to imidazole treatment require maintenance treatment to keep them symptom free (Ketoconazole 200 mg daily or fluconazole 50 mg daily).

*Tumours*

Kaposi's sarcoma often affects the soft palate and posterior pharynx in homosexuals with AIDS (Hadderingh et al 1987). The tumour may respond

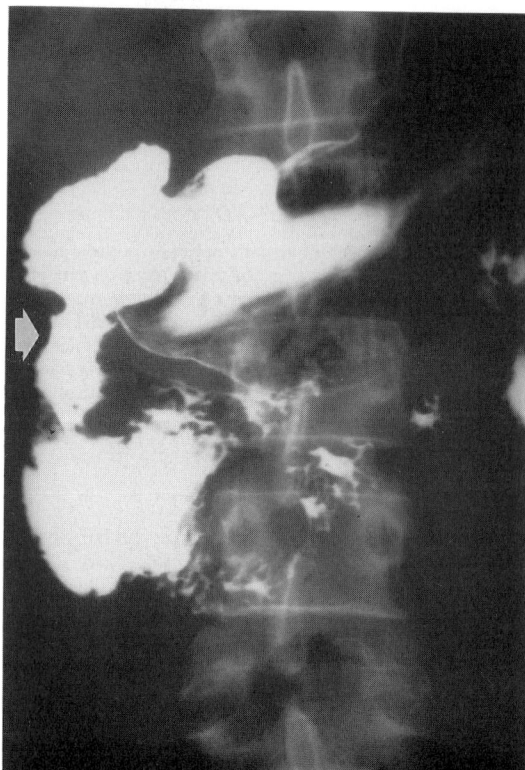

**Fig. 2.2** Barium meal study of an HIV antibody positive patient presenting with weight loss and vomiting. Concentric obstruction of the second part of the duodenum is seen which was due to Kaposi's sarcoma. The patient's vomiting was controlled and nutrition was supplied by bypassing the obstruction with a fine bore naso-duodenal tube and liquid feeds. The patient died 3 months after presenting with vomiting.

initially to radiotherapy and/or chemotherapy but often fungates and symp-tomatic management is all that can be offered.

*Viral causes of odynophagia/dysphagia*

Both cytomegalovirus (CMV) and herpes simplex virus-1 (HSV-1) cause ulceration of the oesophagus and pain. It is thought that CMV is more likely to cause dysphagia than odynophagia. The predominant clinical feature of HSV-1 ulceration is severe odynophagia (Agha et al 1986). Treatment with Ganciclovir is indicated in the management of CMV odynophagia/dysphagia with improvement in clinical symptoms (Chachoua et al 1987). Clinical trials of acyclovir for herpetic lesions of the oropharynx or oesophagus are currently in progress.

There appears to be little doubt that another viral agent, possibly HIV, is responsible for some oral and oesophageal ulcers in HIV sero-conversion illness. Enveloped virus-like particles were demonstrated in transmission electron microscopic examination of eight patients with oral ulceration as part of an HIV seroconversion illness (Rabenek et al 1986). Morphological evidence strongly suggested that these particles were not CMV or HSV and it is tempting to speculate that HIV itself may be responsible.

## Diarrhoeal disease

Chronic diarrhoea is one of the most disabling clinical manifestations of HIV disease and is a source of great discomfort and misery for patients. Diarrhoea is a common presenting symptom of AIDS (Modigliani et al 1985). The diarrhoea is often associated with progressive weight loss and malnutrition which can be disabling. HIV infected subjects who become infected with an enteropathogen may become chronically infected, and are unable to eliminate microorganisms which classically cause transient gastroenteritis in immuno-competent people. However the frequency and consistency of AIDS-related diarrhoea varies considerably (Smith et al 1988) but at its worst can be the dominant clinical problem.

## Infectious diarrhoea

Many enteropathogens have been described as causing diarrhoeal disease in HIV infected homosexuals (Table 2.1). A careful search for these entero-pathogens using stool microscopy and culture is mandatory. The figures reported for isolation of an enteropathogen from AIDS patients vary considerably with the highest figure being 85% (Smith et al 1988). The problem with such studies is determining whether or not the enteropathogen detected is implicated in the aetiology of the diarrhoea. This can often only be determined by therapeutic trials, if drugs are available, and such trials may be very difficult to interpret particularly if the aetiology of the diarrhoea is multifactorial.

**Table 2.1**   Gastrointestinal problems encountered in HIV diseases.

| Clinical problem | Aetiology | Management |
|---|---|---|
| Odynophagia and dysphagia | Sero conversion illness | Supportive |
| | Candidiasis (oral) | Nystatin mouthwash |
| | Candidiasis (oesophageal) | fluconazole (100mg/day) (plus prophylaxis— dose to be determined) |
| | Herpes simplex ulceration | Acyclovir (5mg/kg, 8hrly; 7 days) |
| | Cytomegalovirus ulceration | Ganciclovir (5mg/kg, 12-hrly; 14 days) |
| | Kaposi's sarcoma | Fine bore nasogastric feeding, radiotherapy, chemotherapy, supportive |
| Diarrhoea | Opportunistic entero-infections Cryptosporidia | Symptomatic |
| | *Isospora belli* | Trimethoprim 160 mg Sulphamethiazole 800 mg 800mg (qds) (Septrin) |
| | Microsporidia | Symptomatic |
| | *Giardia lamblia* | Metronidazole, tinidazole 250 mg tds, 5 days |
| | Salmonella | Appropriate antibiotics (plus continued prophylaxis) |
| | Cytomegalovirus colitis | Ganciclovir |
| | Enteropathy | Dietary advice, symptomatic |
| Mechanical internal problems | Tracheo-bronchial fistula | Fine bore nasogastric feeding Treatment of under lying cause, e.g. tuberculous mediastinal lymphadenopathy |
| | Intestinal obstruction, perforation (Kaposi's sarcoma, lymphoma) | Bypass of obstruction using fine bore tube or surgery |
| Weight loss and malnutrition | Anorexia, malabsorption, cytokines | Dietary advice and supplementation Zidovudine |

## Protozoal enteropathogens

*Cryptosporidia.*   Cryptosporidia are coccidian entero-parasites well known by veterinarians to cause diarrhoeal disease in animals and transient enteritis in humans (Pitlik et al 1983). The Centre for Disease Control (USA) now includes in its clinical definition of AIDS those patients who have intestinal cryptosporidiosis for longer than 1 month and for whom no other cause of immunosuppression is apparent.

The main clinical problem experienced by AIDS patients with cryptosporidiosis is severe watery diarrhoea, often associated, particularly terminally, with abdominal pain and weight loss. The hallmark of diagnosis rests with the detection of oocysts in stool using modified Ziehl-Neelsen stain (Connolly et al 1988). Up to six stool specimens may be required to demonstrate the presence of the oocytes. There is as yet no effective chemotherapy for cryptosporidiosis, despite early hopes for the use of Spiramycin in AIDS. However, symptomatic treatment and motility inhibitors, and the longer-acting morphine derivatives, may be useful, particularly in the later stages of the disease. Trials are awaited to determine the efficacy of azidothymidine in suppressing cryptosporidiosis.

Cryptosporidia may also affect the mucosa of the biliary tree and acute cholecystitis and ascending cholengitis have been reported with this infection (Gross et al 1986).

*Isospora belli.* Isospora belli is well documented as an opportunistic enteropathogen in AIDS, particulary evident in tropical and subtropical climates (DeHovitz et al 1986). Chronic watery diarrhoea and weight loss are the main clinical presentations of isosporiasis in AIDS. The diagnosis is made on modified Ziehl-Neelsen staining of stool smears by detection of acid fast oocysts. Organisms can also be detected in jejunal biopsy material. It has recently been demonstrated that oral treatment with a combination of trimethoprim (160mg) and sulphamethoxazole (800mg) (Septrin, Burroughs Wellcome) given four times a day for 10 days successfully treats the condition but that prophylaxis is required to effectively prevent recurrence (Pope et al 1989). Unfortunately, as with Septrin prophylaxis of pneumocystis pneumonia, there is a significant incidence of drug related side effects and alternative prophylactic regimens, e.g. sulphadoxine-pyrimethamine may be required.

Isosporiasis is a veterinary problem, particularly in piglets and calves, and successful eradication of the infection has been achieved in this field using non-absorbable antibiotic agents (May and Baker) which need to be evaluated in humans.

*Microsporidia.* Microsporidia are protozoal coccocidian parasites, some genera of which infest enterocytes (Dobbins & Weinstein 1985) and which seem to be associated with diarrhoeal disease and malabsorption. The organism cannot be detected in stool with ease since spores are very small and its diagnosis rests with its demonstration in intestinal biopsy specimens using light microscopy (Brown-Bennin stain) or transmission electron microscopy. Currently there is no effective chemotherapy and treatment is supportive.

*Giardia lamblia.* Giardia lamblia is detected in 4-15% of symptomatic AIDS patients in the USA (Smith et al 1988) and causes an acute diarrhoeal illness which is readily amenable to conventional antimicrobial treatment with metronidazole or tinidazole.

*Bacterial enteropathogens*

Many species of enteropathogenic bacteria have been described as causing diarrhoeal disease in AIDS patients (Smith et al 1988, Smith & Janoff 1988). Salmonella species causing transient gastroenteritis syndrome in immuno-competent subjects may give rise to bacteraemia preceding AIDS and characterised by relapse (Glaser et al 1985). Such patients require antibiotic therapy to control the initial disease and appropriate prophylaxis to prevent relapse, as in other T cell deficiency syndromes.

*Mycobacterium avium* intracellulare have been found in duodenal biopsies of American homosexuals with weight loss and diarrhoea (Gillin et al 1985) and may be associated with weight loss and fever (Roth et al 1985). The very high incidence of multiple drug resistance to antituberculous therapy makes this condition virtually untreatable.

*Viruses*

CMV can be identified histologically in intestinal biopsies taken throughout the gastrointestinal tract in many AIDS patients, but gastrointestinal disease is only clinically apparent in about 3% of cases (Jacobson & Mills, 1988). The hallmark of CMV infection is the presence of viral inclusion bodies, however the degree of inflammatory infiltrate and vasculitis surrounding these inclusions appears to be a marker of the severity of clinical symptoms. CMV colitis may be severe and progress to serious ulceration and perforation. Treatment of CMV colitis with Ganciclovir reduces symptoms but does not otherwise influence the clinical progression of HIV disease (Jacobson et al 1988). In a prospective study of the presence of enteric viruses in the stool of Australian HIV seropositive patients a high excretion rate of rota and adenoviruses was found (Cunningham et al 1988). The frequency of detection of enteroviruses appeared to increase with the degree of clinically apparent immunosuppression. The clinical significance of these viruses was however not clear in terms of inducing gastrointestinal syndromes. In addition viral particles, morphologically unlike viruses of any currently recognised taxonomic group, have been detected in intestinal mucosa of two patients (Chandler et al 1984).

*Enteropathy*

In many HIV infected patients with diarrhoea and malabsorption no enteropathogen is detected despite a meticulous search. It has therefore been suggested that an enteropathy exists which might be due to HIV per se in some way altering small intestinal function and causing malabsorption. The first reports of partial villous atrophy (PVA) (Gillin et al 1985) in endoscopic biopsies were from AIDS patients with diarrhoea and malabsorption. In this particular study five patients were found to have *Mycobacterium avium intracellulare* and it was suggested that this might be an important aetiological factor. In a more detailed study of malabsorption and jejunal villous architecture it has been shown that in the absence of detectable enteropathogens partial villous atrophy (Fig. 2.3) is present at all clinical stages of HIV disease and that the degree of fat absorption is proportional to the degree of villous atrophy (Fig. 2.4, Miller et al 1988). In addition the subjective presence of diarrhoea in patients of this study correlated with the presence of fat malabsorption. Similar findings of enteropathy associated with HIV have been reported from 45 HIV infected patients in West Berlin (Ullrick et al 1989). Detailed histological analysis of jejunal biopsies (Batman et al 1989) showed that crypt hyperplasia was present (indicating a physiological regenerative response to malabsorption) and that enterocytes were normal in height and transmission electron microscopy confirmed normal microvillous architecture (Mathan et al 1989).

Partial villous atrophy is a common end point of damage to the jejunal mucosa, however the PVA seen in HIV disease appears to be different from

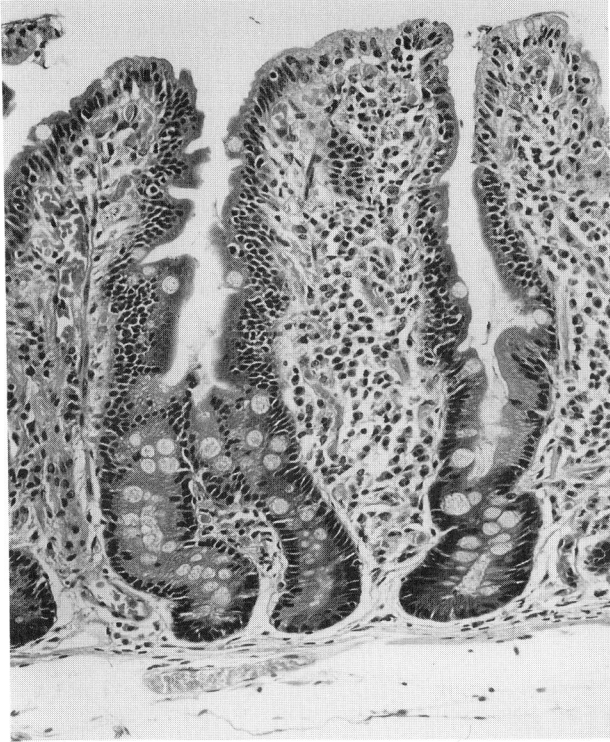

**Fig. 2.3** Photomicrograph of haematoxylin and eosin stained jejunal biopsy (x100) from a male homosexual with AIDS presenting with diarrhoea and weight loss in the absence of a detectable enteropathogen. Partial villous atrophy with crypt hyperplasia is seen and the enterocytes appear normal in height. From Miller et al, 1988 Jejunal mucosal architecture and fat absorption in male homosexuals infected with human immunodeficiency virus. Quarterly Journal of Medicine 69:1009-1119. (Reproduced with permission of Quarterly Journal of Medicine.)

the two classical types of gluten sensitive enteropathy or sprue (Batman et al 1989), but has some similarities with graft versus host disease (GVHD) seen following bone marrow transplantation. This similarity raises the question of the aetiology of PVA seen in HIV disease. The similarity with GVHD and other immunoproliferative small intestinal diseases (Manousos et al 1987) raises the possibility that an immune response within the mucosa may be responsible for the PVA. In addition *in vitro* stimulation of jejunal explant tissue with lectins has been shown to induce PVA.

Another possible explanation for the aetiology of PVA is the direct action of HIV on the mucosa of the intestinal tract. HIV genome has been detected by *in situ* hybridisation in crypt cells thought to be of the argentachromaffin lineage of duodenum and large intestine of patients infected with HIV (Nelson et al 1988). A more recent study has failed to confirm these findings (Fox et al 1989) but showed the presence of HIV genome by *in situ* hybridisation in cells resembling macrophages in the lamina propria. It may be possible to combine both theories of the aetiology of PVA by postulating that infected macrophages within the lamina propria may release cytokines which induce PVA. This is an attractive testable hypothesis.

## Terminal ileal function

Since diarrhoeal disease may result from the malabsorption of bile acids and the subsequent action of these bile acids on the colonic mucosa we have investigated the possibility that malabsorption of bile acids may be partly responsible for diarrhoeal symptoms in HIV diease (Kapembwa et al 1989b). Normal terminal ileal absorptive function (bile acid and vitamin B12) was detected even in the presence of jejunal enteropathy in three subjects with AIDS. However in two subjects suffering from AIDS complicated by intestinal cryptosporidiosis and *Isospora belli* infection, terminal ileal absorptive function was virtually non existent. Thus it appears that the terminal ileum is not a target for HIV enteropathy but that opportunistic infection with cryptosporidia or *Isospora belli* causes a panenteritis severely reducing terminal

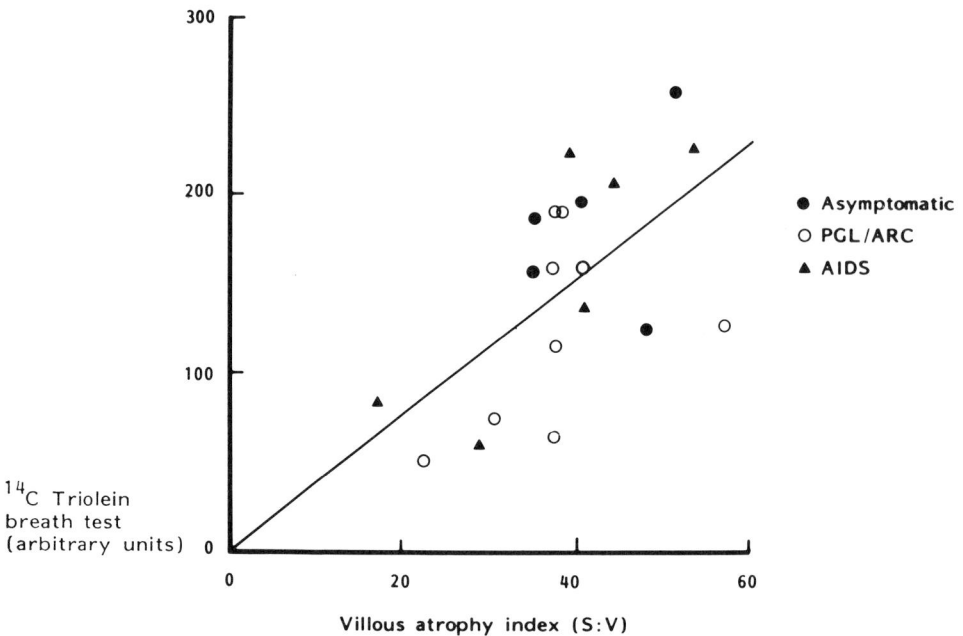

**Fig. 2.4** Fat absorption ($^{14}$C Triolein) and the degree of villous atrophy (S:V) were measured and correlated in two HIV positive male homosexuals. Five were asymptomatic, 9 were classified as persistent generalised lymphadenopathy or AIDS related complex and 6 had AIDS. There is a significant correlation between villous architecture and the degree of fat absorption, i.e. the greater the degree of villous atrophy the lower the absorption of fat. Subjects with fat absorption ( <140 units $^{14}$C Triolein) complained of the presence of diarrhoea. (From Miller et al 1988 Jejunal mucosal architecture and fat absorption in male homosexuals infected with human immunodeficiency virus. Quarterly Journal of Medicine 69:1009-1119. Reproduced with permission of Quarterly Journal of Medicine.)

ileal function. This study suggests that clinical trials of bile acid binding agents e.g. cholestyramine are warranted in such patients.

*Exocrine pancreatic function*

Reduced exocrine pancreatic function (EPF) may lead to diarrhoea, malabsorption and weight loss. Since there was some evidence that intestinal neuroendocrine cells may be affected by HIV disease (Nelson et al 1988) and that the intestinal autonomic system may be affected (vide infra), it was attractive to postulate that EPF may be reduced. A detailed study of 25 HIV infected subjects (20 group IV disease) showed reduced EPF was present to a minor extent in only three subjects and was unlikely to play a significant role in HIV related fat malabsorption (Kapembwa et al 1989a). Similar findings were also documented for Ugandan patients with slim disease. Pancreatitis may be caused by infectious agents in HIV disease e.g. CMV (Torre et al 1987) or cryptosporidia species (Hawkins et al 1987).

*Intestinal autonomic neuropathy*

Autonomic neuropathy of the gut is thought to result in diarrhoeal disease, presumably by affecting motility, and absorption of nutrients. Autonomic neuropathy affecting the cardiovascular system has been demonstrated indirectly using the Valsalva manoeuvre (Craddock et al 1987). Using transmission electron microscopy it has been demonstrated that there is severe degeneration of autonomic neurones and Schwann cells within the lamina propria of the jejunum of HIV infected male homosexuals (Griffin et al 1988). This study has now been extended and confirmed using quantitative histochemistry of intrinsic jejunal autonomic neurones detected with PGP 9.5 neurone specific monoclonal antibody (Batman & Griffin 1989). Thus autonomic denervation of the intestinal tract may play a role in the aetiology of diarrhoeal disease.

## INTESTINAL IMMUNITY IN HIV INFECTION

The presence of chronic opportunistic infections in HIV disease strongly suggests that intestinal immunity is defective at least in the later clinical stages of HIV infection. Indeed there is accumulating evidence documenting such reduced intestinal immunity (Rodgers & Kagnoff 1988). The most convincing evidence from *in vivo* studies shows that the acute serum antibody responses to wild type infection with *Giardia lamblia* is depressed in patients with AIDS (Jaffe et al 1988) in that AIDS patients had significantly depressed serum IgA and IgG response to *Giardia lamblia* trophozoites and an absent IgM response.

Histological analysis of haemotoxylin and eosin stained small intestinal mucosa has revealed a small increase in mononuclear cells in Group III and

IV HIV infected patients and a reduction in CD4 positive T lymphocytes (Rodgers & Kagnoff 1988). Correlation with CD4:CD8 ratios in peripheral blood however suggested that these changes clinically preceded those detected within the intestinal mucosa. IgA containing plasma cells are reduced in numbers in the lamina propria of rectal and small intestinal biopsies from patients with AIDS related complex or AIDS (Kotler et al 1987), however the depletion of IgA containing plasma cells did not correlate with the presence of opportunistic enteric infections. Abnormalities of the intestinal mucosal immune system in addition to predisposing patients to enteric infection may also permit systemic access to the body to cause disseminated infection, e.g. cryptosporidiosis, salmonellosis.

## NUTRITION IN HIV INFECTION

Nutritional status and intestinal function are intimately linked. Wasting of lean tissue mass is a major clinical feature of HIV disease (Hickey & Weaver 1988) and is seen principally during the later clinical stages of the disease. The aetiology of the wasting is multifactorial; malabsorption, intercurrent infections, fever, failure to utilise nutrients and anorexia, have all been suggested as possible factors and clearly all will have a role to play at different clinical stages of HIV infection.

Assessment of nutritional intake of subjects is a notoriously difficult procedure and currently the best accepted method is to prospectively weigh and record all food consumed in a 7 day period. Such records can then be analysed using computers and, for example, daily energy and protein intake can be calculated. This method has been shown to give an accuracy of 10% for such measurements. Using this technique we have measured energy and protein intake in 13 HIV constitutionally well antibody positive homosexuals, and 10 control subjects. In addition fat absorption was assessed using $^{14}$C Triolein method and various anthropometric nutritional indices were measured. The results (Table 2.2) showed that whilst HIV antibody positive male homosexuals ate the same number of calories and the same amount of protein, all of their anthropometric nutritional indices (body mass index, mid arm muscle circumference and grip strength) were reduced. There was little evidence of serious fat malabsorption in the HIV antibody positive group. These data strongly suggest that there may be a failure to utilise nutrients in Group IV HIV disease and that this may be one of the factors responsible for loss of lean body mass. It has recently been demonstrated that plasma levels of a cytokine tumour necrosis factor-alpha (TNF-alpha, also known as cachectin) are constitutively elevated in AIDS patients (Lahdevita et al 1988). TNF-alpha has been implicated as one of the systemic factors responsible for the loss of lean body mass seen during infection. Another possibility is that in the face of normal absorption and nutritional intake there are increased metabolic needs of HIV infected subjects and there is some evidence to support this (Hommes et al 1989).

**Table 2.2** Prospectively measured energy and protein intake and anthropometric nutritional indices in 13 HIV constitutionally well HIV antibody positive male homosexuals and 10 male control subjects. *Key:* (BMI, body mass index; MAMC, mid arm muscle circumference; GS, grip strength.) All anthropometric nutritional indices are reduced in the HIV infected group even though energy and protein intake is the same as control subjects. (Students' two tailed t test)

|  | Food intake Energy (kcal) | Protein (g) | BMI (kg/m$^2$) | MAMC (mm) | GS (kg) | Fat absorption (14CArbitrary Units)[b] |
|---|---|---|---|---|---|---|
| Control (n = 9) | 2408 ± 580 | 81.4 ± 23.6 | 23.1 ± 2.3 | 295.9 ± 25.3 | 44.01 ± 8.7 | >140 |
| HIV antibody positive (n = 13) | 2570 ± 411 | 90.6 ± 17.0 | 21.1* ± 2.2 | 34.3* ± 31.3 | 24.3* ± 10.6 | 149 ± 14 |

*p>0.05

In total intestinal failure due to any reason (infection or intestinal obstruction principally) the question of nutritional support using parenteral nutrition (TPN) arises. In addition to all of the practical problems involved in the administration of TPN, clearly ethical considerations apply as to instituting such treatment since it is difficult to stop. In addition the efficacy of intravenous nutrition in reversing malnutrition and perhaps immunological deficit must be addressed (Hopefl 1988). Refeeding non-HIV infected patients with protein energy malnutrition can reverse abnormalities of lymphocyte function and reverse energy to common skin antigen. However such a restoration of immunological function cannot be achieved in AIDS patients. In addition it is difficult to replete body cell mass in AIDS patients despite adequate calorie and protein intake (Kotler et al 1985). Such findings correlate well with the results shown in Table 2.2. Thus the use of TPN in HIV disease must be carefully assessed for individual patients.

## CONCLUSION

The gastrointestinal tract is a major target in HIV infection either directly or indirectly. The clinical syndromes produced by abnormalities of intestinal function are a source of chronic morbidity and misery for some HIV infected patients and may be a cause of mortality. Fortunately some of the gastrointestinal manifestations of HIV disease can be treated with success, e.g. candidiasis, and a careful diagnostic evaluation of HIV infected patients presenting with gastrointestinal symptoms is warranted.

REFERENCES

Agha F P, Horchang H L, Nostrant T T 1986 Herpetic oesophagitis: a diagnostic challenge in immunocompromised patients. Americal Journal of Gastroenterology 81: 246–253
Barone J E, Wolkomir A F, Muakkassa F F, Fares L G 1988 Abdominal pain and anorectal

rectal disease in AIDS. Gastroenterology Clinics of North America 17: 631–638

Batman P, Griffin G E 1989 Autonomic denervation in jejunal mucosa of male homosexuals infected with HIV. Quarterly Journal of Medicine (submitted)

Batman P, Miller A, Forster S M, Harris J P W, Pinching A, Griffin G E 1989 HIV jejunal enteropathy: quantitative histology. Journal of Clinical Pathology 42: 275–281

Chachoua A, Dieterich D, Kasinski K 1987 9-(1,3-dihydroxy-2-propoxymethyl) guanine (Gancyclovir) in the treatment of cytomegalovirus gastrointestinal disease with acquired immunodeficiency syndrome. Annals of Internal Medicine 107: 133–136

Chandler F W, White E H, Callaway C S, Spria T J, Ewing E P 1984 Unidentified virus-like particles in the intestine of patients with acquired immunodeficiency syndrome. Annals of Internal Medicine 100: 851–853

Colebunders R, Francis H, Mann J M 1987 Persistent diarrhoea, strongly associated with HIV infection in Kmshasa, Zaire. American Journal of Gastroenterology 82: 859–864

Connolly G M, Dryden M S, Shanson D C, Gazzard B G 1988 Cryptosporidial diarrhoea in AIDS and its treatment. Gut 29: 593–597

Craddock C, Pasvol G, Bull R, Protheroe A, Hopkin J 1987 Cardiorespiratory arrest and autonomic neuropathy in AIDS. Lancet ii: 16–18

Cunningham A L, Grohman G S, Harkness J et al 1988 Gastrointestinal viral infections in homosexual men who were symptomatic and seropositive for human immunodeficiency virus. Journal of Infectious Diseases 158: 386–391

DeHovitz J A, Pope J W, Boncy M, Johnson W D Jr 1986 Clinical manifestations and therapy of Isospora belli infection in patients with the acquired immunodeficiency syndrome. New England Journal of Medicine 315: 87–90

Dobbins W O, Weinstein W M 1985 Electron microscopy of the intestine and rectum in acquired immunodeficiency syndrome. Gastroenterology 88: 738–749

Farman J, Tavitian A, Rosenthal L E 1986 Focal oesophageal candidiasis in acquired immunodeficiency syndrome (AIDS). Gastrointestinal Radiology 11: 213–220

Fox C H, Kotler D, Tierney A, Wilson C S, Fauci A S 1989 Detection of HIV-1 RNA in the lamina propria of patients with AIDS and gastrointestinal disease. Journal of Infectious Diseases 159: 467–471

Friedman-Kein A E, Laubenstein J L, Rubenstein P 1982 Disseminated Kaposi's sarcoma in homosexual men. Annals of Internal Medicine 96: 693–700

Gillin J S, Shike M, Alcock N 1985 Malabsorption and mucosal abnormalities of the small intestine in the acquired immunodeficiency syndrome. Annals of Internal Medicine 102: 619–622

Glaser J B, Kute-Morton L, Berger S R 1985 Recurrent Salmonella typhimurium bacteraemia associated with the acquired immunodeficiency syndrome. Annals of Internal Medicine 102: 189–193

Griffin G E, Miller A, Batman P, Pinching A, Harris J R W, Mathan M 1988 Damage to intrinsic jejunal autonomic nerves in HIV infection. AIDS 2: 379–382

Gross T L, Wheat J, Bartlett M 1986 AIDS and multiple system involvement with cryptosporidium. American Journal of Gastroenterology 81: 456–458

Hadderingh R J, Tange R A, Danner S A, Eeftinck Schattenkerk J K 1987 Otorhinolaryngological findings in AIDS patients: a study of 63 cases. Archives Otorhinolaryngology 244: 11–14

Hawkins S P, Thomas R P, Teasdale C 1987 Acute pancreatitis: a new finding in cryptosporidial enteritis. British Medical Journal 294: 483–484

Hickey M S, Weaver K E 1988 Nutritional management of patients with ARC or AIDS. Gastroenterology Clinics of North America 17: 545–561

Hommes M, Romijn J A, Godfried M H, Endert E, Danner S A, Sanerwein H P 1989 Increased resting energy expenditure in HIV-infected men In: Abstracts 5th International Conference on AIDS p218

Hopefl 1988 What is the role of parenteral nutrition in AIDS. Clinical Pharmacy 7: 512–513

Jacobson M A, Mills J 1988 Serious cytomegalovirus diease in the acquired immunodeficiency syndrome (AIDS)– clinical findings, diagnosis and treatment. Annals of Internal Medicine 108: 585–594

Jacobson M A, O'Donnell J J, Porteus D, Brodie H R, Feigal D, Mills J 1988 Retinal and gastrointestinal disease due to cytomegalovirus in patients with the acquired immunodeficiency syndrome; prevelance, natural history and response to Gancyclovir therapy. Quarterly Journal of Medicine 67: 473–486

Jaffe H W, Bregman D J, Selik R M 1983 Acquired immunodeficiency syndrome in the United States: the first 1000 cases. Journal of Infectious Diseases 148: 339–345

Jaffe E N, Smith P D, Blaser M J 1988 Acute antibody responses to Giardia lamblia are depressed in patients with AIDS. Journal of Infectious Diseases 157: 798–804

Kapembwa M S, Fleming S C, Griffin G E, Caun K, Pinching A J, Harris J R W 1989a Fat absorption and exocrine pancreatic function in human immunodeficiency virus infection. Quarterly Journal of Medicine (in press)

Kapembwa M S, Joseph A E, Fleming S C, Griffin G E 1989b Ileal absorptive function in acquired immunodeficiency syndrome (AIDS). A2170, 5th International Conference on AIDS, Montreal 1989

Klein R S, Morris C A, Small C B 1984 Oral candidiasis in high risk patients as the initial manifestation of the aquired immunodeficiency syndrome. New England Journal of Medicine 311: 354–358

Kotler D P, Wang J, Pierson R N 1985 Body composition studies in patients with acquired immunodeficiency syndrome. Journal of Clinical Nutrition 1255–1265

Kotler D P, Scholes J V, Tiernay A R 1987 Intestinal plasma cell alterations in acquired immunodeficiency syndrome. Digestive Diseases and Sciences 32(2): 129–138

Lahdevita J, Mawry C P J, Tepp A-M, Repo H 1988 Elevated levels of circulating cachectin/tumour necrosis factor in patients with acquired immunodeficiency syndrome. American Journal of Medicine 85: 289–291

Lake-Bakaar G, Tom W, Lake-Bakaar D et al 1988 Gastropathy and ketoconazole malabsorption in the acquired immunodeficiency syndrome (AIDS). Annals of Internal Medicine 109: 471–473

Lemlich G, Schwamm L, Lebwohl M 1987 Kaposi's sarcoma and acquired immunodeficiency syndrome: post mortem findings in 24 cases. Journal of American Academy of Dermatology 16: 319–325

McLoughlin L C, Nord K S, Joshi V V, Oleske J M, Connor E M 1987 Severe gastrointestinal involvement in children with the acquired immunodeficiency syndrome. Journal of Paediatric Gastroenterology and Nutrition 6: 517–524

Malebranche R, Arnoux E, Guerin J M et al 1983 Acquired immunodeficiency syndrome with severe gastrointestinal manifestations in Haiti. Lancet 2: 873–877

Manousos O, Economidou, Papademetriou C H, Triantaphyllidis J, Constandinidou A, Stathopoulos A 1987 Malabsorption associated with non malignant immunoproliferative small intestinal disease. Digestion 36: 182–188

Mathan M, Griffin G E, Miller A 1989 Ultrastructure of the human jejunal mucosa in human immunodeficiency virus infection. British Journal of Pathology (in press)

Miller A, Griffin G E, Batman P et al 1988 Jejunal mucosal architecture and fat absorption in male homosexuals infected with human immunodeficiency virus. Quarterly Journal of Medicine 69: 1009–1119

Modigliani R, Bories C, le Charpentier Y et al 1985 Diarrhoea and malabsorption in acquired immune deficiency syndrome: a study of four cases with special emphasis on opportunistic protozoan infestations. Gut 26: 179–187

Nelson J A, Wiley C A, Reynolds-Kohler C, Reese C E, Margaretten W, Levy J A 1988 Human immunodeficiency virus detected in bowel epithelium from patients with gastrointestinal symptoms. Lancet i: 259–262

Pitlik, Faunstein V, Garza D 1983 Human cryptosporidiosis: spectrum of disease. Archives of Internal Medicine 143: 2269–2275

Pope J W, Verdier R-I, Johnson W D 1989 Treatment and prophylaxis of Isospora belli infection in patients with the acquired immunodeficiency syndrome. New England Journal of Medicine 320: 1043–1047

Potter D A, Danforth D N, Macher A B, Longo D L, Stewart L, Masur H 1984 Evaluation of abdominal pain in the AIDS patient. Annals of Surgery 199: 332–339

Quinn T C 1985 Gastrointestinal manifestations of AIDS. Practical Gastroenterology 9: 23–24

Quinn T C 1986 Clinical approach to intestinal infections in homosexual men. Medical Clinics of North America 70: 611–634

Quinn T C, Stamm W E, Goodell S E et al 1983 The polymicrobial nature of intestinal infections in homosexual men. New England Journal of Medicine 309: 576–582

Rabeneck L, Bogko W J, McLean D M, McLeod W A, Wong K K 1986 Unusual oesophageal ulcers containing enveloped virus-like particles in homosexual men. Gastroenterology

90(6): 1882–1889

Rauffmann J-P 1988 Odynophagia/dysphagia in AIDS. Gastroenterology Clinics of North America 17: 599–613

Rauffmann J P, Travitian A, Straus E W 1986 Diagnostic, therapeutic and prognostic implications of oral candidiasis in patients with AIDS or AIDS-related complex. Digestive Diseases and Sciences 31: 4765

Rodgers V D, Kagnoff M F 1988 Abnormalities of the intestinal immune system in AIDS. Gastroenterology Clinics of North America 17: 487–494

Roth R I, Owen R L, Keren D F 1985 Intestinal infection with mycobacterium avium in acquired immunodeficiency syndrome (AIDS). Histological and clinical comparison with Whipple's disease. Digestive Diseases and Sciences 30: 497–504

Serwadda D, Mugerwa R D, Sewankambo N K et al 1985 Slim disease: a new disease in Uganda and its association with HTLVIII infection. Lancet ii: 850–852

Smith P D, Janoff E N 1988 Infectious diarrhoea in human immunodeficiency virus infection. Gastroenterology Clinics of North America 17: 587–598

Smith P D, Lane C, Gill V J et al 1988 Intestinal infections in patients with acquired immunodeficiency syndrome (AIDS) etiology and response to therapy. Annals of Internal Medicine 108: 328–333

Steinberg J J, Bridges N, Feine H D 1985 Small intestinal lymphoma in three patients with acquired immunodeficiency syndrome. American Journal of Gastroenterology 80: 21–26

Tavitian A, Rauffman J P, Rosenthal L E 1986 Ketoconazole-resistant candida oesophagitis in patients with acquired immunodeficiency syndrome. Gastroenterology 90: 443–445

Torre D, Montanari M, Fiori P G, Dietz A, Sampieto C 1987 HIV and the pancreas. Lancet ii: 1212

Ullrich R, Zeitz M, Heise W, L'age M, Hoffken G, Riecken E O 1989 Small intestinal structure and function in patients infected with human immunodeficiency virus (HIV): evidence for HIV induced enteropathy. Annals of Internal Medicine 111: 15–21

Wexner S D, Smithy W B, Milsom J W, Dailey T M 1986 The surgical management of anorectal disease in AIDS and pre AIDS patients. Disease of Colon and Rectum 29: 719–723.

# The epidemiology and pathogenesis of the human T-cell leukaemia/lymphoma viruses, types 1 and 2 (HTLV-1, HTLV-2)

*Jonathan Weber*

## INTRODUCTION

Pathogenic human retroviruses are without doubt of some antiquity, but have only become recognised in the past decade. While the human immunodeficiency virus (HIV) has attracted the greatest attention since 1982, owing to its rapid pandemic spread and high mortality, the older, widespread endemic human T-lymphotropic viruses (HTLV) have been relatively neglected. After an early period of enthusiastic sero-epidemiology in 1982–1984, many of the details of the distribution of HTLV around the world are still obscure. However, there is enough data on the distribution of these human retroviruses to believe that there are currently more subjects infected by HTLV-1 in the UK than are infected by HIV-1. The HTLV viruses are transmitted vertically probably through maternal milk, and by horizontal transmission by blood transfusion and sexual intercourse. After long periods of latency, the HTLV viruses are causally associated with a form of acute leukaemia termed the adult T-cell leukaemia (ATL), and with a progressive form of lower limb paralysis known for historical reasons as tropical spastic paraparesis (TSP).

As HTLV is spread in a similar manner to HIV, it is likely to currently exist, or become prevalent in patients attending STD clinics; this will be particularly true if the patients also derive from an area of the world where HTLV infection is particularly common, which for the UK population implies the Caribbean islands and West Africa. The recognition of the clinical syndromes associated with HTLV infection, and a knowledge of the sero-epidemiology and diagnosis will therefore be important to controlling the virus, and to counselling patients found to be infected by HTLV.

## TAXONOMY AND NOMENCLATURE

All retroviruses are RNA-containing, enveloped viruses which replicate through reverse transcription and the integration of a DNA intermediate into the host cell genome (Weiss 1989). They are widely distributed in vertebrates, and affect most classes of animals from reptiles through to primates. Retroviruses are broadly divided by their effects, and their morphology on electron microscopy:

## Lentiviruses (e.g. human immunodeficiency virus – HIV)

These are characterised by their budding at the cell surface, and the long latency between infection and disease. They are associated with chronic immunodeficiency (HIV, SIV, FIV, BIV), neurological disease (Maedi) and joint disease (CAEV).

## Spumaviruses, (e.g. human foamy virus – HFV)

These viruses cause foamy vacuolation of cells in culture, and have been isolated from primates, monkeys and man. They have at present no clear disease association.

## Oncornaviruses (e.g. HTLV)

These viruses may be endogenous (non-oncogenic, found in human and all other genomes; endogenous sequences represent fossil retroviruses, present in the human germ-line as evolutionary remnants), or exogenous (i.e. infectious). Exogenous retroviruses are associated with cancer in a wide range of animals, and now in humans (HTLV). They are divided by electron microscopic morphology into types A–D. Type D is one of the monkey immunodeficiency viruses, similar to the Mason-Pfizer monkey virus. B-type are the avian viruses, and the C-type cover all of the mouse, rat and cat leukaemia viruses, now also including the sole example of an oncogenic human tumour retrovirus, HTLV-1.

## HISTORY OF THE HTLV'S

Tumour viruses were first recognised in chickens in 1909 by Peyton Rous, who demonstrated the acute development of a sarcoma in chicken through the transmission of a filtrable agent, i.e. a virus. This work was contrary to contemporary dogma, and was consequently ignored for over 40 years. In the 1950's, Ludwig Gross confirmed Rous' work with mouse leukaemia virus and in the 1960's, Bill Jarrett in Glasgow isolated the feline leukaemia virus (FeLV). The life cycle of these viruses was poorly understood until the crucial work of Baltimore and Temin in 1970, who demonstrated that these viruses were capable of reverse transcription of viral RNA to DNA. They then characterised the viral enzyme responsible for this phenomenon, the RNA directed DNA polymerase enzyme, now universally known as reverse transcriptase. Once the mechanism of viral DNA production was known, it was clear that this group of RNA tumour viruses were best characterised by their unique possession of reverse transcriptase, and hence they were renamed 'retroviruses'.

Subsequent searching for a human equivalent of these widespread animal tumour viruses involved many groups in the 1970's. The search for endogenous tumour virus sequences (as opposed to exogenous, infectious virus) preoccupied many researchers, as there was so little evidence to suggest that cancer in humans had an infectious aetiology. After many false starts and alarms, these putative human tumour viruses were unofficially renamed 'human tumour viruses'. Through that decade, Gallo and others generated the techniques required for the long-term culture of human lymphocytes, through the isolation and cloning of the T-cell growth factor (TCGF, now reclassified as interleukin-2, IL-2). Eventually, and by chance, one of the many hundreds of transformed T-cell lines derived from human leukaemia and lymphomas generated by Gallo's lab was found in 1981 to contain a novel retrovirus, which was termed the human T-cell leukaemia/lymphoma virus (HTLV) (Poiecz 1982). The patient from which this virus was isolated had been originally diagnosed as having the cutaneous lymphoma, mycosis fungoides; this was to prove a misdiagnosis. In parallel to Gallo's work, Japanese investigators were studying a newly recognised adult T-cell leukaemia (ATL) found in Japan (Uchiyama et al 1977). This leukaemia had a distribution suggesting a possible infectious aetiology, and cell lines grown from ATL patients expressed an antigen (ATL-antigen) which was recognised by antibodies in all ATL patients serum. Simultaneously to Gallo's work, and in isolation, Miyoshi (Miyoshi et al 1981) and others showed that there was a novel retrovirus in these cell lines responsible for the ATL-antigen (Hinuma et al 1982), and this virus, ATL-virus reported in 1981, was subsequently shown in 1984 to be identical to the human T-leukaemia/lymphoma virus (Watenabe et al 1984). The final turn of the wheel led to the original patient from which Gallo had isolated HTLV being reclassified as a case of ATL. In 1982, a related virus termed HTLV-2 was isolated from a patient with hairy cell leukaemia (Kalyanaraman et al 1982); this virus is close to HTLV-1 and serologically cross-reacts. The role of this virus in the causation of hairy cell leukaemia is still uncertain, but it is clear that the very great majority of hairy cell leukaemia cases are not infected by HTLV-2.


## THE VIRUSES

The HTLV virus is similar in structure to HIV, and to other retroviruses; two identical strands of the 9032 nucleotide viral RNA are contained in an inner core structure, within an outer lipid containing envelope. As with all retroviruses, there are three basic structural genes, termed *gag*, *pol* and *env*, sandwiched between the two long terminal repeats (LTR) which contain the control and promoter sequences for the virus (Seiki et al 1983). The *gag* gene codes for a 53 kilodalton (kd) precursor protein which is cleaved to form both inner core (p24, p15) and outer shell proteins (p19). The *pol* gene codes for a large 99 kd precursor protein, which generates three protein products: the reverse transcriptase enzyme, an endonuclease (integrase) to cut the host DNA, and a protease to cleave the *gag* and *pol* precursor proteins into their mature products. The *env* gene codes for a 65 kd precursor, which is cleaved by cellular enzymes to form the outer viral envelope glycoprotein (gp46) which is expressed through the envelope, attached by a short transmembrane glycoprotein (p20E). All of these structural gene products, both precursors and mature proteins are immunogenic in natural infection, and like with HIV, immunoblots or immunoprecipitations with human antiserum reveal multiple viral bands. In addition, there are regulatory genes in alternate reading frames from a region of the virus known as the pX region. These regulatory genes produce proteins called tax (p40) and rex (p27). As with HIV, these regulatory gene products are responsible for fine control over HTLV gene expression, capable of acting also on non-viral genes in the nucleus and the cytoplasm.

## Pathogenesis

HTLV-1 will infect a broad range of animals and their cells. Although initially grown in $CD4^+$ T-cell lines, HTLV-1 will infect many haematopoetic and non-haematopoetic human cells with ease (Clapham et al 1983). However, only $CD4^+$ T-cells are capable of being transformed by HTLV-1, that is made capable of infinite growth in culture (Yoshida et al 1984). The receptor for HTLV is unknown at present, although studies of mice/human hybrid cells suggest that the gene for the receptor is lying on the long arm of chromosome 17 (Sommerfeld et al 1989). Rabbits may be infected with HTLV-1, and these are an important animal model for infection, but these animals do not appear to develop disease (Kotani et al 1986). It is also possible to infect old and new world primates with HTLV-1, although it is still unclear whether they develop any HTLV related disease.

   The mechanism of leukaemagenesis by HTLV-1 is unclear; the virus appears to integrate randomly, rather than in association with any known proto-oncogene (Seiki et al 1984). The observation that leukaemic cells are clonal suggests that a second event is necessary for maligancy to occur in virally infected cells, and that this second event is rare (Yoshida et al 1984). Suggestions for this second event are unfocussed, and Strongyloides stercoralis co-infection has been put forward as a co-factor, more in hope, it would seem (Nakada et al 1984). HTLV transformed T-cells express high numbers of IL-2 receptors, and grow independently of IL-2 (autocrine stimulation) (Greene 1986). It is therefore possible that if one of the IL-2 genes were to mutate in an HTLV-1 infected cell, this cell may become tumorous under the influence of the transactivating gene of HTLV (tax). This concept of a multi-step process involving the presence of the virus and a second mutational event occurring spontaneously is in keeping with current ideas on carcinogenesis. It certainly explains the long latency from infection to disease, and the observation that only a small proportion of infected subjects develop disease.

   The pathogenesis of HTLV-1 is far from resolved; it is interesting to speculate that transgenic animals may provide a key to rapid understanding of these viruses. Transgenic mice expressing only the HTLV-1 tax gene have been made which develop lesions indistinguishable from neurofibromatosis (von Recklinghausen's disease) (Hinrichs et al 1987). The significance of this is unknown !

## SEROLOGY AND SERO-EPIDEMIOLOGY

Infection by HTLV leads to an antibody response which is of high titre and persists life long; this is the basis for the identification of infection in the individual subject, and in populations. As with HIV, the options for diagnosis begin with simple, sensitive and inexpensive serological screening assays such as the ELISA or particle agglutination assay. Progression to assays of greater specificity such as the immunoblot, radio-immuno-precipitation (RIPA) or neutralisation assay may be required, and finally molecular assays are being developed which now mean the amplification of the HTLV genome by the polymerase chain reaction (PCR) or more laboriously of all, growth of HTLV by cell culture techniques.

### HTLV assays

*High sensitivity, low specificity screening assays*

1. ELISA
2. Particle agglutination
3. Immunofluorescence

*Higher specificity, lower sensitivity*

1. Competitive ELISA or RIA
2. Neutralising antibody
3. Immunoblot
4. RIPA

*Definitive assays for virus*

1. Culture
2. PCR

The screening assays currently all use cell lysates of HTLV on the solid phase for the test antibody binding. However, HTLV is a very cell associated virus, with little free virus generated into the culture supernatant. This means that the viral antigens are heavily contaminated with lymphocytic antigens, and this is a major cause of non-specific false positivity. In some populations, the false positive rate may be as high as 10% (Weber et al 1989). This could be overcome by using recombinant antigen on the solid phase, and although this may be achieved in the future, it is not available presently. The immunoblot is currently used as the gold standard for HTLV serology, but the human sera may react with any number of bands (Weber et al 1989). In addition, there is a practical problem of the sera which react with one or two *gag* bands only on immunoblot, without other reactivity. At the moment, these indeterminate reactivities are a considerable problem, particularly for blood transfusion directors, but equally for the subject involved.

The distinction between HTLV-1 and HTLV-2 is also difficult, as in serological terms they are very similar; neutralising assays will distinguish them as there is no cross neutralisation, but these assays are highly specialised (Weiss et al 1985). Wider use of the PCR technique will be valuable, but the two problems of contamination and reaction to endogenous retroviruses remain to be overcome (Bangham et al 1988). Until PCR has been better validated, it cannot be used with confidence on human material.

Serology for HTLV-1 at present uses a commercial direct antiglobulin ELISA (Dupont, Abbott) or a latex or gelatin particle agglutination assay (Serodia) as an initial screen, followed by immunoblot, or a competitive assay, currently only available in-house to one or two laboratories (Tedder et al 1984). Every effort should be made to confirm HTLV serology through the Virus Reference Laboratory at the Central Public Health Laboratory Service, Colindale, London NW9, before any information is given to the patient.

## EPIDEMIOLOGY

With the caveats given above as to the problems with serology, and the lack of attention to HTLV owing to the AIDS epidemic, the distribution and transmission are not as reliably known as would be wished. Below we attempt to list those areas where HTLV-1 is known to exist, associated with ATL or TSP; areas where sero-positivity is reported, but no disease is apparent; and areas where results lack confirmation, and no disease reported.

### Distribution of HTLV-1

*Category 1: definite virus and disease*

Japan
Caribbean islands
Caribbean immigrants to UK and elsewhere
South-eastern USA
West Africa

*Category 2: definite virus, ? disease*

East, Central Africa
South India

Eastern Siberia
Colombia and South America

*Category 3: ? virus, no disease*

Papua New Guinea
Other African countries
Australian aboriginals
Eskimo / Inuit / Aleuts

The distribution of HTLV-1 through south-western Japan and the northern island, Hokkaido (Hinuma et al 1982) and through the Caribbean is now beyond reasonable doubt (Blattner et al 1982). Prevalence ranges from 6–12% in these locations, and the sero-prevalence increases with increasing age, suggesting either that transmission is now less common than previously in these areas, or that there is delayed sero-conversion to HTLV-1 over time (Miller et al 1986).

In the USA, HTLV-1 infection is found in the south eastern states, in the black population who, one assumes, share the same risk as the Caribbean population. This must reflect ancient infection from their origin in West Africa (Gallo 1987). Testing of blood donors in the USA shows rates of between 0–0.1% (Williams et al 1988); however, the Sloan Kettering Hospital showed that multiply transfused oncology patients had a significant rate of HTLV-1 sero-positivity, suggesting that blood borne HTLV contamination was a problem in clinical practice, even at the low sero-prevalence rates noted above (Minamoto et al 1988).

In the UK, HTLV-1 has been detected in up to 6% of asymptomatic Caribbean immigrants (Catovsky et al 1982, Robert-Guroff et al 1984), including second generation children born in the UK, although this situation is considerably less common than for children born in the Caribbean. 4–5% of male homosexuals at risk for AIDS were HTLV-1 positive, and 6% of i.v. drug users were HTLV-2 infected (Tedder et al 1984). One bizarre feature of the epidemiology of HTLV-1 to emerge recently is the sporadic cases. In the UK, two clusters of family infections with HTLV-1 have been described, in white caucasian men and their families who have never left the country, nor had exposure to any endemic area or contact. These small foci have been reported from the Fjords of Norway, Southern Italy and Sicily, France and from northern states of the USA (Levine et al 1988, Manzari et al 1984, Goldman Leikie et al 1987). As vertical transmission of this virus is the major path of spread, and silent asymptomatic infection life-long is the rule, one can imagine that HTLV-1, introduced into a family by a traveller several generations previously, could remain present indefinitely.

## SPECIAL PROBLEMS WITH HTLV-2

As mentioned above, HTLV-2 was described first in 1982 from a patient with an unusual T-cell variant of an unusual leukaemia, the hairy cell leukaemia

(Kalyanaraman et al 1982); only one further isolate has ever been reported from this disease, and only five isolates are described in total (Rosenblatt et al 1986). There is complete serological overlap between these two viruses, but no cross-neutralisation (Weiss et al 1985). Competitive assays may distinguish HTLV-1 and 2, and data from these surveys has shown that i.v. drug users have a 4–6% prevalence of HTLV-2 in both the UK and the USA (Tedder et al 1984, Robert - Guroff et al 1984). It may be the most pragmatic solution to consider HTLV-2 as a sero-type of HTLV-1. The distribution of HTLV-2 around the world is not known, but no endemic group other than i.v. drug users has yet been described. Unpublished work by Blattner suggests that 40% of HTLV-1 sero-positive New Orleans i.v. drug abusers are in fact HTLV-2 infected when analysed by more specific PCR analysis. As the association of HTLV-2 with disease is so tenuous, it may be best to think of HTLV's in general, rather than HTLV-1 with its diseases and HTLV-2 possibly being non-pathogenic. If one accepts that the full natural history of these viruses remains unstudied in terms of prospective follow-up, one should consider life-long follow-up of all infected subjects in order to investigate the natural history further.

## TRANSMISSION OF HTLV-1

The exact modes(s) of transmission of HTLV-1 are unknown. The earlier work from Japan suggested that transmission by sexual contact occurred (Tajima et al 1982). The increased prevalence of HTLV-1 in women in endemic areas has been explained by the greater relative efficiency of male-to-female transmission at intercourse, than vice versa. Sexual transmission is corroborated by the relatively higher rates of HTLV-1 in sexually active male homosexuals at risk for HIV (Tedder et al 1984, Robert-Guroff et al 1984) and by the finding of an increased risk of HTLV-1 sero-positivity in sexually promiscuous i.v. drug users matched for needle sharing (Rezza et al 1988). However, a limited study of London prostitutes at risk for HTLV-1 through unprotected sexual intercourse with their West Indian boyfriends has shown no cases of HTLV-1 infection (Weber, unpublished). Mother to child transmission was reported in utero (Komuro et al 1983), and later via breast milk (Nakano et al 1984). The latter route is favoured by the rabbit HTLV-1 model, where breast feeding transmits HTLV-1 efficiently, but the trans-placental route does not lead to infection in the offspring (Hirose et al 1988). Blood transfusion has been repeatedly shown to be a significant route of transmission (Hino et al 1984), and has been thought to account for up to 16% of all HTLV-1 infections in an endemic area in Southern Japan (Okochi et al 1984).

However, closer examination of the details of HTLV-1 distribution in the Caribbean pose questions to this tidy view of the world. Miller (Miller et al 1986) has shown that rates of HTLV-1 sero-positivity rise with age, and that female infection is always more common than male; this has been confirmed by large serological studies (Levine et al 1988, Agius et al 1988). Infection was related to the quality of housing, with inferior social conditions significantly producing more infection; proximity to water and poor housing may implicate insect borne transmission. Certainly, the distribution of HTLV-1 around the world is confined largely to the humid tropical belt, and within these areas, HTLV-1 seropositivity is found predominantly in the coastal regions, where arthropod-borne diseases are more common (Weber et al 1989). Intriguingly, many have noted that mother to child transmision of HTLV-1 is more common in children born to sero-positive mothers in the Caribbean, than in children of sero-positive Caribbean immigrant mothers, born in the UK (Greaves et al 1984). Some factor applying to the tropics, and not to the UK, enhances transmission dramatically; this may be the social factors of poor housing and hygiene noted as independent risk factors in the Caribbean. Changes in these social factors may explain why the sero-prevalence of HTLV-1 appears to be declining in endemic areas (Ueda et al 1988).

Beyond the observation that HTLV-2 is more common in drug abusers than homosexual men, one may suppose that transmission by blood is more efficient than by sex (Robert - Guroff et al 1984). No other transmission data on HTLV-2 is available.

## DISEASES ASSOCIATED WITH HTLV INFECTION

### Adult T-cell leukaemia (ATL)

The first clinical description of ATL was published in 1977 by Uchiyama and Takatsuki (Uchiyama et al 1977). It is a rapidly progressive acute leukaemia of T-cell phenotype, which is unusual for the acute leukaemias (where over 95% are B-cell or Null cell phenotype). Patients present acutely, frequently have fever, generalised lymphadenopathy, hypercalcaemia and disseminated grade IV disease is often present on presentation; prognosis is poor. The skin is often involved, with lesions varying from discrete or confluent nodules to plaques, patches and erythroderma, and this accounted for the initial confusion with mycosis fungoides. The systemic complications include pleural effusion, aseptic meningitis and gastrointestinal tract involvement. The hypercalcaemia, which is almost invariable, is associated with skeletal lesions, a high alkaline phosphatase and normal phosphate. Patients in the leukaemic phase are more susceptible to opportunist infections, and *Pneumocystis carinii* pneumonia, CMV, cryptococcosis and candidiasis have been described (Cappell & Chow et al 1987).

The leukaemic cells have a particular morphology which is characteristic, and biopsy of the lymph node, but rarely the skin lesions, also gives diagnostic information. Peripheral blood lymphocytes from ATL patients will grow indefinitely in cell culture, without requiring IL-2. HTLV genome can be demonstrated in these cells, which are clonal. It is possible that pre-leukaemic stages of ATL exist and asymptomatic carriers may have small numbers of abnormal circulating lymphocytes (Yamaguchi et al 1983).

## Tropical spastic paraparesis

While studying the sero-prevalence of HTLV-1 on Martinique, Gessain, then a medical student, observed that there was a strong association between HTLV-1 infection and tropical spastic paraparesis (Gessain et al 1985), a syndrome first described by Montgomery and Cruikshank in 1964 (Montgomery et al 1964). Further studies by Newton in London, Rodgers-Johnson et al (Newton et al 1987, Rodgers-Johnson et al 1985) in the Caribbean and others have confirmed this epidemiological association. Moreover, Japanese investigators have noted a syndrome termed the HTLV-associated myelopathy (HAM) which is clinically indistinguishable from TSP (Osame et al 1986). HAM cases have been observed following transfusion associated HTLV-1 infection in Japan, as well as with perinatally or horizontally acquired infection (Osame et al 1987). HTLV-1 associated TSP has now also been described from temperate zones, including Santiago in Chile (Cartier - Rovirosa et al 1989) and southern Italy (Annunziata et al 1987) and so a change of nomenclature is clearly desirable.

The virological association of TSP/HAM with HTLV-1 is now far from circumstantial. In addition to the serological association of HTLV-1 antibodies to TSP, which approaches 100% correlation in some series (Newton et al 1987), HTLV-1 virus has been isolated from the CSF of these patients (Imamura et al 1988). CSF isolates from TSP have recently been shown to be closely related by nucleotide sequence and restriction enzyme polymorphism to the virus found in lymphocytes in ATL cases (Bangham et al 1988, Yoshida et al 1987). There is intra-thecal synthesis of anti-HTLV-1 IgG in the CSF (Ceroni et al 1988) and it is possible to find abnormal, pleomorphic lymphocytes in the peripheral blood of TSP/HAM patients which resemble the abnormal lymphocytes seen in the pre-leukaemic stage of ATL (Dalgleish et al 1989, Morgan et al 1987). One case has been reported of an HTLV-1 sero-positive patient with both TSP and ATL (Bartholomew et al 1986). The pathogenesis of HTLV in the CNS is unknown; there are very high antibody titres to HTLV-1 in the CSF and serum of TSP patients compared to ATL patients, and this may possibly reflect an immunological basis to TSP, whereby cross-reacting antibodies between HTLV-1 and a host protein such as myelin basic protein leads to auto-immune damage to the CNS (Dalgleish 1989).

The clinical features of TSP/HAM are distinctive, and quite separate from multiple sclerosis (MS). The disease presents initially between the ages of 20 and 50 years, with lumbar back pain, radiating down the legs as the commonest presenting symptom. The criteria for diagnosis are :

In patients with no childhood history of weakness, 2 of the following must be present within 2 years of onset;

1. Low back and leg pain
2. Urinary frequency, nocturia and/or retention of urine
3. Symmetrical weakness within 6 months
4. Dysaesthesiae/anaesthesiae of the lower limbs

Clinical examination should show spasticity of the lower limbs, with increased patellar reflexes, no sensory level and no pupillary changes; upper limb signs may occur later in disease. There must be no history of relapse or remission, which is the characteristic of the MS presentation in the older patient, where lower limb long tract signs may predominate.

CSF examination characteristically shows a lymphocytic pleocytosis with raised protein levels, normal glucose and oligoclonal bands. In the Tropics, the major differential diagnoses are:

1. Meningovascular syphilis
2. Syringomyelia
3. Spinal schistosomiasis
4. Transverse myelitis

In the West, the major differential diagnosis is MS, and so the history of chronic progression against relapse and remission are of some importance. The neurophysiological parameters of MS may also be found to be abnormal in TSP, and the visual and auditory evoked potentials may be identical. Magnetic resonance imaging (MRI) may show the extensive plaques associated with MS which are not a feature of TSP, but CT scanning may be less useful (Newton et al 1987, Tournier - Lasserve et al 1987). MRI abnormalities may also be seen in the brain of asymptomatic HTLV-1 carriers (Mattson et al 1987). Pathologically, TSP shows a lymphocytic perivascular cuffing in the spinal cord, and meningeal inflammation.

It is clear from the above discussion that the finding of a virus associated with an MS-like disease is of interest to the possible aetiology of MS itself. Despite several encouraging reports, it is extremely unlikely that HTLV is associated with MS in any causal manner. However, this is a rapidly moving field, and interested clinicians are advised to watch this space.

## OTHER DISEASE ASSOCIATIONS OF HTLV

As risk groups for HTLV and HIV are shared, it is not surprising that doubly infected subjects have been found. Studies in Trinidad have suggested that doubly infected patients, who have antibodies to both HTLV-1 and to HIV-1, have a higher rate of conversion to AIDS after infection by HIV (Bartholomew et al 1987). This requires further study. Two reports of dual infection leading to a CD8 + T-cell lymphoproliferative disease have been published (Harper et al 1988, Mulin et al 1988), and the importance of continued vigilance for the development of new clinical syndromes in dual infection must be stressed. A recent report suggests that ATL patients have a high rate of multiple primary malignancies (Immamura et al 1989), and further oncological sequelae of HTLV infection need to be sought.

Other, rare clinical associations of HTLV-1 include Sjogren's syndrome (Vernant et al 1988), T-cell alveolitis (Sugimoto 1987) and large granular lymphocyte proliferative disorders (Pandolfi 1987), and a case report of HTLV-1 associated chronic inflammatory arthropathy (Nishioka et al 1989). Reports of the association of HTLV-1 with MS and with mycosis fungoides must be treated with caution at this time.

## COUNSELLING THE HTLV INFECTED PATIENT

The natural history of HTLV-1 suggests that there is a 4.5% cumulative life-time risk of ATL development for males, and a 2.6% lifetime risk of ATL in an infected female (Tokudome et al 1989). Similar figures, though without the male bias, of a cumulative lifetime risk of ATL of 4.0–4.2% in those infected by HTLV-1 before the age of 20 years have been found by computer modelling (Murphey et al 1989). The lifetime chance of TSP/HAM developing is not yet known but may be slightly higher. It is not yet known whether there are any other consequences of infection, nor whether HTLV-2 infection has these or different sequelae. The prevalence of a pre-leukaemic stage is unknown, but all subjects should have a blood film examination (bone marrow only if abnormal cells seen in the film) and a neurological history and examination.

The chance of horizontal transmission from male to female is apparently higher than for female to male, and both are much lower than for hepatitis B virus, and probably for HIV. Vertical transmission occurs as the major mode of transmission of HTLV, and breast milk is clearly implicated as the principal route of infection to the child. No HTLV-infected mother should be allowed to breast-feed. There is no evidence to suggest that HTLV infected pregnancies should be terminated, providing there is no breast feeding. As vertical transmission is the dominant feature of this virus, screening and counselling should be offered to the family of subjects, in all generations. A family history should be sought, to check for elderly relatives with unexplained paraparesis, as this may respond to therapy.

HTLV-infected subjects should never give blood, bone marrow, breast milk, semen or any organ, and should not carry organ donor cards.

Infected subjects must be encouraged to carry on their lives as before. This virus has been around for a long time, and causes little disease. Awareness of this agent should not lead to panic, and it is especially important to avoid confusion with HIV and AIDS. However, my personal experience with screening geriatric paraparesis at the RPMS is that many families with HTLV are found, and that the number of unknowns in this infection make counselling almost impossibly difficult. Unfortunately, the USA have decided to screen blood donors for HTLV-1, and threat of litigation will doubtless cause the UK to follow suit. Now is the time to practise the management of the asymptomatic HTLV carrier; I have no feelings on pre-test counselling, except that the lack of hard knowledge about HTLV precludes rational advice prior to testing. Our knowledge will only increase with more widespread screening, but as ever, the individual may well be better off in ignorance of this virus. A more broad based consensus from the Caribbean population in particular is required urgently to defuse this situation.

Finally, concurrent HTLV and HIV may worsen the progression of both. As these viruses share many epidemiologic features, HTLV infection in a subject who is not from an endemic area should precipitate screening for HIV, HBV, syphilis and other sexually transmissable and blood borne agents.

## Acknowledgement

I would like to thank Mr Craig Barr for his assistance in the preparation of this manuscript.

REFERENCES

Agius G, Biggar R, Alexander S et al 1988 HTLV-1 antibody patterns: evidence of difference by age and sex. Journal of Infectious Diseases 158: 1235.

Annunziata P, Fanetti G, Giarratana M et al 1987 HTLV-1 associated TSP in an Italian woman. Lancet ii: 1393.

Bangham C, Daenke S, Phillips R et al 1988 Enzymatic amplification of exogenous and endogenous retroviral sequences from DNA of patients with TSP. EMBO Journal 7: 4179.

Bartholomew C, Cleghorn F, Charles W et al 1986 HTLV-1 and TSP. Lancet ii: 99.

Bartholomew C, Blattner W, Cleghorn F et al 1987 Progression to AIDS in homosexual men co-infected with HIV-1 and HTLV-1 in Trinidad. Lancet ii: 1469

Blattner W, Kalyanaraman V, Robert-Guroff M et al 1982 The human C-type retrovirus, HTLV, in blacks from the Caribbean and their relationship to ATL. International Journal of Cancer 30: 257

Cappell M, Chow J 1987 HTLV-associated lymphoma affecting the entire alimentary tract and presenting as an acquired immunodeficiency. American Journal of Medicine 82: 649

Cartier-Rovirosa L, Mora C, Araya F et al 1989 HTLV-1 positive TSP in a temperate zone. Lancet i: 556

Catovsky D, Rose M, Goolden A et al 1982 ATL in blacks from the West Indies. Lancet i: 639

Ceroni M, Piccardo D, Rodgers-Johnson P et al 1988 Intra-thecal synthesis of IgG antibodies to HTLV-1 supports an aetiological role for HTLV-1 in TSP. Annals of Neurology 235: 785

Clapham P, Nagy K, Cheingsong-Popov et al 1983 Productive infection and cell free transformation of HTLV in a non-lymphoid cell line. Science 222: 1125

Dalgleish AG, Richardson J, Sinclair A, Newell A 1989 HTLV-1 infection in TSP in the UK. AIDS Res. Hum. Retrovir. 1988 4: 475–485

Gallo RC 1987 HTLV-1 — the first human retrovirus. Scientific American 77–88

Gessain A, Barin F, Vernant J et al 1985 Antibodies to HTLV-1 in patients with tropical spastic paraparesis. Lancet ii: 1247

Goldman-Leikie R, Verst C, Kiev M et al 1987 HTLV-1 associated ATL in an atypical host. Archives of Pathology and Laboratory Medicine 111: 1054

Greaves M, Verbi W, Tilley R et al 1984 HTLV in the UK. International Journal of Cancer 33: 795

Greene W 1986 Deregulated IL-2 receptor expression in ATL. In: Greene W (moderator) The human Interleukin 2 receptor. Annals of Internal Medicine 105: 560

Harper M, Kaplan M, Marselle et al 1988 Concommittant infection with HTLV-1 and HTLV-III in T8 lymphoproliferative disease. New England Journal of Medicine 315: 1073

Hino S, Kawamichi T, Funakoshi M et al 1984 Transfusion mediated transmission of ATL virus. Gann 75: 1070

Hinrichs S, Nerenberg M, Reynolds K et al 1987 A transgenic mouse model for human neurofibromatosis. Science 237: 1340

Hinuma Y, Komoda H, Chosa T et al 1982 Antibody to adult T-cell leukaemia virus associated antigen (ATLA) in sera from patients with ATL and controls in Japan. International Journal of Cancer 29: 631

Hirose S, Kotani S, Uemura Y et al 1988 Milk borne transmission of HTLV-1 in rabbits. Virology 162: 487

Imamura J, Inada T, Kuramoto A 1989 Multiple primary malignant neoplasms in patients with ATL. Lancet i: 219

Imamura J, Tsujimoto A, Ohta Y et al 1988 DNA blotting analysis of HTLV in CSF of spastic paraparesis patients. International Journal of Cancer 42: 221–224

Kalyanaraman V, Sarngadharan M, Robert-Guroff M et al 1982 A new subtype of human T-cell leukaemia virus (HTLV-2) associated with a T-cell variant of hairy cell leukaemia. Science 218: 571

Komuro A, Hayami M, Fujii H et al 1983 Vertical transmission of ATL virus. Lancet i: 240

Kotani S, Yoshimoto S, Yamoto K et al 1986 Productive infection of the rabbit by HTLV-1. International Journal of Cancer 37: 843

Levine P, Blattner W, Clark J et al 1988 Geographic distribution of HTLV-1. International Journal of Cancer 42: 7

Manzari V, Gradilone A, Barillari G et al 1984 HTLV-1 is endemic in Southern Italy: detection of the first cluster in a white population. International Journal of Cancer 34: 501

Mattson D, McFarlin D, Mora C, Zaninovic V 1987 CNS lesions detected by MRI in an HTLV-1 antibody postive symptomless individual. Lancet ii: 49

Miller G, Pegram S, Kirkwood B et al 1986 Ethnic composition, age and sex together with location and standard of housing as determinants of HTLV-1 infection in an urban Trinidadian community. International Journal of Cancer 38: 801

Minamoto G, Gold J, Scheinberg D et al 1988 Infection with HTLV-1 in patients with leukaemia. New England Journal of Medicine 318: 219

Miyoshi I, Kubonishi I, Yoshimoto S et al 1981 Type C retrovirus in a cord blood T-cell line derived by co-cultivating normal human leukaemic T-cells. Nature (London) 294: 770

Montgomery R, Cruickshank E, Robertson W, McKenemy W 1964 Tropical spastic paraperesis. Brain 87: 425

Morgan O, Rodgers-Johnson P, Gibbs W et al 1987 Abnormal peripheral lymphocytes in TSP. Lancet ii: 403

Mulin G, Sheppell A, Mayer L et al 1988 Infection with HTLV-1 and HTLV-III in T8 lymphoproliferative disease. New England Journal of Medicine 316: 1343

Murphey E, Hanchard B, Figueroa J et al 1989 Modelling the risk of ATL in patients infected by HTLV-1. International Journal of Cancer 43: 250

Nakano S, Ando Y, Ichjio M et al 1984 Search for possible routes of transmission of ATL virus. Gann 75: 1044

Nakada K, Kohakura M, Komoda H, Hinuma Y 1984 High incidence of HTLV antibodies in carriers of Strongyloides stercoralis. Lancet i: 633

Newton M, Miller D, Rudge P et al 1987 Antibody to HTLV-1 in west Indian born UK residents with spastic paraparesis. Lancet i: 415

Nishioka K, Maruyama I, Sato K et al 1989 Chronic inflammatory arthropathy associated with HTLV-1. Lancet ii: 441

Okochi K, Sato H, Hinuma Y 1984 A retrospective study on transmission of ATL virus by blood transfusion: seroconversion in recipients. Vox Sanguinis 46: 245

Osame M, Usuku K, Izumo S et al 1986 HTLV-1 associated myelopathy, a new clinical entity. Lancet i: 1031

Osame M, Igata A, Usuku K et al 1987 Mother to child transmission in HAM. Lancet i: 106

Pandolfi F, Schriver K, Scarselli E et al 1987 HTLV-1 antibodies and lymphoproliferative disease of granular lymphocytes. Lancet ii: 1527

Poiecz B, Ruscetti F, Gazdar A et al 1982 Detection and isolation of retroviruses from cell lines of adult T-cell leukaemia and its implications in the disease. Proceedings of the National Academy of Sciences of the USA 79: 2031

Rezza G, Titti F, Rossi G et al 1988 Sex as a risk factor for HTLV-1 spread among IV drug abusers. Lancet i: 713

Robert-Guroff M, Blayney D, Safai B et al 1984 HTLV-1 antibodies in AIDS patients and others at risk. Lancet ii: 128

Robert-Guroff M, Weiss SH, Girou JA et al 1986 HTLV 1 2 & 3 in IV drug users in the USA. Journal of the Americal Medical Association 255: 3133–3137

Rodgers-Johnson P, Gajdusek D, Morgan O et al 1985 HTLV-1 and HTLV-2 antibodies and TSP. Lancet ii: 1247

Rosenblatt J, Golde D, Wachsman W et al 1986 A second isolate of HTLV-2 associated with atypical hairy cell leukaemia. New England Journal of Medicine 315: 372

Seiki M, Hattori S, Hirayami Y, Yoshida M 1983 Human adult T-cell leukaemia virus: complete nucleotide sequence of the provirus genome integrated in leukaemia cell DNA. Proceedings of the National Academy of Sciences 80: 3618

Seiki M, Eddy R, Shous T, Yoshida M 1984 Non-specific integration of the HTLV genome into adult T-cell leukaemia cells. Nature (London) 309: 640

Sommerfeld M, Clapham P, Goodfellow P, Weiss RA 1989 Gene for the receptor for HTLV-1 maps to chromosome 17. Science 1988 242: 1557–1559

Sugimoto M, Kakashima H, Watanabe S et al 1987 T-lymphocyte alveolitis in HTLV-1 associated myelopathy. Lancet ii: 1220

Tajima K, Tominaga S, Suchi T et al 1982 Epidemiological analysis of the distribution of antibody to ATLV-antigen: possible horizontal transmission of ATLV. Gann 73: 893

Tedder RS, Shanson DC, Jeffries D et al 1984 Low prevalence in the UK of HTLV-1 and HTLV-III infection in subjects with AIDS, lymphadenopathy syndrome and at risk of AIDS. Lancet ii: 125

Tokudome S, Tokunaga O, Shiramoto S et al 1989 Incidence of ATL among HTLV-1 carriers in Japan. Cancer Research 49: 226

Tournier-Lasserve E, Gout O, Gessain A et al 1987 HTLV-1, Brain abnormalities on MRI and relation with MS. Lancet ii: 49

Ueda K, Kusuhara K, Tokugawa K 1988 Transmission of HTLV-1. Lancet i: 1163

Uchiyama T, Yodi J, Sagama K et al 1977 Adult T-cell leukaemia; clinical and haematological features of 16 cases. Blood 59: 451

Vernant J, Buissson G, Magdeleine H et al 1988 T lymphocyte alveolitis, TSP and Sjogren's syndrome. Lancet i: 177

Watenabe T, Seiki M, Hinuma Y et al 1984 Human T-lymphotropic (US isolate) and adult T-cell leukaemia virus (Japanese isolate) are the same species of human retrovirus. Virology 133: 238

Weber J, Banatvala N, Clayden S et al 1989 False positive HTLV-1 serology in Papua New Guinea. Journal of Infectious Diseases (in press)

Weiss RA 1984 In: Weiss RA, Coffin, Teich (eds) RNA tumor viruses, Cold Spring Harbour

Weiss RA, Clapham P, Nagy K, Hoshiro H 1985 Envelope properties of the human T-cell leukaemia viruses. Current Topics in Microbiology and Immunology 115: 235

Williams A, Fang C, Slamm D et al 1988 Sero-prevalence and epidemiologic correlates of HTLV-1 infection in US blood donors. Science 240: 643

Yamaguchi K, Nishimura H, Kohrogi H et al 1983 A proposal for smouldering ATL. Blood 63: 758

Yoshida M, Osame M, Usuku K et al 1987 Viruses detected in HTLV-1 associated myelopathy and ATL are identical on DNA blotting. Lancet i: 1085

Yoshida M, Seiki M, Yamagudi K, Takatsuki K 1984 Monoclonal integration of HTLV provirus in all primary tumours of ATL suggests causative role of HTLV in the disease. Proceedings of the National Academy of Sciences 81: 2534

# Kaposi's sarcoma, aetiology and management

*J. Armes   S.M. Forster*

## INTRODUCTION

Kaposi's sarcoma (KS) is present in approximately 28% of AIDS patients at the time of their first medical presentation and a further 10% develop KS during the course of their illness. Along with pneumocystis pneumonia, it was one of the original manifestations of the severe immunodeficiency seen in homosexual males, which heralded the beginning of the AIDS epidemic.

AIDS-related KS has many similarities with the classical form of KS which was first described over a century ago (Kaposi 1872). This recent epidemic has served to renew interest in KS and to highlight many unanswered and intriguing questions which surround the disease.

At present the aetiology of KS is unresolved and is confounded by the fact that KS is associated with distinct epidemiological categories which have a wide spectrum of disease severity. KS can be divided into four epidemiological categories, which are described below:

### Epidemic KS

Epidemic KS is the term used to describe HIV-related KS. 'Epidemic' emphasises the enormous increase in the incidence of KS seen in the last decade, which has arisen in parallel to the epidemic of HIV infection. Interestingly, amongst the different population groups at risk of developing HIV infection, KS is much more commonly seen in homosexual males (36%) and African patients. In fact only 1% of haemophiliacs with AIDS have been reported to develop KS. In addition, KS is extremely rare in HIV-infected women or children.

HIV-related KS covers a spectrum of severity of disease. Patients may present with only one, or a few of the characteristic red-brown macules or papules on the skin. However this may progress to severe, disseminated KS, with widespread and confluent skin lesions, multiple lymph node and visceral lesions, including involvement in the lungs and gastrointestinal tract. The prognosis of AIDS patients is poor, although the cause of death in AIDS patients is likely to be directly related to infection rather than KS. Nonetheless, KS has been found in skin, viscera and lymph nodes in approximately 50% of AIDS patients at autopsy (Niedt & Schinella 1985,

Marmor et al 1982), and hence KS must contribute considerably to their morbidity.

## Classical KS

The first documented cases of KS (Kaposi 1872) would be included in the classical epidemiological subtype. It is a rare disease, but prior to the AIDS epidemic, it was the commonest form of KS seen in Europe and the USA. The annual rate of KS in the United States from 1973 until 1979 (before the outbreak of AIDS) was 0.29 per 100 000 population of men, and 0.07 per 100 000 population of women (Biggar et al 1984). Thus the male:female ratio ranges from 4:1, as reported above, to 10:1, and the patients are usually in their fifth to eighth decade. The underlying conditions which predispose to the development of classical KS are not known, although it has been suggested that these patients may have some non-specific deficit in their immune function, perhaps related to ageing. There appears to be some increased incidence of classical KS in men of Jewish or Mediterranean extraction (DiGiovani & Safai 1981), although the reason for this observation is again unclear.

Classical KS is not usually a severe disease and is often limited to a single skin lesion on the lower limb. The mortality from classical KS is correspondingly low.

## Endemic KS

KS is a common disease in central, sub-Saharan Africa, particularly Uganda, Rwanda and Zaire. KS had been described in this location before the onset of the AIDS epidemic and is distinct from HIV-related KS seen in Africa. Like classical and epidemic KS, endemic KS has a pronounced male predominance when seen in adults (male:female ratio approximately 10:1). However, unlike most other categories of KS, it is relatively common in children, where the sex incidence is approximately 2 male:1 female.

The clinical spectrum of disease in adult endemic KS is broad and can be limited, locally aggressive or disseminated. The limited form is usually confined to a single lesion on the lower limb. Oedema is often associated with the KS lesion and it may even affect the limb before the KS lesion is visible macroscopically. Locally aggressive KS is usually a single lesion, but may ulcerate and erode underlying tissue, including bone. If left untreated the prognosis of locally aggressive KS is poor, although chemotherapy is usually effective at prolonging survival. The disseminated form of endemic KS is rapidly progressive, with KS involving lymph nodes and viscera as seen in disseminated HIV-related KS. In children, a lymphadenopathic variant of KS may occur, when there is massive involvement of the lymph nodes, although, in contrast to other forms of KS, skin involvement is insignificant or absent. These children usually die within 1 year of onset of their disease.

Apart from the endemic forms of KS described above, in which patients have no other manifestations of AIDS and, when tested, are HIV negative, there is an increasing incidence of HIV-related KS in Africa. This new category of African KS is known as atypical, African KS (Bayley et al 1985) and the male:female ratio is approximately 5:1. It is a more acute disease than endemic African KS, which rapidly progresses, with early involvement of lymph nodes and other viscera. The outlook for these patients is poor, with over 50% mortality within 1 year of onset of disease.

### Immunosuppression-associated KS

It has been known for some time that patients may develop KS whilst immunosuppressed for reasons other than HIV infection. This form of KS has been most commonly seen in renal transplant recipients. Penn (1979) reported an incidence of 3% in a series of 600 renal transplant recipients. These patients are generally younger than those with classical KS (the most common age being in the fourth decade) and KS in these patients is often related to the onset of immunosuppression. The male:female ratio is reported to be 2:1 (Dictor 1987). Apart from patients with iatrogenic immunosuppression, there is also an increased incidence of KS in patients immunosuppressed for other reasons, notably in association with primary malignancies, especially lymphoma.

Immunosuppression-associated KS affects the skin and the viscera and is more often related to the cause of death than classical KS. Fortunately, KS may respond to withdrawal or reduction of immunosuppressive therapy, if the underlying immunosuppression is iatrogenic.

## PATHOGENESIS OF KAPOSI'S SARCOMA

### Pathological appearances

There are two main components of KS lesions when seen microscopically. One is a proliferation of spindle cells, the other is the development of abnormal endothelial elements. Although both components are present in most KS lesions, their proportions vary with the histological spectrum of the disease.

Early KS lesions show only very subtle microscopic differences from surrounding tissues and when seen in the dermis may bear a striking resemblance to early scar tissue or non-specific inflammatory changes. The characteristic appearance of these early 'patch' lesions is a predominance of abnormal endothelial elements. These form vessels which are thin-walled, excessively dilated and irregular and are lined by flattened endothelium. The spindle cell component in this histological form of KS is inconspicuous.

Plaque lesions are thought to be a more advanced stage of KS than patch lesions. Spindle cells are present either diffusely or in aggregates and are seen together with the abnormal endothelial elements, which gives the plaque lesion a much more cellular appearance than the patch stage of KS. Many biopsies taken from AIDS patients show plaque-like pathological appearances (Francis et al 1986), although these changes have also been reported in patients without HIV infection (Ackerman 1979).

KS is also seen in a nodular form, when there are well-defined aggregates of spindle cells making up an easily-recognisable tumour. The spindle cells are usually surrounded by dilated, abnormal vessels, commonly seen in the patch and plaque KS lesions. It is not known whether this type of histological appearance is a more advanced stage of KS, or whether it arises de novo. Biopsies of the classical epidemiological form of KS usually have a nodular appearance. However the association of this histological form with classical KS may be due to these lesions being biopsied at a relatively late stage of disease development, when compared to HIV-related KS.

It is rare to see signs of cellular atypia in either the endothelial elements or the spindle cells of KS. However, in the locally aggressive form of endemic KS, cellular and nuclear pleomorphism, and a high mitotic rate of the spindle cells have been reported. These cytological indicators of aggressive behaviour have not been reported in HIV-related KS.

## The cell of origin of KS

The nature of the cell of origin of KS has been the subject of some debate. Although the histological appearance of KS would suggest that abnormal endothelium constitutes part of the lesions, the relation of the endothelial elements to the spindle cells is not well defined. Nonetheless, several studies have attempted to elucidate whether both spindle cell and endothelial elements are of similar origin and also whether they show lymphatic rather than vascular endothelial differentiation. These studies have primarily used immunohistochemcial and related techniques.

Beckstead et al (1985) and Russell-Jones et al (1986) concluded that KS had properties similar to lymphatic endothelium, rather than vascular endothelium, due to the profile of staining of cells within the KS lesion with a panel of endothelial markers which was compared to the staining profiles obtained with these endothelial markers on normal vascular or lymphatic endothelium. In both studies staining of the spindle cell component was absent or stained only poorly. The endothelial cells did not stain with vascular endothelial markers, such as Factor VIII and it was proposed that the profile of staining was suggestive of lymphatic origin. However, since a good histological marker which positively identified lymphatic endothelium was not available, the lack of endothelial staining could not identify lymphatic differentiation conclusively.

In contrast, two other studies have reported that KS has features of vascular endothelium rather than lymphatic endothelium. Rutgers et al (1986) described an immunochemical study in which both the endothelial and the spindle cell component stained with markers which also identified vascular, but not lymphatic endothelium. In addition, Suzuki et al (1986) used antibodies to HLA-A, B and C antigens, which are usually detected on normal blood vessels and found positive staining in KS tissue, thus concluding that KS shows vascular endothelial differentiation.

In addition to using immunohistochemical techniques, the spindle cells of KS have been examined for Wiebal-Palade bodies, using electron microscopy (these bodies are an ultrastructural feature of vascular endothelium). However, in the study by McNutt et al (1983), Weibal-Palade bodies were not detected.

The results of the studies described above are conflicting and the cell of origin of the KS lesion is proving difficult to define by immunocytochemical methods. This may reflect the paucity of endothelial markers specifically raised against endothelial antigens and also the altered sensitivity of some markers, such as Factor VIII antibodies, as a result of the different tissue processing procedures carried out in different laboratories. Alternatively, the lack of reproducibility of staining in both the endothelial and spindle cell elements of KS may reflect a relatively immature stage of development of the cellular component of KS. If this were so, one would not expect to find staining profiles similar to differentiated endothelium of either vascular or lymphatic origin.

## KS, a neoplasia or hyperplasia?

KS has many features which appear different from common malignant tumours, ranging from its sometimes slow growth to its histological appearance. Thus the hypothesis has been proposed that KS may be a hyperplastic rather than a neoplastic lesion (Costa & Rabson 1983, Brooks 1986). Several features seem to implicate the hyperplastic nature of KS. The clinical presentation of KS is not typical of other malignant tumours, in which development of a primary tumour is classically followed by development of metastatic lesions. In KS, crops of skin lesions may arise simultaneously. Furthermore, it has been reported that lesions occuring late in a patient's disease may not resemble pre-existing lesions histologically and may have the appearances of an early patch-like lesion (Reynolds et al 1965). Furthermore, KS lesions of the gastrointestinal tract, which may become apparent after the development of skin lesions, usually occur in the mucosa and submucosa rather than in the serosa, where most metastatic lesions in the gastrointestinal tract occur.

Most neoplasias are thought to be clonal and thus primary explant cultures of cells derived from one lesion should have an identical genetic constitution. Delli-Bovi et al (1986) cultured cells derived from KS material which were identified as likely to originate from KS rather than supporting stromal cells, due to their staining profile with endothelial cell markers. The cells showed identical chromosomal rearrangements within individual cultures, but the rearrangements differed between cultures, even though each culture was propagated from the same KS lesion. This genetic heterogeneity was interpreted as suggesting that the original tissue did not form by clonal expansion and hence was more likely to be of hyperplastic rather than neoplastic origin.

Another phenomenon associated with KS is its ability to regress which, although not seen commonly in KS lesions, is well documented and occurs with much greater frequency than is seen in most malignant tumours. It would seem likely that regression could occur in a hyperplastic rather than truly neoplastic lesion since, in the former, growth is not completely autonomous, and thus regression could be explained by removal of the external stimulus to proliferation, or alternatively, the reimposition of a state of growth inhibition.

In some cases of KS the clinical progression is one of a non-malignant and rather indolent disease, even in HIV-infected patients. At this stage the KS lesions may be hyperplastic rather than neoplastic and presumably proliferating under the control of an external stimulus. However, other patients may be severely debilitated by disseminated KS and in these patients the KS appears to be behaving in a malignant fashion. One model of the pathogenesis of KS, accounting for the extremes of behaviour of this disease, could be proposed in which KS is initially a hyperplastic lesion dependent on external stimuli to proliferation. Sustained proliferation could then lead onto further genetic events which may result in some elements becoming truly neoplastic and thus independent of the original stimulus to growth.

## AETIOLOGY OF KAPOSI'S SARCOMA

Various factors have been proposed as aetiological agents of KS and are described below:

### An infectious agent

An infectious aetiology for KS has been proposed for some time. This proposal was mostly based on the peculiar geographical distribution of African endemic KS. A tumour belt of KS exists in Central Africa, where the disease is extremely common, and can include up to 12% of all malignancies. This high incidence declines sharply north of the Sahara and more gradually to the east and west. There are also some areas within Central Africa where time-space clustering of cases of endemic KS have occurred (Owor & Hutt 1977, Bland et al 1977). McHardy et al (1984) have reported endemic cases from the West Nile district of Uganda, where most patients live in isolated communities at altitudes above 800 meters. Interestingly, KS was not found in all populations living in this district at high altitude, suggesting that the lifestyle adopted when living at high altitude did not itself predispose to the development of KS, rather the high incidence seen in certain communities compared to the general population reflected their relative isolation.

There are several features of epidemic KS which are compatible with the view that KS develops following infection with a second agent, other than HIV. Epidemic KS is usually seen in the homosexual population of Western AIDS patients and also in African AIDS patients. KS is much less common amongst drug abusers than homosexual patients and is still a rare occurrence in haemophiliacs with AIDS. African and homosexual AIDS patients are largely thought to acquire HIV infection via sexual transmission. One explanation for their particular susceptibility to KS, may be their increased exposure to sexually transmitted infections, in addition to HIV, when compared to patients at risk of HIV for other reasons. It is therefore interesting to note the recent decline in the proportion of homosexual AIDS patients who present with KS (Des Jarlais et al 1987). This fact has been interpreted as suggesting that the decline in KS is the result of some modification of behaviour in this AIDS subgroup, since there has been a parallel decline in both KS and the incidence of sexually transmitted disease other than HIV, such as gonnorhoea and syphilis.

*Cytomegalovirus infection*

The most frequently proposed, and also the most studied candidate for a KS-related infectious agent, is the Herpes virus, Cytomegalovirus (CMV). Giraldo et al (1972) described Herpes virus-like particles in five out of eight tissue culture lines derived from different cases of African KS. The virus isolated from one of these cultures was later characterised and found to have some of the properties of CMV (Glaser et al 1977). A further association between CMV and KS was noted when sero-epidemiological studies showed a high incidence of CMV antibodies in both European and American patients with KS (Giraldo et al 1975, 1978). It was also known that other members of the Herpes virus group were linked to development of malignancies, eg. Epstein Barr virus was associated with the development of Burkitt's lymphoma and nasopharyngeal carcinoma and, at this time, Herpes simplex virus was thought to be associated with the development of cervical carcinoma. Therefore, it was reasoned that CMV may be involved in KS oncogenesis. Giraldo et al (1980) then reported the presence of CMV DNA in KS tissue biopsies using DNA:DNA reassociation kinetics, when purified CMV virion DNA was used as a probe to search for CMV genome in KS cells. The finding of CMV DNA in KS tissue appeared to support the hypothesis that CMV infection was associated with the development of KS.

However, since these studies were performed, evidence for a direct link between CMV and the development of KS has become less convincing. Ruger et al (1984) showed that CMV genome had sequences which were homologous to parts of the human genome, thus raising the possibility that the DNA reassociation techniques used by Giraldo et al (1980) to detect CMV genome in KS tissue could have produced spuriously positive results. Ruger et al (1984) and Delli-Bovi et al (1986) have looked for CMV DNA in KS tissue using cloned CMV probes which lack the sequences which share homology with normal human DNA. In both cases CMV DNA was detected in some KS lesions, but since CMV DNA was also detected occasionally in normal skin from the same patients, the relevance of CMV to the development of KS could not be established.

Indeed, it is relatively difficult to prove an aetiological relation between CMV and KS, since both are commonly found in immunosuppressed patients. Homosexual men have an extremely high incidence of CMV reactivation or re-infection and the prevalence of CMV antibody in this population may be as high as 94% (Drew et al 1981). Thus, since KS is seen in only a small fraction of this population, it is obvious that CMV infection must be at most only one of a complex set of contributing factors leading to the development of KS.

*HIV infection*

HIV has not been detected in KS lesions from AIDS patients by Southern blot analysis (Delli-Bovi et al 1986). This fact, together with the apparent irrelevance of HIV to the development of non-HIV-related KS, had led to its dismissal as an aetiological agent for KS, other than as a cause of immunosuppression. However, a recent study by Vogel et al (1988) has renewed interest in a direct link between HIV and the development of KS.

In this study, the *tat* gene of HIV was introduced into the germline of mice, under the control of the HIV LTR (long terminal repeat). Various tissues from the transgenic progency of these mice were screened for *tat* gene mRNA expression, however, such expression was only found in skin, where it occurred in both male and female mice. Interestingly, 33 of the 37 male transgenic mice went on to develop skin tumours which were histologically similar to human KS (such tumours did not arise spontaneously in the same strain of non-transgenic mice). In contrast none of the female transgenic mice developed these skin tumours, despite *tat* gene expression in skin. Thus, not only did the tumours appear similar to KS morphologically, but they also shared the same predisposition for development in males. Cells were cultured from some of the skin tumours. However, *tat* gene expression could not be detected in these tumour cells, using Northern blot analysis, despite examining cells from early culture passages.

Thus these data indicate that although the *tat* gene appeared critical to the development of skin tumours in the transgenic mice, *tat* gene mRNA was not produced in the tumour cells themselves. One possible explanation for this finding is that the tumour cells proliferated in response to stimuli from neighbouring non-tumour cells and that the stimuli may have been produced in response to *tat* gene expression. If this hypothesis were to be extended to human KS in HIV-infected individuals, one would not expect to find evidence of HIV infection in the KS tumour cells themselves. Rather, as proposed for the development of skin tumours in transgenic mice, KS cells could be proliferating in response to products of neighbouring cells infected by HIV. Hence, if this model of KS pathogensis is correct, HIV nucleic acid would not be detected in KS tissue by conventional Southern or Northern blot analysis.

The study described above does not explain why KS develops in patients who are not infected with HIV, nor why HIV-related KS is most commonly seen in patients with sexually transmitted HIV infection. It may be that gene products from other infectious agents could produce similar effects as HIV, or that HIV gene expression only effectively induces KS growth in conjunction with other factors. The development of skin tumours in the male transgenic mice and not female mice does imply that, like KS, the hormonal environment may be important for tumour development.

*Other viruses*

KS tissue has been examined for Epstein Barr virus (Giraldo et al 1975) and Hepatitis B virus (Siddiqui 1983, Delli-Bovi et al 1986) infection. Although evidence of infection with these viruses has occasionally been found, there is little evidence to suggest a causal relationship between these viruses and KS. However, Nakamura et al (1988) found that cell cultures derived from KS tissue proliferated in response to growth factors produced by T-cell lines transformed by human T-cell leukaemia viruses (HTLV). Although it is unlikely that infection with HTLV alone are responsible for the maintenance of KS, this finding may indicate the dependence of KS growth on factors secreted by virally-infected cells. This model of KS growth is consistent with the data described above (Vogel et al 1988), in which HIV *tat* gene expression was found in skin tissue of transgenic mice, but not tumour tissue itself. Hence, it may be that looking for viral genes in KS tumour material, rather than neighbouring cells will be unrewarding and that the role of virus infection in the development of KS may be via production of factors conducive to KS growth by a different cell population.

**Angiogenic factors**

Although there is indirect evidence for an infectious aetiology of KS, it is unlikely to be the only factor leading to the development of this disease. The association of most types of KS with immunodeficiency could suggest that immunodeficiency itself may be important to KS development, regardless of the accompanying infections. However, reduced immunosurveillance alone cannot account for the prevalance of KS in immunosuppressed patients since, if this were so, one would not expect KS to be particularly common in immunosuppressed patients, when compared to other tumours, such as lung and gastrointestinal tumours.

There is evidence that factors involved in the immune response may affect endothelial cell function. Activated T-cells have been shown to release lymphokines which stimulate angiogenesis (Auerbach & Sidky 1979) and activated macrophages produce soluble factors responsible for neovascularisation of the guinea-pig cornea (Polverini et al 1977). Lymphokines have also been shown to cause expression of HLA-DR antigens on endothelial cells (reviewed by Baldwin 1982) and also inhibition of endothelial cell migration (Cohen et al 1982). Many of the factors affecting endothelium have not been characterised, although heparin and prostaglandin $E_1$ have been implicated in angiogenesis.

It seems that the relationship between the immune system and endothelial function is complex and our knowledge of their interaction is far from complete. However, it is possible to envisage that a disruption in the immune system may lead to an imbalance in the secretion of these angiogenic factors, or alternatively, a decrease in factors which inhibit angiogenesis. It is interesting that enhanced angiogenesis is compatible with the histological appearance of KS.

In addition to cells of the immune system secreting angiogenic factors, it is possible that angiogenic factors may be produced by KS cells themselves. It has been shown that cell cultures derived from AIDS KS tissue produce a profusion of cytokines, many of which have been identified and are known to evoke angiogenesis. Basic fibroblast growth factor and interleukin-2 have been detected in the medium conditioned by KS cell cultures (Ensoli et al 1989) and have been shown to be biologically effective angiogenic factors, acting in both a paracrine and autocrine manner. However, although production of cytokines by KS cells may contribute to growth of KS, it does not explain how KS development is initiated.

## Oncogenes

Oncogene expression has been linked to the development of several neoplastic tumours. Oncogene expression has also been examined in KS lesions. Indeed, a transforming DNA sequence has been identified in KS tissue (Lo & Liotta 1984), following extraction of DNA from KS tissue taken from skin and a lymph node of a homosexual AIDS patient with disseminated KS. A standard DNA transfection assay was performed in which KS DNA was transfected into mouse fibroblasts (NIH 3T3 cells), which were grown in culture. Transformed colonies of the NIH 3T3 cells were identified, which were shown to contain human repetitive DNA sequences (ie. the transformed colonies had taken up human DNA). DNA was then extracted from these transformed primary colonies and transfected again into more NIH 3T3 cells, following which secondary transformed colonies were generated. The DNA from the primary and secondary colonies were injected into immunodeficient mice, which went on to develop angiosarcomatous tumours.

Thus the above data indicate that the DNA originally extracted from the KS tissue contained sequences which were both capable of transforming cells in culture and were oncogenic in immunosuppressed mice. In order to characterise the transforming sequence further, DNA from transformed colonies were hybridised to probes derived from known oncogenes ($ras^H$, $ras^N$, $ras^K$, v-sis, v-src, v-fes). However, following Southern blot analysis, the identity of the transforming sequence could not be demonstrated and therefore it seemed that the oncogenic sequence found in this study had not been previously characterised.

Other studies have since reported the presence of an oncogenic sequence in AIDS-related KS (Delli-Bovi & Basilico 1987, Delli Bovi et al 1987). DNA from KS lesions from a number of AIDS patients were transfected into NIH 3T3 cells. Only one transformed colony developed, and all subsequent experiments were performed on cells derived from this clone. Again human repetitive DNA sequences were detected in DNA from the transforming colony and secondary transformants were established following further transfection of DNA from the primary colony into NIH 3T3 cells. In addition, DNA extracted from both primary and secondary colonies were capable of producing tumours in immunodeficient mice.

Therefore this data supported that of Lo & Liotta (1984), since it appeared that an oncogenic sequence had again been identified in KS tissue. In the more recent studies the transforming DNA sequence was isolated and found to be 11KB long, from which two mRNA transcripts were made (1.2 and 3.2 KB). The protein translated from the 1.2 KB transcript could promote growth in NIH 3T3 cells. Interestingly, the amino acid sequence of this protein showed significant homology to basic and acidic fibroblast growth factors, which are known to be strongly angiogenic. Thus it was proposed that the production of a possible angiogenic growth factor in KS tissue might be responsible for the vascular appearance and proliferation of KS cells.

Unfortunately the oncogenic sequence described above was only isolated from one of several KS specimens. It may be that this transforming sequence is difficult to isolate, or that it was absent from the other KS lesions. The other possibility is that the transforming sequence was generated by the experimental procedure itself, especially since the putative oncogene was not detectable in the original KS tissue. Further comparison of the transforming sequence has shown it to be homologous to the *hst* oncogene, which has been detected in human stomach cancer (Sakamoto et al 1986, Taira et al 1987). However, since the presence of the *hst* oncogene has also been found in normal gastric mucosa by similar transfection techniques, it is possible that this particular sequence is prone to generation by the transfection assay. Indeed, in a recent study the *hst* oncogene was not detected in KS cell cultures (Ensoli et al 1989), which again raises the possibility that this transforming sequence found in KS may have arisen during the transfection assay.

## Hormonal influence

It has been noted for some time that the incidence of KS is increased in males compared to females of the same age. This situation is also seen in epidemic KS, which is a relatively rare manifestation of HIV infection in females of either Western or African origin. This male bias suggests that some protection may be gained from hormones such as oestrogen. However, since there is no accentuated increase in the number of KS cases in postmenopausal women compared to premenopausal women, when increased age is taken into account, protection by female sex hormones is not obvious (Templeton 1972). Reversal of the hormonal environment in male patients with non-epidemic KS with oestrogen therapy has been attempted, but has had little effect on KS progression (Templeton 1972). The possibility remains that a male trait may actively promote the development of KS.


CONCLUSION

KS remains a clinical and biological enigma. The relationship between HIV-associated KS and KS seen in other epidemiological categories has not been clearly established. Neither is there a definitive explanation for the large excess of HIV-related KS in homosexual patients when compared to patients in other AIDS-risk groups. Although several suggestions have been proposed to account for the aetiology of KS, none are at present entirely satisfactory. However, it does seem that the recent epidemic of KS has led to renewed interest and research into this fascinating disease.


MANAGEMENT OF KAPOSI'S SARCOMA IN PATIENTS WITH AIDS

In the past this has been governed by the assumption that treating the Kaposi's sarcoma (KS) does not improve the prognosis of the underlying disease (AIDS), the patients ultimately dying from other opportunist disease, usually infection. Treatment has therefore, been aimed at ameliorating symptoms without producing undue side effects or further immunosuppression. By and large this premise still stands, however, as our treatment and prophylaxis of the opportunistic infections seen in AIDS has improved, and with the advent of effective anti-HIV drugs such as Zidovudine, there is no doubt that we are seeing more patients for whom disseminated KS is their most serious and ultimately terminal condition. Perhaps we should be treating KS more agressively and earlier in view of this trend and more work into the role of combination chemotherapy in these patients is urgently needed (see below).

The assessment of any form of therapy in KS is difficult for two main reasons, the great variation in the extent and natural history of the disorder between different patients, and the lack of any meaningful staging system in KS as is used in other forms of cancer.


### The clinical course of Kaposi's sarcoma

The natural history of KS in AIDS patients may vary widely. Some may present with a smaller number of cutaneous lesions that progress very slowly over a period of many years, occasionally lesions even regressing. In others the disease accelerates rapidly over a period of months or even weeks. Most patients present with relatively slowly progressive cutaneous lesions, the disease accelerating with the development of systemic symptoms as the patient becomes more immunosuppressed. However, the pattern of cutaneous disease may not reflect what is happening internally, and symptomatic gastrointestinal or respiratory disease can occur with no cutaneous KS at all (Barrison et al 1988). Virtually every organ of the body may be involved with KS, but CNS disease is rare. Occasionally disease affects predominantly the lymph nodes. Involvement of the dermal lymphatics can produce severe localised oedema and cellulitis especially of the legs or face.

## Staging of Kaposi's sarcoma

Several attempts have been made to stage the disease in a way comparable to that used in other malignancies (Krigel et al 1983, Laubenstein 1984, Mitsuyasa et al 1986, Mitsuyasa 1987) but this has been fraught with difficulty. Mortality and response to treatment seem to be more linked to the state of the patient's immune system (as assessed by parameters such as the absolute T4 count, presence of P24 antigenaemia etc.) and the presence or absence of opportunistic infection, than the extent of the KS or the presence of systemic symptoms (indeed it is difficult in many cases to determine if these are due to KS, infection or HIV itself) (Vadhan Raj et al 1986, Taylor et al 1986). The location of KS does affect prognosis however. Those patients with predominantly cutaneous or lymph node involvement fare better than those with systemic disease. Patients need to be assessed and treatment selected and monitored using a combination of:

1. Rate of development of new lesions
2. Number, extent and size of lesions
3. Appearance of lesions (as a result of therapy lesions may flatten, fade in colour and become less nodular although remaining the same size)
4. Presence of systemic symptoms, and systemic involvement with KS
5. Immunological profile (T4 counts etc)
6. Presence and nature of other opportunist disease

## Support

KS is often the first major disease experienced by an AIDS patient, and is a diagnosis that many HIV infected patients dread because of the disfigurement it can cause. All patients need support, counselling and reassurance when first diagnosed. Many are surprised that the lesions are not surgically removed or treated more aggressively. The role of camouflage cosmetics should not be underestimated and expert advice on this should be sought.

## Anti-retroviral drugs

Zidovudine, the reverse transcriptase inhibitor, will prolong the life of patients with KS, and reduce the frequency of other opportunistic disease occurring. In some patients KS lesions may regress within a few weeks of taking Zidovudine, and it is quite common to see the rate of new lesions appearing drastically reduce after Zidovudine has been started. In other patients no benefit to the KS is seen at all, and unfortunately in the majority of patients any benefit seen is only temporary, and the KS ultimately progresses. In general, however, Zidovudine should be offered to all patients with AIDS-related KS.

## Local therapy

Surgical excision is not usually used unless there is a need for a diagnostic biopsy or in rare cases where it is essential that a mass is removed e.g. a large polypoid lesion at risk of causing obstruction in the naso-pharynx. Apart from the risk of haemorrhage, KS lesions tend to recur at the site of the scar (and indeed it is common for new lesions to appear at the site of previous trauma). Intralesional bleomycin, vincristine and etoposide have been used, but are painful and produce tissue necrosis. Other local treatments used by some centres include cryosurgery, topical application of 2, 4-dinitrochlorobenzene and intralesional injection of recombinant human tumour necrosis factor. None of these techniques have widespread usage at present.

## Radiotherapy

Fortunately, as with classical KS, cutaneous AIDS-related KS lesions are radio-sensitive and usually respond to a dose in the region of 800 rad (Krown 1988a, Harris & Reed 1985, Hill 1987). If treated early the lesion may completely fade. Often it will flatten and become less nodular, fading to leave only a brown patch of pigmentation which the patient finds much more cosmetically acceptable (and of course the lesion has been prevented from growing any larger). Side effects for cutaneous lesions are minimal, and in the early stages of KS cutaneous disease can often be contained using repeated radiotherapy. Unfortunately care must be taken when giving radiotherapy to mucosal surfaces as a severe mucositis often develops, usually complicated by infections such as candidiasis or herpes simplex (prophylactic acyclovir and anti-fungal agents such as fluconazole may be indicated to prevent this). Low dose fractionation should always be used in these areas, and also to avoid exacerbation of localised oedema due to lymphatic involvement.

Subtotal electron beam therapy may be used if there is one part of the body particularly severely affected (eg. a leg). In a very few patients where widespread cutaneous disease is a major problem and chemotherapy cannot be given, total skin electron beam radiotherapy may be used (Nisce & Safei 1985). In general systemic disease is best treated with chemotherapy, but occasionally lymph node involvement and even more generalised respiratory or gastrointestinal disease have been treated with radiotherapy (Nobler et al 1987).

## Interferon therapy

Because of its antiviral, antitumour and immune modulating effect, alpha-interferon was one of the first drugs used in the treatment of AIDS-related KS

(Krown et al 1983) and it became obvious that some patients had a dramatic response to the drug (Groopman et al 1984, Volberding et al 1985, Real et al 1986). However, it was difficult to compare these studies as widely different dose regimes were used to treat patients in different stages of the disease. In studies using higher doses regimes major responses were seen in up to 40% of patients, but these doses produced significant side effects (flu-like febrile illness, depression, lethargy, myelo- and hepatotoxicity etc) and many clinicians felt that the large treatment failure group did not warrant the morbidity as a result of side effects. However, studies performed in the last few years have greatly clarified the situation, and a good response to interferon is strongly associated with:

1. High T4 counts (>400)
2. Absence of prior opportunistic infections
3. Absence of systemic symptoms
4. Absence of P24 antigen

Patients in this category may have a response rate far greater than 50% (Volberding et al 1987, De Wit 1988, Lane et al 1988).

Interferon alpha has been shown to have an anti-HIV effect in vitro (Ho et al 1985) and in vivo, although its use clinically as an anti-HIV drug is still under investigation. It may be that it has more effect in early patients and that a degree of 'resistance' to interferon develops as HIV disease progresses, possibly associated with down regulation of interferon receptors or the development of anti-interferon antibodies, as it is known that levels of endogenous 'acid labile' interferon becomes progressively elevated as HIV disease progresses. Recent work suggests (De Wit et al 1988) that those patients whose KS responds to alpha interferon are also more likely to show evidence of a response to interferon as an anti-HIV drug in terms of a fall in P24 antigen. Controlled studies are necessary to show whether patients treated with interferon have a better long-term survival or not.

It would seem that interferon therapy does have a place for the treatment of a certain group of patients with KS who are prepared to tolerate its side effects for a limited period of time. The fever chills and malaise can be reduced by starting at lower doses and increasing the dose gradually, giving the injection at night and giving concurrent paracetamol. Tolerance to the drug does develop after the first few weeks. The patient must be monitored carefully for myelo or hepato toxicity. Most patients learn to inject themselves. In those patients who have responded the interferon can be continued at a lower maintenance dose. In those that respond, remission may last for many months even years. However, it is important that patients realise the limitations of therapy, and the extent of the side effects of the drug.

Although alpha-interferon is used frequently in the treatment of KS in the USA, it has never been a popular treatment in the UK, most centres relying on radio and chemotherapy.

Studies with Zidovudine and alpha-interferon in combination are also showing promising results, response rates with much lower doses of interferon being seen (Mulin et al 1988). Interferon in high doses exacerbates the haematological toxicity of Zidovudine. When given in combination with other chemotherapeutic agents such as etoposide or vinblastine the risk of haematological toxicity is also increased with no apparent benefit.

## Chemotherapy

Chemotherapeutic agents have been used successfully in Kaposi's sarcoma not associated with AIDS, particularly the endemic African form, with a good but often short lived response (Olweny 1981). A number of agents have been used in AIDS-associated KS (see Table 4.1) either as a single agent or combination chemotherapy. However, for the reasons outlined above, namely the problems in accurately staging the disease or defining a response to therapy it is difficult to compare these studies and none of them have been compared in terms of long term mortality to untreated controls. There is no right or wrong therapeutic regime at present, therefore, each major centre tending to have its own preference. The best course is to be flexible, adapting the therapy according to the needs of the patient (e.g. intravenous versus oral) the side effects incurred (e.g. for some patients hair loss is a more serious problem than for others who tolerate it well) and the other drugs the patient may be taking (particular care being taken with those that suppress the bone marrow or are neurotoxic).

Response rates as high as 84% have been reported (Laubenstein 1984) with a median remission of about 8 months, however, other studies are less successful than this and in general those regimes with the greatest efficacy are usually the most toxic (Volberding et al 1987).

Chemotherapy is indicated in those patients with evidence of systemic disease (e.g. respiratory or gastrointestinal KS) but will also slow down or even halt the appearance of cutaneous lesions and may alter the appearance of

Table 4.1   Chemotherapeutic agents used in AIDS-associated KS

| CHEMOTHERAPEUTIC | REFERENCES |
|---|---|
| Etoposide | Laubenstein et al 1984 |
| Vincristine | Mintzer et al 1985 |
| Vinblastine | Volberding et al 1985 |
| Bleomycin | Wernz et al 1986 |
| Doxorubicin | Fischl et al 1988 |
| Doxorubicin, Vincristine & Bleomycin | Laubenstein et al 1984 |
| Vinblastine & Vincristine | Kaplan et al 1986 |
| Vinblastine & Bleomycin | Wernz et al 1986 |
| Vincristine & Bleomycin | Glaspy et al 1986 |
| Vinblastine & Methotrexate | Minor et al 1986 |
| Actinomycin, Bleomycin & Vincristine | Gill et al 1986 |
| Interferon α 2b & Etoposide | Krigel et al 1988 |
| Interferon α, Actinomycin D, | |
| Vinblastine & Bleomycin | Shepherd et al 1988 |
| Actinomycin D, Vincristine & | |
| Bleomycin | Latif et al 1989 |

existing ones, causing them to flatten and fade. Occasionally they may completely regress although there is usually some residual pigmentation. In those patients with extensive disease and evidence of profound immunosuppression response is less likely and may not justify the inconvenience and side effects of the drugs. In all cases the use of chemotherapy should be regarded as palliative.

Each drug has its own individual problems. Vinblastine, one of the most effective drugs used, produces bone marrow suppression which limits its use in most patients. Given as an IV injection weekly the white cell count usually drops at 4–10 days and may not recover for some weeks. Neurological toxicity is less marked than with vincristine where a mixed sensorimotor neuropathy may occur in 1/3 of patients or more (although bone marrow suppression is less marked). Nerve conduction studies may be helpful in differentiating this from the other causes of neurological disease in HIV infection, although these may potentiate each other. Etoposide has the advantage that it can be given (in higher doses) orally, although alopecia is common and bone marrow suppression usually limits the dose given. Bleomycin produces minimal bone marrow toxicity but is commonly associated with rashes and the total dose given should be limited to 300 mg (possibly less in those patients with pre-existing lung disease) because of its association with the development of intestinal pneumonitis and fibrosis (difficult to differentiate from that seen in AIDS due to other causes). Doxorubicin produces alopecia, gastrointestinal, cardiac and bone marrow toxicity (the cardiac toxicity may have a delayed onset) and is less frequently used.

We favour at present a regime of vincristine and bleomycin, as these drugs have demonstrated efficacy against KS with minimal myelotoxicity. Zidovudine can be given with this regime safely (Brunt et al 1989) although if neutropenia occurs the Zidovudine should be stopped until recovery has occurred and restarted at a lower dose until the course of chemotherapy has finished.

As in other fields of oncology, it is hoped that the new haematopoietins, in particular granulocyte colony stimulating factor (GCSF) will allow us to give higher and longer doses of chemotherapy safely. Preliminary studies indicated that GCSF will increase the circulating neutrophil count in AIDS patients with neutropenia and that these neutrophils function normally, however work on GCSF and GMCSF (granulocyte macrophage colony stimulating factor) is still in progress and at the time of writing they are not yet available for clinical use.

REFERENCES

Ackerman A B 1979 Subtle clues to diagnosis by conventional microscopy: the patch stage of Kaposi's sarcoma. American Journal of Dermatopathology 1: 165–172
Auerbach R, Sidky Y A 1979 Nature of the stimulus leading to lymphocyte-induced angiogenesis. Journal of Immunology 123: 751–753

Baldwin W M 1982 The symbiosis of immunocompetent and endothelial cells. Immunology Today 3: 267–269

Barrison I G, Forster S M, Harris J W et al 1988 Upper gastrointestinal KS in HIV-antibody-positive patients in the absence of cutaneous disease. British Medical Journal 296: 92–93

Bayley A C, Downing R G , Cheinsong-Popov R, Tedder R S, Dalgleish A G, Weiss R A 1985 HTLV-III serology distinguishes atypical and endemic Kaposi's sarcoma in Africa. Lancet i: 359–361

Beckstead J H, Wood G S, Fletcher V 1985 Evidence for the origin of Kaposi's sarcoma from lymphatic endothelium. American Journal of Pathology 119: 294–300.

Biggar R J, Horm J, Fraumeni J F Jr, Greene M M, Goedert J J 1984 Incidence of Kaposi's sarcoma and mycosis fungoides in the United States including Puerto Rico, 1973–1981. Journal of the National Cancer Institute 73: 89–94

Bland J M, Mutoka C, Hutt M S R 1977 Kaposi's sarcoma in Tanzania East Africa. Journal of Medical Research 4: 47–53

Brooks J J 1986 Kaposi's sarcoma: a reversible hyperplasia. Lancet ii: 1309–1311.

Brunt A M, Goodman A B, Phillips R H, Youle M S, Gazzard B G 1989 The safety of intravenous chemotherapy and zidovudine when treating epidemic Kaposi's sarcoma. AIDS 3: 457–460.

Cohen M C, Picciano P T, Douglas W J, Yoshida T, Kreutzer D L, Cohen S B 1982 Migration inhibition of endothelial cells by lymphokine-containing supernatants. Science 215: 301–303.

Costa J, Rabson A S 1983 Generalised Kaposi's sarcoma is not a neoplasm. Lancet i: 58

Delli-Bovi P, Basilico C 1987 Isolation of a rearranged human transforming gene following transfection of Kaposi's sarcoma DNA. Proceedings of the National Academy of Sciences of the USA 84: 5660–5664

Delli-Bovi P, Donti E, Knowles D M II et al 1986 Presence of chromosome abnormalities and lack of AIDS retrovirus DNA sequences in AIDS-associated Kaposi's sarcoma. Cancer Research 46: 6333–6338

Delli-Bovi P, Curatola A M, Kern F G, Greco A, Ittmann M, Basilico C 1987 An oncogene isolated by transfection of Kaposi's sarcoma DNA encodes a growth factor that is a member of the FGF family. Cell 50: 729–737

Des Jarlais D C, Stoneburner R, Thomas P, Friedman S R 1987 Declines in proportion of Kaposi's sarcoma among cases of AIDS in multiple risk groups in New York City. Lancet ii: 1024–1025

De Wit R, Schattenberk J, Boucher C A B et al 1988 Clinical and virological effects of high dose recombinant interferon alpha in disseminated AIDS-related Kaposi's sarcoma. Lancet ii: 1214–1217

Dictor 1987 Kaposi's sarcoma: a trifactorial model. Medical Hypothesis 22: 429–441

DiGiovani J J, Safai B 1981 Kaposi's sarcoma: retrospective study of 90 cases with particular emphasis on the familiar occurrence, ethnic background and prevalence of other diseases. American Journal of Medicine 71: 779–783

Drew W L, Mintz L, Miner R C, Sands M, Ketterer B 1981 Prevalence of Cytomegalovirus infection in homosexual men. Journal of Infectious diseases 143: 188–192

Ensoli B, Nakamura S, Salahuddin S Z et al 1989 AIDS-Kaposi's sarcoma-derived cells express cytokines with autocrine and paracrine growth effects. Science 243: 223–226

Fischl M A, Krown S, Mitsuyasu R et al 1988 Weekly doxorubicin in the treatment of patients with AIDS related Kaposi's sarcoma (abstract). The IV International Conference on AIDS, Stockholm

Francis N D, Parkin J M, Weber J, Boylston A W 1986 Kaposi's sarcoma in acquired immune deficiency syndrome (AIDS). Journal of Clinical Pathology 39: 469–474

Gill P, Deyton L, Radick C et al 1986 Results of a prospective trial of adriamycin, bleomycin and vincristine in the treatment of epidemic Kaposi's Sarcoma (abstr) Proceedings of the American Society of Clinical Oncology 6:5

Giraldo G, Beth E, Coeur P, Vogel C L, Dhru D S 1972 Kaposi's sarcoma: a new model in the search for viruses associated with human malignancies. Journal of the National Cancer Institute 49: 1495–1507

Giraldo G, Beth E, Kourilsky F M et al 1975 Antibody pattern to Herpes viruses in Kaposi's sarcoma: serological association of European Kaposi's sarcoma with Cytomegalovirus. International Journal of Cancer 15: 839–848

Giraldo G, Beth E, Henle W et al 1978 Antibody patterns to herpes viruses in Kaposi's sarcoma II. Serological association of American Kaposi's sarcoma with cytomegalovirus. International Journal of Cancer 22: 126–131

Giraldo G, Beth E, Huang E-S 1980 Kaposi's sarcoma and its relationship to cytomegalovirus (CMV) III. CMV DNA and CMV early antigens in Kaposi's sarcoma. International Journal of Cancer 26: 23–29

Glaser R, Geder L, St. Jeor S, Michelson-Fiske S, Haquenau F 1977 Partial characterisation of a herpes-type virus (K9V) derived from Kaposi's sarcoma. Journal of the National Cancer Institute 59: 55–60

Glaspy J, Miles S, McCarther S, Carden J, Mitsuyashu R 1986 Treatment of advanced stage Kaposi's sarcoma with vinblastine and bleomycin. Proceedings of the American Society of Clinical Oncology 5:3

Groopman J E, Gottlieb M S, Goodman J et al 1984 Recombinant alpha-2 interferon therapy for Kaposi's sarcoma associated wtih AIDS. Annals of Internal Medicine 100: 671–676

Harris J R W, Reed T A 1985 Kaposi's sarcoma in AIDS: the role of radiation therapy. Frontiers of Radiation Therapy and Oncology 19: 126–132

Hill D R 1987 The role of radiotherapy for epidemic Kaposi's sarcoma. Seminars in Oncology 14 (suppl) 3: 19–22

Ho D D, Hartshom K L, Rota T R et al 1985 Recombinant human interferon, alpha-A suppresses HTLV-III replication in vitro. Lancet i: 602–604

Kaplan L, Abrams D, Volberding P 1986 Treatment of Kaposi's sarcoma in AIDS with an alternating vincristine and vinblastine regime. Cancer Treatment Reports 70: 1121–1122

Kaposi M 1872 Idiopathigches multiples pigment sarcom der Haut Archives Dermatologie und Syphilis 4: 265–273

Krigel R L, Laubenstein L J, Muddia F M 1983 Kaposi's sarcoma: a new staging classification. Cancer Treatment Reports 67: 531–534

Krown S E 1988a AIDS-associated Kaposi's sarcoma: pathogenesis, clinical course and treatment. AIDS 2: 71–80

Krown S E, Real Fx, Cunningham-Rundles S et al 1983 Preliminary observations on the effects of recombinant leukocyte A interferon in homosexual men with Kaposi's sarcoma. New England Journal of Medicine 308: 1071–1076

Krown S E et al 1988b Proceedings of the American Society of Clinical Oncology (abstract)7:1

Lane H C, Kovacs J A, Feinberg J et al 1988 Anti-retroviral effects of interferon alpha in AIDS-associated Kaposi's sarcoma. Lancet ii: 1218–1223

Latif A, Houstan S, Neill P, Bassett M, Thornton C, Sitima J et al 1989 Kaposi's sarcoma in patients with HIV infection, (abstract MBP289) V International Conference on AIDS, Montreal

Laubenstein L 1984 Staging and treatment of KS in patients with AIDS. In Friedman Kien A E, Laubenstein L J (eds) AIDS, the epidemic of Kaposi's sarcoma and opportunistic infection. Massan USA New York pp 51–55

Lo S-C, Liotta L A 1984 Vascular tumours produced by NIH/3T3 cells transfected with human AIDS Kaposi's sarcoma DNA. American Journal of Pathology 110: 7–13

McHardy J, Williams E H, Geser A, De-The G, Beth E, Giraldo G 1984 Endemic Kaposi's sarcoma: incidence and risk factors in the West Nile district of Uganda. International Journal of Cancer 33: 203–212

McNutt N S, Fletcher V, Conant M A 1983 Early lesions of Kaposi's sarcoma in homosexual men. American Journal of Pathology III: 62–77

Marmor M, Friedman-Kien A E, Lauberstein L et al 1982 Risk factors for Kaposi's sarcoma in homosexual men. Lancet i: 1083–1087

Minor D R, Brayer T 1986 Velban and methotrexate combination chemotherapy for epidemic Kaposi's sarcoma. Proceedings of the American Society of Clinical Oncology 5:1

Mintzer D M, Real Fx, Jorino L, Krown S E 1985 Treatment of Kaposi's sarcoma and thrombocytopenia with vincristine in patients with AIDS. Annals of Internal Medicine 102: 200–202

Mitsuyasu R T 1987 Clinical variants and staging of Kaposi's sarcoma. Seminars in Oncology 14 (suppl 3): 13–18

Mitsuyasu R T, Taylor J M G, Glaspy J, Fahey J L 1986 Helerogeneity of epidemic Kaposi's sarcoma. Implications for therapy. Cancer 56: 1657–1661

Mulin M et al 1988 (abstract). Proceedings of the American Society of Clinical Oncology 7:1

Nakamura S, Salahuddin S Z, Biberfeld P et al 1988 Kaposi's sarcoma cells: long-term culture with growth factor from Retrovirus-infected CD4 + T cells. Science 242: 426–433

Niedt G W, Schinella R A 1985 AIDS. Clinicopathological study of 56 autopsies. Archives of Pathology and Laboratory Medicine 109: 727–734

Nisce L Z Safai B 1985 Radiation therapy of Kaposi's sarcoma in AIDS. Frontiers of Radiation Therapy and Oncology 19: 133–137

Nobler M P. Leddy M E, Huh S H 1987 The impact of palliative irradiation on the management of patients with AIDS. Journal of Clinical Oncology 5: 107–112

Olweny C L M 1981 Management of Kaposi's sarcoma. Antibiotics and Chemotherapy 29: 88–95

Owor R, Hutt M S R 1977 Kaposi's sarcoma in Uganda: further epidemiological observations. East African Journal of Medical Research 4: 55–57

Penn I 1979 KS in organ transplant recipients: report of 20 cases. Transplantation 27: 8–11

Polverini P J, Cotran R S, Gimbrone M A Jr, Unanue E R 1977 Activated macrophages induce vascular proliferation. Nature 269: 804–806

Real Fx, Oettger H F, Krown S E 1986 Kaposi's sarcoma and AIDS: treated with high and low doses of recombinant leucocyte A interferon. Journal of Clinical Oncology 4: 544–551

Reynolds W A, Winkelmann R K, Soule E H 1965 Kaposi's sarcoma: a clinicopathological study with particular reference to its relationship to the reticuloendothelial system. Medicine 44: 419–441

Ruger R, Burmester G R, Kalden J R et al 1984 Search for human cytomegalovirus DNA in Kaposi's sarcoma and haematopoietic cells from homosexual men with AIDS or unexplained lymphadenopathy. Acquired Immune Deficiency Syndrome. Liss, New York, pp 127–137

Russell-Jones R, Spaull J, Spry C, Wilson Jones E 1986 Histogenesis of Kaposi's sarcoma in patients with and without acquired immune deficiency syndrome (AIDS). Journal of Clinical Pathology 39: 742–749

Rutgers J L, Wieczorek R, Bonetti F et al 1986 The expression of endothelial cell surface antigens by AIDS-associated Kaposi's sarcoma. American Journal of Pathology 122: 493–499

Sakamoto H, Mori M, Taira M et al 1984 Transforming gene from human stomach cancers and a noncancerous portion of stomach mucosa. Proceedings of the National Academy of Sciences of the USA 83: 3997–4001

Siddiqui A 1983 Hepatitis B virus DNA in Kaposi's sarcoma. Proceedings of the National Academy of Sciences of the USA 80: 4861–4864

Stambuk D, Youle M, Hawkins D et al 1989 The efficacy and toxicity of azidothymidine (AZT) in the treatment of patients with AIDS and AIDS-related complex (ARC); an open uncontrolled treatment study. Quarterly Journal of Medicine 70: 161–174

Suzuki Y, Hashimoto K, Crissman J, Kanzaki T, Nishiyama S 1986 The value of blood group-specific lectin and endothelial associated antibodies in the diagnosis of vascular proliferations. Journal of Cutaneous Pathology 13: 408–419

Taira M, Yoshida T, Miyagawa K, Sakamoto H, Terada M, Sugimura T 1987 cDNA sequence of human transforming gene *hst* and identification of the coding sequence required for transforming activity. Proceedings of the National Academy of Sciences of the USA 83: 2980–2984

Taylor J, Afrasiabi R, Fahey J L et al 1986 Prognostically significant changes in AIDS with Kaposi's sarcoma. Blood 67: 666–671

Templeton A C 1972 Studies in Kaposi's sarcoma. Cancer 30: 854–967

Vadhan-Raj S, Wong G, Gnecco C et al 1986 Immunological variables as predictors of prognosis in patients with Kaposi's sarcoma and AIDS. Cancer Research 46: 417–425

Vogel J, Hinrichs S H, Reynolds R K, Luciw P A, Jay G 1988 The HIV *tat* gene induces dermal lesions resembling Kaposi's sarcoma in transgenic mice. Nature 35: 606–611

Volberding P A, Abrams D I, Conout M, Kaslow K, Vranizan K, Ziegler J 1985 Vinblastine therapy for Kaposi's sarcoma in AIDS. Annals of Internal Medicine 103: 335–338

Volberding P A, Mutsuyasu R T, Golando J P, Spiegel R J 1987 Treatment of Kaposi's sarcoma with interferon alpha 2b. Cancer 59: 620–625

Wernz J, Laubenstein L, Hynes K, Walsh C, Muggia F 1986 Chemotherapy and assessment of response in epidemic Kaposi's sarcoma with bleomycin and velban. Proceedings of the American Society of Clinical Oncology 5:4

# 5

# The radiology of HIV infection

*Susan Barter*

Initial reports of the acquired immunodeficiency syndrome (AIDS) were first made in the United States in 1981 and followed in the United Kingdom several years later. Since then the epidemic has spread in this country with numbers of reported cases following the projected rising trend.

This chapter aims to describe the more important radiological manifestations of AIDS and HIV infection. Whilst it would be impossible in a text of this size to describe every conceivable radiological complication, it is hoped to present the more important findings and relate them to clinical practice.

The revised case definition of AIDS published by the Centres for Disease Control (CDC) in 1987, allows for the presumptive diagnosis of indicator diseases, for example *Pneumocystis carinii* pneumonia (PCP) based on clinical and radiographic findings without confirmatory laboratory evidence. This places a larger emphasis on the place of radiology, not only in the diagnostic role of pattern recognition but also in techniques for obtaining tissue diagnosis and monitoring response to treatment. In discussing the radiology of HIV infection, it is convenient to adopt a system orientated approach.

## NEURORADIOLOGY OF HIV INFECTION AND AIDS

Neurological abnormalities in patients with HIV infection have become common features of the disease affecting up to 33% of AIDS victims. Neuroradiological studies are, therefore, frequently requested in these patients in order to identify potentially treatable conditions thus prolonging the time a patient spends outside hospital.

It has long been recognised that a large number of patients with AIDS have neurological complaints and that up to 10% of patients may present with neurological symptoms prior to other manifestations of HIV infection (Levy et al 1986).

More recently, however, Ho et al (1985) examined specimens of brain, spinal cord and cerebrospinal fluid in 45 patients who were sero-positive for HIV. 33 of these patients had neurological symptoms and HIV was cultured from 24 of them. These and other results suggest virus attacks CNS tissue and that there may be CNS disease irrespective of opportunistic infections or tumours.

The most common indications for neuroimaging in HIV positive patients include decreased mental status, altered level of consciousness, headache, fits, focal neurological defects and cranial nerve palsies. Because clinical features are often non-localising, even in the presence of focal abnormalities such as abscesses, CT (or if available magnetic resonance imaging, MRI) has a valuable role to play.

The neuroradiological findings generally fall into four patterns. The most common finding is cerebral atrophy. The second pattern is single or multiple mass lesions that may be caused by infection or neoplastic disorders. The third pattern is focal or diffuse white matter disease and the fourth least frequently observed abnormality is leptomeningeal disease (Table 5.1)

**Table 5.1**   Neuroradiological abnormalities in AIDS

| | Cause | |
| | Common | Uncommon |
| --- | --- | --- |
| Atrophy | HIV<br>CMV | |
| Mass lesions | Toxoplasma<br>Lymphoma | Candida<br>TB<br>Cryptococcus<br>Kaposi's sarcoma |
| White matter disease<br>Focal<br>Diffuse | Ischaemia<br>HIV<br>CMV<br>Ischaemia | PML<br>Herpes zoster<br>Herpes simplex |
| Leptomeningeal disease | HIV<br>CMV<br>Cryptococcus<br>Lymphoma | Histoplasmosis<br>Candida<br>Aspergillus<br>Coccidiomycosis<br>Mycobacteria |

**Cerebral atrophy**

This is evident on CT which demonstrates enlarged sulci and ventricles, often striking in these generally young patients (Fig. 5.1). There is no enhancement following the administration of contrast. The aetiology of the diffuse cerebral atrophy is unclear but there is close correlation between the AIDS dementia complex (ADC) and development of cerebral atrophy on CT imaging.

It seems probable the atrophy results from the direct cytopathic effect of HIV on brain tissue. CT is indicated in patients with ADC to exclude a treatable space occupying lesion. Cytomegalovirus (CMV) is seen pathologically in the brain of 25% of AIDS victims. CMV causes a diffuse encephalitis that may also lead to loss of brain tissue producing atrophy on CT imaging (Petito et al 1986).

**Mass lesions**

Intracranial mass lesions are common in patients with AIDS occurring in about 22% (Levy et al 1986). Toxoplasmosis and CNS lymphoma account for

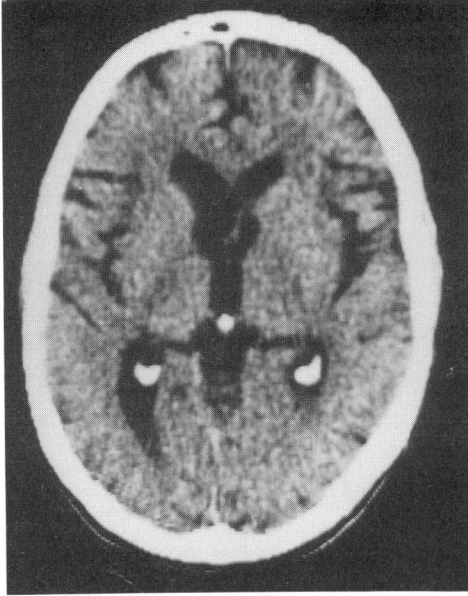

**Fig. 5.1** CT of brain in 23-year-old male patient with AIDS dementia complex showing evidence of cerebral atrophy. Note widened sulci and enlarged lateral ventricles.

the large majority of mass lesions (Navia & Price 1986). Less commonly seen are abscesses due to Candida, TB and Cryptococcus. Even more rare are metastatic Kaposi's sarcoma (KS) and bacterial infections.

Toxoplasmosis occurs in approximately 10% of patients. Clinically, there may be subacute headache, fever and focal neurology but non-focal findings of confusion and decreased mental state are common. One or more poorly circumscribed lesions with either ring or nodular enhancement typically occurring in the grey/white matter interface or basal ganglia, surrounded by oedema may be demonstrated. Solitary lesions are less common, and some lesions have low attenuation centres which are probably more mature abscesses with necrotic centres (Fig. 5.2A).

Because cerebral toxoplasmosis is the most common cause of focal abnormality, and treatable with effective therapy, it is the general practice to give a trial of antitoxoplasma treatment to such cases, reserving brain biopsy for those who fail to respond. There is generally marked clinical improvement in one week and CT appearances are dramatically improved on follow-up scans 10–14 days after treatment (Fig. 5.2B).

Patients with atypical findings on CT such as solitary, solid or non-enhancing lesions are still usually empirically treated with antitoxoplasma therapy.

After toxoplasmosis the next most common mass lesion found in HIV positive patients is primary CNS lymphoma occurring in up to 6% (Petito et al

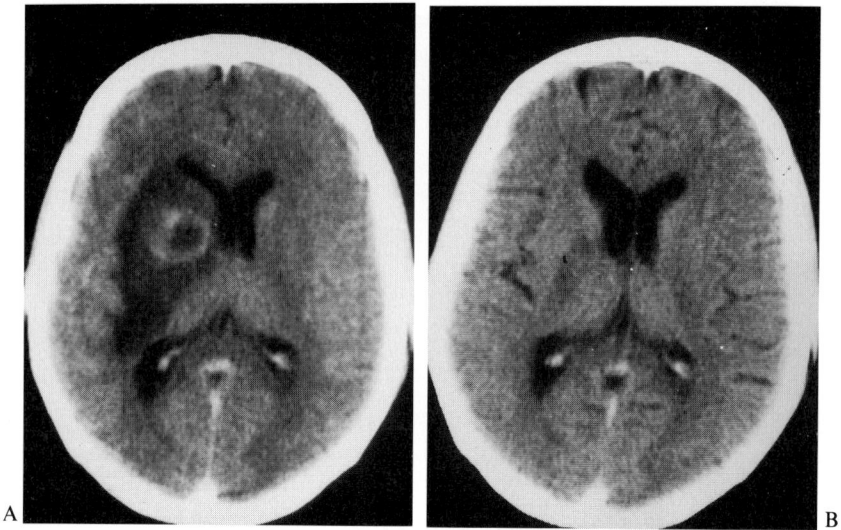

**Fig. 5.2** **A,** Typical toxoplasma abscess **B,** Showing resolution after several weeks of treatment.

1986). The clinical findings are variable including encephalopathy, fits, cranial nerve palsies and focal neurological symptoms. The prognosis is very poor with most patients surviving less than 2 months.

The CT appearance is of a solitary mass that enhances homogenously after contrast. Ring enhancement is seen in up to 50% of primary CNS lymphoma lesions, an unusual appearance that does not occur in non-AIDS CNS lymphoma. The lesions may be multiple (Fig. 5.3).

### White matter disease

This is common in HIV positive patients although often only seen at autopsy. The cause is usually due to viral infection, often HIV itself. Other agents that attack the white matter include CMV, JC Papova virus which causes progressive multifocal leucoencephalopathy (PML), herpes zoster and herpes simplex. Ischaemia may also play a part in white matter disease, particularly if the patient is hypoxic from pneumonia.

MRI is much more sensitive to white matter changes than CT but is not widely available in the UK. CT shows diffuse low density in the periventricular white matter commonly in AIDS patients and although unproven in most cases this is probably secondary to HIV encephalitis (Fig. 5.4).

PML causes necrosis and demyelination of white matter. CT shows destructive zones of decreased density in the white matter which enlarge without mass effect, or contrast enhancement. The absence of these latter features and non-vascular distribution distinguish the lesions from ischaemia, focal infection and neoplastic disease.

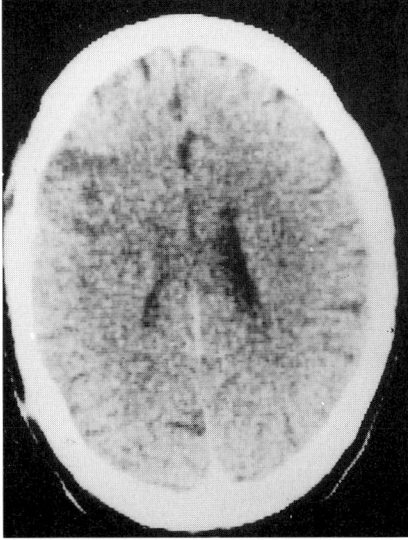

**Fig. 5.3**  Primary CNS lymphoma. Note solitary mass which enhances homogeneously.

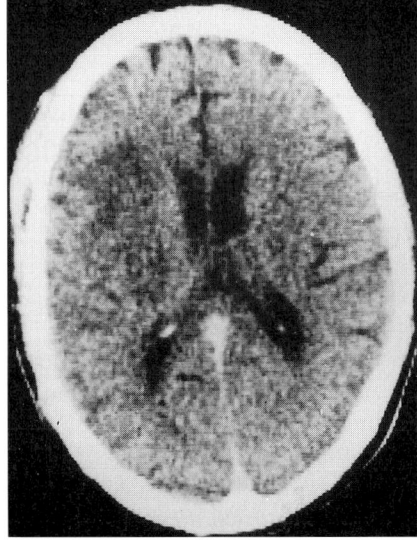

**Fig. 5.4**  CT of the brain showing diffuse low density in the peri-ventricular white matter due to white matter disease.

## Leptomeningeal disease

Although common pathologically in AIDS, this is not usually visible on imaging. Contrast CT may show abnormal enhancement of the meninges or mild hydrocephalus, or atrophy. The most important role of CT in such cases is excluding mass lesions or other pathology which would preclude lumbar puncture.

The causes of leptomeningeal disease are summarised in Table 5.1.

## Myelopathy

The occurrence of myelopathic symptoms in AIDS patients has become another of the initially overlooked, but now more obvious components of the disease.

It may be caused by cord compression from tumour such as non-Hodgkins lymphoma, or more commonly by intrinsic cord pathology. The latter is probably the result of direct infection by HIV which has been cultured from the spinal cord in some patients (Ho et al 1985).

Myelography in these patients is usually normal but CT scans performed after a 12–24 hour delay following intrathecal contrast, may demonstrate mild to moderate uptake of contrast in the cord. This is thought to represent a collection of contrast in areas of vacuolation in the cord similar to that seen in post-traumatic myelomalacia.

MR studies have not yet been reported in this situation. If there is extrinsic cord compression, CT or MRI will demonstrate an extradural mass causing compression.


## PULMONARY MANIFESTATIONS

Pulmonary complications were the first to be stressed in the radiological literature and more than 50% of AIDS patients develop pulmonary disease at some time. Radiographic evaluation plays an important role in the diagnosis and management of these patients, despite considerable overlap in the clinical and radiological findings (Naidich et al 1987, Goodman & Gamsu 1987).

*Pneumocystis carinii* pneumonia (PCP) is the most common life-threatening pulmonary infection, occurring in up to 84% of patients with pulmonary disease (Murray et al 1984).

In this country other common organisms giving rise to pulmonary pathology include mycobacteria, especially *Mycobacterium tuberculosis* (MTB), cytomegalovirus and pyogenic bacteria.

In the United States, however, infection with *Mycobacterium avium-intracellulari* (MAI), *cryptococcus neoformans* and *Histoplasma capsulatum* occur relatively frequently whilst MTB is seen less frequently except in the Hiatian immigrant population.

Neoplastic disorders, especially KS and lymphoma may also cause radiographic abnormalities in the lung.


### *Pneumocystis carinii* pneumonia

The earliest visible change on a chest x-ray in PCP is peribronchial and perivascular cuffing caused by infiltration of the peribronchial and perivascular sheaths giving rise to inflammatory exudate, oedema and connective tissue proliferation (Fig. 5.5B).

More typically, PCP presents radiographically, as bilateral perihilar and/or basal reticular or reticular-nodular infiltrates resembling pulmonary oedema which progress rapidly over 3–5 days to diffuse air space consolidation involving the entire lung (Fig. 5.6).

This appearance is caused by the inflammatory process moving centrifugally and spilling into the alveolar spaces. Organisms may be detected in the alveolar exudates using appropriate stains. Thin slice CT has also been used to detect airspace disease but is not widely utilised for this purpose in this country (Naidich et al 1989).

Ultimately, the lungs may become massively consolidated and relatively airless with respiratory failure indistinguishable from other forms of the adult respiratory distress syndrome, despite adequate initial therapy.

Gallium 67 lung scans have been shown to be a very sensitive although non-specific, test for the presence of PCP, showing bilateral diffuse uptake in

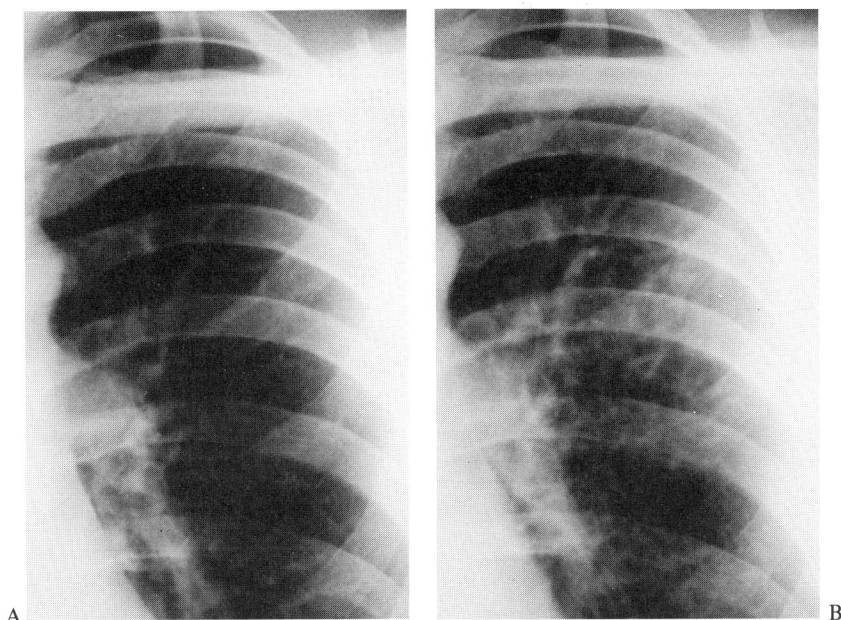

**Fig. 5.5**   26-year old male HIV positive homosexual patient with a 2 day history of cough and pyrexia. **A**, Normal CXR. **B**, Early changes of PCP can be seen with loss of the normal definition of the hilar structures and early peribronchial and perivascular cuffing.

the lungs (Coleman et al 1984). The test is expensive and not widely used in the UK.

Organisms other than PCP are far less likely to cause widespread diffuse consolidation, an important sign in differential diagnosis (Hopewell & Luce 1986).

CMV pneumonitis results in a radiologically identical picture to PCP and is a common postmortem finding. However, it is very rarely the sole causative pathogen of such appearances (Wallace & Hannah 1987).

Appropriate therapy for PCP usually results in gradual clearing of the infiltrates over a period of 13–15 days. The radiographic improvement often lags behind clinical improvement. Sometimes there is significant worsening of appearances 3–5 days after initiation of therapy, this usually results from alterations in fluid balance due to the large volume of intravenous fluid required for administration of treatment. Improvement is usually noted after diuretic therapy and fluid restriction.

Chest radiography, in conjunction with arterial blood gas measurement has been shown to be of value in follow-up patients with potentially recurrent disease. If there is a deterioration in both parameters, recurrent PCP is likely, but if there is only a change in one or none, recurrent disease is much less

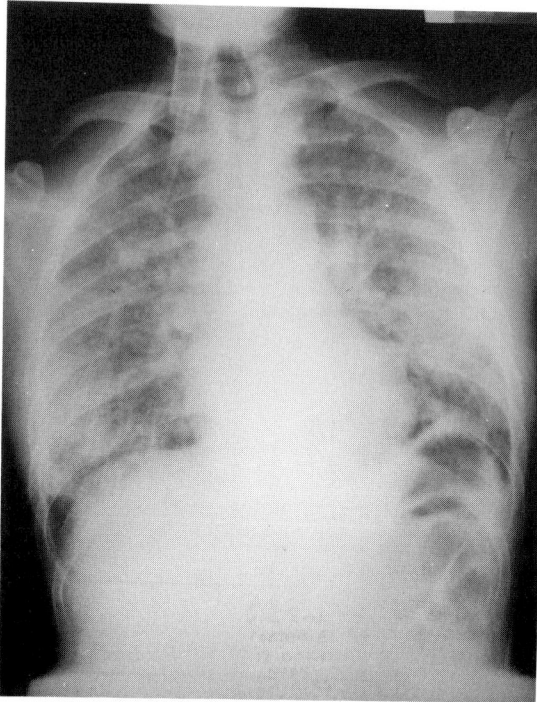

**Fig. 5.6** Typical appearances of advancing PCP with widespread bilateral alveolar shadowing.

likely (Naidich et al 1989). This may allow empiric therapy without the need for invasive diagnostic procedures.

Unfortunately, despite good initial response to therapy in patients with PCP, relapse and recurrence is frequent, and prophylaxis is now routinely prescribed. In up to 20% of patients with acute PCP, respiratory failure develops despite adequate therapy. Mortality is about 90% for those patients requiring endotracheal intubation and mechanically assisted ventilation.

It is important to realise that a normal or minimally abnormal chest radiograph does not exclude the diagnosis of PCP, especially since radiographic changes often lag behind the symptoms. These patients appear to manifest the best prognosis and it is generally agreed that bronchoscopy and biopsy are recommended in the HIV positive patient with respiratory illness despite a normal chest x-ray to ensure prompt diagnosis.

### Radiographic features not typical of PCP

Several radiological changes are now well recognised to occur only rarely, if at all, in association with PCP and their presence implies infection with another or additional organism, or the development of malignancy.

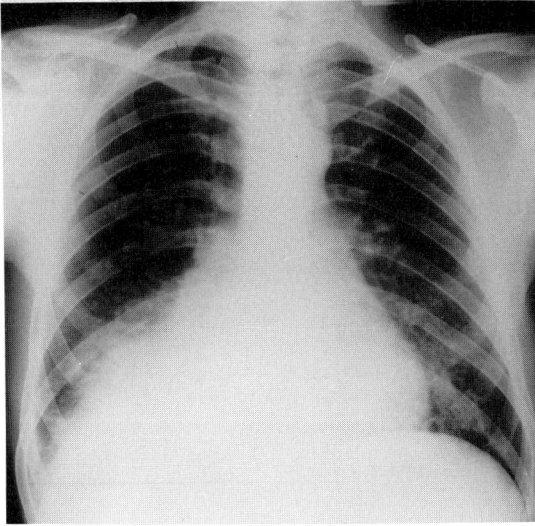

**Fig. 5.7**  Segmental consolidation which has developed in a patient undergoing treatment for PCP. *Strep. pneumoniae* subsequently cultured from sputum. There was a good response to therapy.

*Focal airspace consolidation*

Unilateral, segmental or lobar distribution of consolidation has been described in patients with AIDS, including upper lobe involvement simulating TB (Fig. 5.7). However, bacterial infection whether in conjunction with PCP or alone is often implicated. MTB may also give rise to segmental consolidation.

*Pleural effusions*

Small pleural effusions may occur in uncomplicated PCP, especially if there is relative fluid overload during treatment, but large effusions are strongly suggestive of intrathoracic KS. Effusions have also been noted in association with bacterial, tuberculous and fungal infections.

*Hilar and mediastinal lymphadenopathy*

This should always be interpreted as indicative of serious intrathoracic disease, and is most often caused by mycobacterial infections, KS and lymphoma. It is a distinctly unusual manifestation of PCP (Fig. 5.8).

*Coarse nodular opacities*

Fine, nodular opacities with an almost miliary appearance may occur in PCP when there is diffuse interstitial infiltration, but coarse nodules are not a

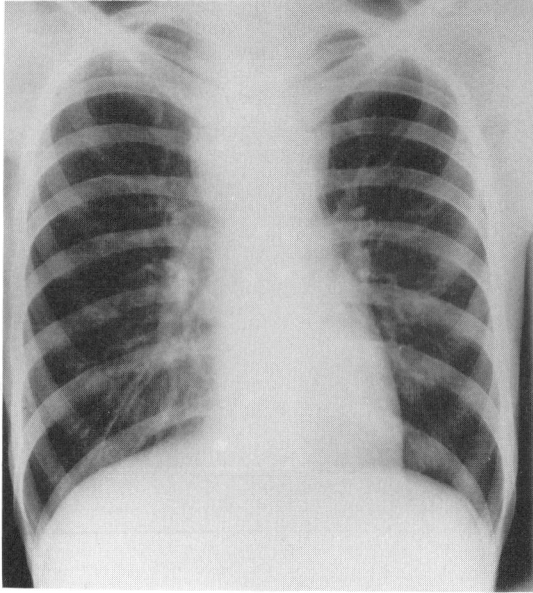

**Fig. 5.8**  Marked paratracheal lymphadenopathy due to MAI. Intrathoracic lympadenopathy is a rare feature of PCP.

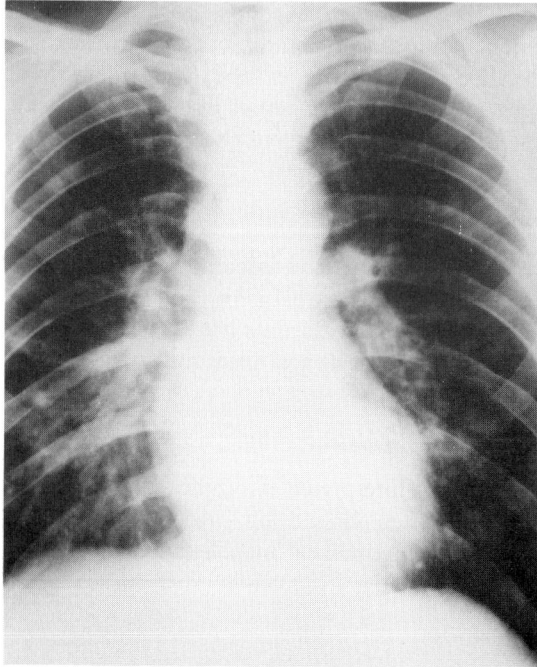

**Fig. 5.9**  Multiple coarse nodules in the lung due to Kaposi's sarcoma.

feature and are most likely to be caused by Kaposi's sarcoma (Fig. 5.9). In the United States, nodular lesions have been described in association with endemic fungal diseases.

*Cavitating opacities*

Air-filled, cystic parenchymal changes complicating otherwise unremarkable PCP are rare (Milligan et al 1985, Goodman et al 1986).

The mechanism by which these cysts develop is unknown but concurrent bacterial, fungal or viral infection may play a role. These cysts pose a risk for the development of pneumothoraces, both spontaneous and following biopsy. Frank cavitation may be seen in bacterial pneumonia, in fungal infections and in TB.

## Mycobacterial infection

Pulmonary infection with MTB is common in AIDS patients in the UK and occurs in about 10% of patients in the United States (Murray et al 1984, Hopewell & Luce 1986, Pitchenik & Rubison 1985), when it may precede the diagnosis of AIDS by several months. In the United States MTB is common in the Hiatian population and in IV drug abusers. It may be typical in appearance with segmental patchy consolidation, or may resemble primary TB, with intrathoracic adenopathy and pleural effusions (Pitchenik & Rubison 1985).

Atypical mycobacteria, particulary MAI, may be isolated from patients with a normal chest x-ray, or there may be pleural effusions, lymphadenopathy, diffuse infiltrates or cavitating lesions (Marinelli et al 1986) (Fig. 5.8).

## Bacterial infections

It is now well recognised that the incidence of bacterial pneumonia in HIV positive patients is increased with *Streptococcus pneumoniae* and *Haemophilus influenzae* most commonly implicated.

The radiological picture is that of focal parenchymal disease. When properly identified bacterial pneumonias respond well to appropriate antibiotics, hence the need for prompt and accurate diagnosis if segmental consolidation is seen (Fig. 5.7).

## Neoplastic disease

A significant number of AIDS patients with pulmonary disease have malignancy either due to disseminated KS (6%) or non-Hodgkins lymphoma (4%) (Cohen et al 1984).

Common findings in KS are coarse nodular opacities and diffuse interstitial shadowing which have been shown to correlate in size, configuration and distribution to nodules of KS and infiltration in interlobar septae at postmortem (Davis et al 1987). Pleural effusions are strongly suggestive of KS and intrathoracic lymphadenopathy may also occur (Onigbene et al 1985, Davis et al 1987).

The nodules are often poorly defined and shaggy and occur in perivascular and bronchocentric distribution. Their appearance is characteristic, especially when seen with CT (Fig. 5.9).

Endobronchial KS lesions are often seen at bronchoscopy but do not give rise to radiological abnormality unless they are large enough to result in bronchial occlusion, giving distal segmental collapse/consolidation.

The postmortem studies by Davis et al (1987) have given a high, positive predictive value to parenchymal nodules, effusions and mediastinal lymphadenopathy, all features distinctly unusual in PCP.

AIDS-related lymphomas are usually extra-nodal in distribution and thoracic involvement is difficult to document. It may manifest as hilar or mediastinal lymphadenopathy, pleural effusions or diffuse parenchymal involvement. Whilst non-specific lymphadenopathy is significant it should be emphasised that enlarged hilar and mediastinal nodes are not present in the diffuse lymphadenopathy syndrome of HIV positive patients.

Lymphoid interstitial pneumonitis is a diffuse pulmonary disease characterised by the accumulation of lymphocytes, plasma cells and recticulo-endothelial cells in the interstitium. It is considered diagnostic of AIDS when confirmed in a child under 13 years of age or, if documented, in a sero positive adult. The radiological findings are non-specific and are indistinguishable from PCP and other causes of diffuse interstitial shadowing.

In summary, whilst there is an overlap in the radiographic appearance of many of the common AIDS-related pulmonary disorders, there are some radiological patterns sufficiently typical or atypical to suggest a diagnosis.

The following guidelines have been found useful in establishing diagnostic priorities (Naidich et al 1989).

1. If there are no pathognomonic radiographic abnormalities, histological and bacterial samples should be obtained at bronchoscopy to expedite therapy.
2. Opportunistic infection or tumour may be present despite a normal chest x-ray. Arterial blood gases, lung function tests, and Gallium 67 scans may be useful in the symptomatic patient with negative radiology.
3. Intrathoracic lymphadenopathy is always indicative of serious intrathoracic disease and is not a feature of the diffuse lymphadenopathy syndrome or AIDS related complex (ARC). It is a distinctly unusual manifestation of PCP and is most often caused by mycobacterial infections, KS and lymphoma.
4. Pleural disease, both unilateral and bilateral, should also be regarded with suspicion and is most often caused by the above disorders.
5. Focal parenchymal disease may be a manifestation of PCP

but the increased incidence of bacterial infection in AIDS patients justifies bronchoscopy and biopsy to identify potentially treatable infections.


## THE GASTROINTESTINAL TRACT

Gastrointestinal radiology has an important role to play in the investigation and management of HIV positive patients. Of the 12 diseases indicative of AIDS without proof of HIV infection, 6 involve the GI tract and many of these entities produce radiographic findings which are virtually pathognomonic. Radiological changes may occur from oesophagus to rectum.


### Oesophagus

Dysphagia due to opportunistic oesophagitis is common in AIDS patients and is usually due to *Candida albicans*, but may also be caused by CMV and herpes infection.

A double contrast barium swallow is the most useful radiological investigation and may distinguish oesophageal candidiasis from CMV infection with expertise.

Candidal infection in the oesophagus is diagnostic of AIDS in HIV positive patients (Centre for Disease Control 1987), so radiological confirmation is extremely significant. There is fine ulceration and plaques particularly in the distal oesophagus and there may be thickened folds (Fig. 5.10). Meticulous double contrast techniques is required to demonstrate early changes.

Similar changes may be produced by herpes simplex (Levine et al 1981). Several distinct changes may be seen in CMV oesophagitis that distinguish it from candidiasis. Focal diamond-shaped ulceration, with a well-defined margin is commonly seen (Balthazar et al 1985). There is a high incidence of ulceration at the gastro-oesophageal junction, sometimes producing thick folds which extend into the gastric fundus. Giant oesophageal ulcers are also a feature of CMV and are thought to be due to a combination of infection and vasculitis.

Kaposi's sarcoma (KS) may be detected on barium studies as discrete submucosal elevations in the oesophagus (Fig. 5.11). KS lesions are often seen at endoscopy as plaque in the oesophageal wall (Rose et al 1982).


### Stomach and small intestine

AIDS related lesions in the stomach do not often produce symptoms and are often discovered during the investigation of oesophagus or small bowel. The radiologist may, therefore, be the first to detect gastric pathology.

KS of the stomach produces intraluminal or intramural polypoid lesions, measuring from 3 mm to 3 cm in diameter. There may be a central collection of barium representing ulceration (Fig. 5.12, Rose et al 1982). As the disease

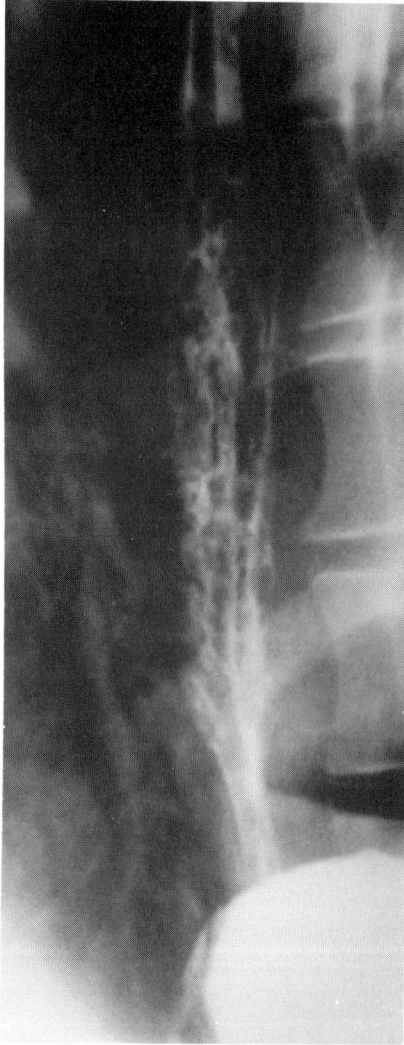

**Fig. 5.10** Barium swallow demonstrating fine ulceration and plaques due to oesophageal candidiasis.

progresses the submucosa becomes progressively infiltrated. In advanced cases CT may demonstrate gross thickening of the stomach wall.

Lymphoma may also occur in the stomach and produces a wide variety of appearances from focal thickening of the gastric wall to ulceration and irregular masses, but more often involves the small bowel and colon.

Thick, irregular folds, particularly at the gastro-oesophageal junction may occur with CMV gastritis. Submucosal involvement produces thickening of the mucosa, giving a 'thumbprinting' pattern. The antrum and pylorus may

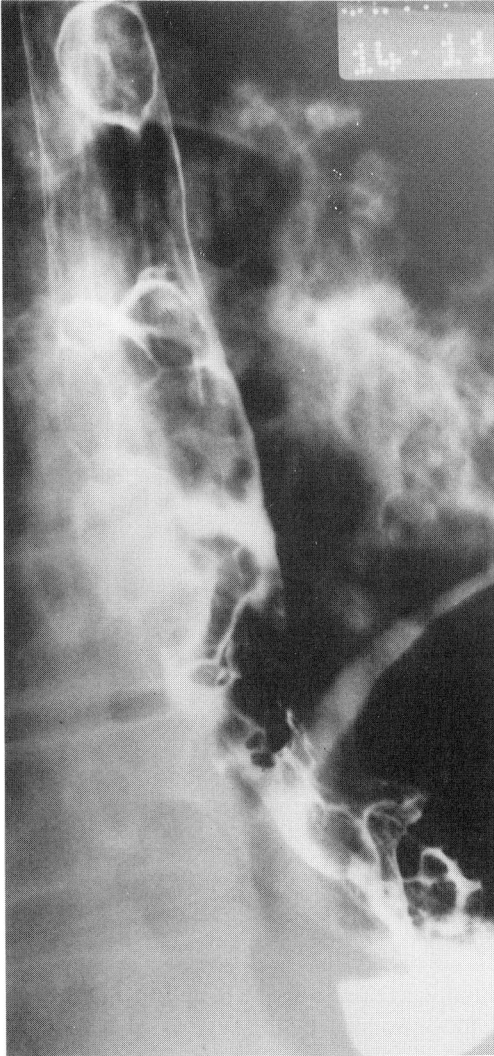

**Fig. 5.11**   Barium swallow showing multiple submucosal filling defects proven on endoscopy to be due to Kaposi's sarcoma.

be involved and show evidence of ulceration and stenosis (Balthazar et al 1985). This appearance has also been reported with Crytosporidial infection and indeed both organisms are often cultured together (Berk et al 1984).

Many AIDS patients suffer from malabsorbtion and severe watery diarrhoea. Cryptosporidial enteritis, mycobacteria, CMV and neoplasms have all been described. There is clinical overlap between the symptoms of neoplastic versus infectious disease in the small bowel and the radiologist is in an important position to suggest a diagnosis.

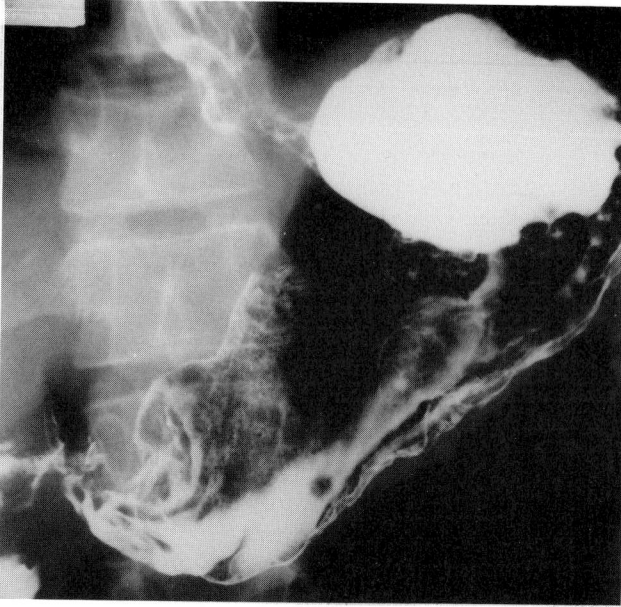

**Fig. 5.12** Barium meal in-patient with Kaposi's sarcoma of the stomach. Note multiple polypoidal filling defects and thickened folds.

Cryptosporidiosis may cause thickening of the mucosal folds, flocculation of barium and mild dilatation (Berk et al 1984). There is high incidence of thickening of folds or nodularity in the duodenum which is of high predictive value.

Mycobacterial infections of the GI tract are common and again may produce thickened folds especially in the ileum which is a most unusual appearance and, if seen, is strongly suggestive of MAI. CT may reveal mesenteric and retroperitoneal lymphadenopathy, splenomegaly and ascites if there is mycobacterial infection (Nyberg et al 1985).

CMV infection may produce a diffuse enteritis but changes are often limited to distal ileum and colon. There may be thickening of folds, narrowing of the lumen and separation of loops (Teixidor et al 1987).

KS lesions may develop in the small intestine of patients with AIDS but small bowel radiography is relatively insensitive to their detection. Lymphoma may cause focal lesions with discrete penetrating ulcers or multiple nodules with bowel thickening. CT scanning has a high detection rate in GI lymphoma and is the imaging modality of choice to exclude this diagnosis in AIDS patients (Nyberg et al 1986).

Findings include variably thickened small bowel loops with loss of mucosal features. Mesenteric lymphadenopathy is not frequently seen and is far more suggestive of an infectious process.

## Colon and rectum

The large bowel is a common site for both infection and KS in AIDS patients. Colitis may be due to a variety of organisms including CMV, Cryptosporidia and MAI.

CMV colitis is a common infection found in AIDS patients. Double-contrast barium examination may show diffuse mucosal granularity in mild cases, with or without apthous ulcers, and in severe disease there may be large discrete ulcers particularly in the right side of the colon. Contiguous involvement of ileum and right colon are variable and distal colitis may be considered virtually diagnostic of CMV in an AIDS patient.

Colitis produced by other organisms have not generated enough radiographic case material so far to allow definition of characteristic features.

The frequency of bowel involvement with KS has been reported as over 50%, and there may be colonic or rectal disease before the development of skin lesions. The diagnosis is usually made at sigmoidoscopy, since double-contrast barium enemas may fail to demonstrate small submucosal plaques, or focal areas of submucosal infiltration of KS. There have been reports where circumferential infiltration of the colonic wall produces an ulcerated, narrow segment of bowel resembling inflammatory colitis.

Colonic lymphoma is more common in the HIV positive population than in non-HIV patients with bowel lymphoma. The appearances are variable. There may be polypoid lesions simulating adenocarcinoma. There is a high predilection of rectal involvement, infiltrating the pelvic floor.

## Biliary disease

Biliary tract disease has recently been recognised as a complication of AIDS and most cases have described an association between Cryptosporidial infection and acalculous inflammation of the biliary tree (Dolmatch et al 1987).

Radiological changes may be demonstrated at ultrasound and at ERCP which are identical to those seen in sclerosing cholangitis (Fig. 5.13). CMV has also been implicated in this pathology. Endoscopic papillotomy has produced variable results with regard to relief of symptoms and biochemical abnormalities in these patients.

## Liver and spleen

In any AIDS patients with an abnormal liver function test, imaging should be performed to evaluate the presence of hepatomegaly or space occupying lesions within the liver. Attention should be paid to the biliary tree as described above.

The liver may be enlarged, as a result of infection, lymphoma or KS. Because AIDS related lymphoma commonly involves multiple abdominal

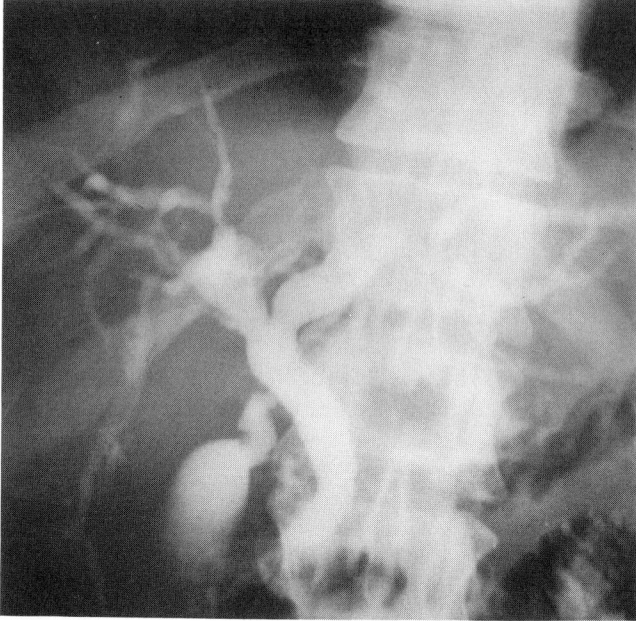

**Fig. 5.13**  ERCP in an AIDS patient with a history of painless jaundice. Ultrasound had demonstrated a dilated and thickened common bile duct. Changes in the biliary tree have been demonstrated which are similar to sclerosing cholangitis with areas of narrowing and stricture formation.

sites, CT is the imaging investigation of choice in HIV-positive patients with hepatomegaly. This will also reveal whether there is any intra-abdominal lymph node involvement, bowel involvement or splenic involvement. The spleen may also be enlarged non-specifically due to Castleman's disease.

A special mention should be made of the role of ultrasound and CT in the investigation of abdominal abnormalities in AIDS patients. Abdominal lymph nodes are commonly involved with AIDS related lymphoma, including the para-aortic and mesenteric lymph node groups (Fig. 5.14). CT and ultrasound are useful for evaluating this lymphadenopathy. Identification of bulky abdominal nodes is important in HIV positive patients since it suggests the presence of a serious complication.

The common causes of bulky lymphadenopathy (greater than 1.5 cm) are lymphoma and infection, particularly MAI. KS less frequently causes lymphadenopathy. Nodes between 1 and 1.5 cm may be seen in patients with PGL and do not necessarily indicate serious pathology.

Since radiographic and CT findings alone are rarely diagnostic, biopsy of enlarged lymph nodes under CT or ultrasound control is often necessary to establish the diagnosis. It should be emphasised that abdominal nodal enlargement greater than 1.5 cm is unusual in PGL and should prompt CT guided biopsy to exclude neoplastic or infectious nodal disease.

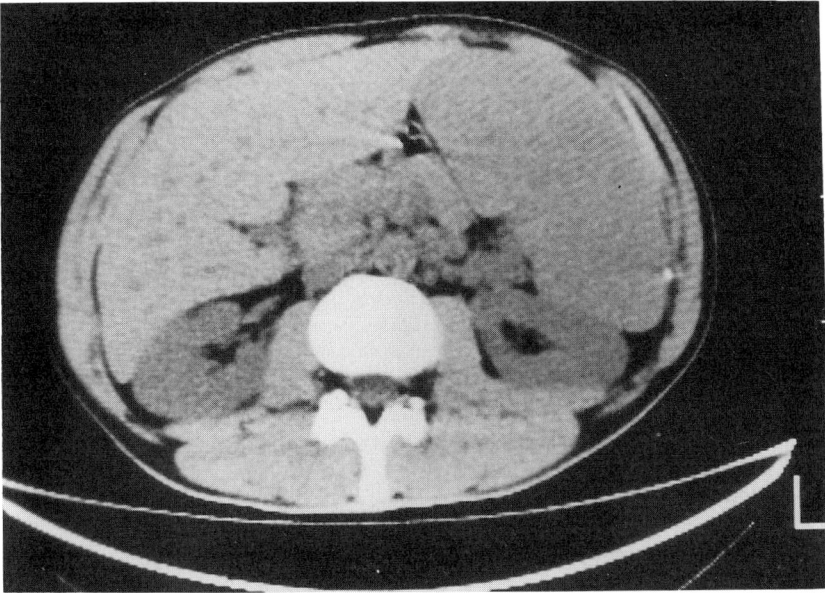

**Fig. 5.14**    Hepato-splenomegaly and abdominal lymphadenopathy due to AIDS related lymphoma.

## CONCLUSION

In conclusion, the increasing frequency of AIDS has presented and will continue to present the medical profession with a great challenge. The variety of radiological abnormalities may be perplexing and confusing but certain findings can prove useful in suggesting a diagnosis, whilst other findings are virtually pathognomonic of AIDS related illnesses. Radiology can also play an important role in monitoring progression or resolution of disease and provide a modality for guided biopsies, often enabling prompt diagnosis and treatment.

**Acknowledgements**

I am most grateful to Miss Jo Burton for typing the manuscript and to the staff of St Mary's Hospital, who performed many of the radiological investigations.

REFERENCES

Balthazar EJ, Megibow AJ, Hulnick DH 1985 Cytomegalovirus esophagitis and gastritis in acquired immune deficiency syndrome. American Journal of Roentgenology 144: 1201–1204
Berk RN, Wall SD, McCardle CB et al 1984 Cryptosporidiosis of the stomach and small

intestine in patients with acquired immunodeficiency syndrome. American Journal of Roentgenology 143: 549–554

Centers for Disease Control 1987 Revision of the CDC Surveillance case definition of acquired immunodeficiency syndrome. Morbidity and Mortality Weekly Report 36 (Suppl 1) 18–48

Cohen BA, Pomeranz S, Rabinowitz J et al 1984 Pulmonary complications of AIDS; radiologic features. American Journal of Roentgenology 143: 115–122

Coleman DL, Hattner RS, Luce JM et al 1984 Correllation between Gallium lung scans and fibreoptic bronchoscopy in patients with suspected *Pneumocystis carinii* pneumonia and the acquired immunodeficiency syndrome. American Review of Respiratory Disease 130: 1166–1169

Davis SD, Henschke CI, Chamides BK, Westcott JL 1987 Intrathoracic Kaposi's sarcoma in AIDS patients: radiographic-pathologic correlation. Radiology 163: 495–500

Dolmatch BL, Laing FC, Federle MP et al 1987 AIDS-related cholangitis: radiographic findings in nine patients. Radiology 163: 313–316

Goodman PC, Daley C, Minagi H 1986 Spontaneous pneumothorax in AIDS patients with pneumocystis carinii pneumonia. American Journal of Roentgenology 147: 29–31

Goodman PC, Gamsu G 1987 Radiographic findings in the acquired immunodeficiency syndrome. Postgraduate radiology 7: 3–15

Hinnant R, Rotterdam HZ, Bell ET, Tapper ML 1986 Cytomegalovirus infection of the alimentary tract: a clinico-pathological correlation. American Journal of Gastroenterology 81: 944–950

Ho DD, Rota TR, Schooley RT et al 1985 Isolation of HTLV-III from cerebrospinal fluid and neural tissues of patients with neurologic syndromes related to the acquired immunodeficiency syndrome. New England Journal of Medicine 313: 1493–1497

Hopewell PC, Luce JM 1986 Pulmonary manifestations of the acquired immunodeficiency syndrome. In: Pinching AJ (ed) AIDS and HIV infection. Clinics in Immunology and Allergy 6(3): 489–518

Levine MS, Laufer I, Kressel HY, Freidman H 1981 Herpes esophagitis. American Journal of Roentgenology 138: 863–866

Levy RM, Rosenbloom S, Perrett LV 1986 Neuroradiologic findings in AIDS: a review of 200 cases. American Journal of Roentgenology 147: 977–983

Marinelli DL, Albelda SM, Williams TM, Kern JA, Iozzo RV, Miller WT 1986 Nontuberculous mycobacterial infection in AIDS: clinical, pathologic and radiographic features. Radiology 160: 77–82

Milligan SA, Stulbarg MS, Gamsu G, Golden JA 1985 Pneumocystis carinii pneumonia radiographically simulating tuberculosis. American Review of Respiratory Disease 132: 1124–1126

Murray JF, Felton CP, Garay SM et al 1984 Pulmonary complications of the acquired immunodeficiency syndrome. New England Journal of Medicine 3120: 1682–1688

Naidich DP, Garay SM, Leitman BS, McCauley DI 1987 Radiographic manifestations of pulmonary disease in the acquired immunodeficiency syndrome (AIDS). Seminars in Roentgenology 22: 14–30

Naidich DP, Garay SM, Goodman PC, Rybak BJ, Kramer EL 1989 Pulmonary manifestations of AIDS. In: Federle M, Megibow A, Naidich DP (eds) Radiology of AIDS Raven Press, New York. p47–76

Navia BA, Price RW 1986 Central and peripheral nervous system complications of AIDS. In: Pinching AJ (ed) AIDS and HIV infection. Clinics in Immunology and Allergy 6 (3): 543–588

Nyberg DA, Federle MP, Jeffrey RB et al 1985 Abdominal CT findings in disseminated mycobacterium avium intracellulare. American Journal of Roentgenology 145: 297–299

Nyberg DA, Jeffrey RB, Federle MP et al 1986 AIDS-related lymphomas: evaluation by abdominal CT. Radiology 159: 59–63

Onigbene FP, Steis RG, Macher AM et al 1985 Kaposi's sarcoma causing pulmonary infiltrates and respiratory failure in the acquired immunodeficiency syndrome. Annals of Internal Medicine 102: 471–475

Petito CL, Cho ES, Lemann W, Navia BA, Price RW 1986 Neuropathology of the acquired immunodeficiency syndrome (AIDS): an autopsy review. Journal of Neuropathology and Experimental Neurology 45: 635–646

Pitchenik AE, Rubison HA 1985 The radiographic appearance of tuberculosis in patients with the acquired immunodeficiency syndrome (AIDS) and pre-AIDS. American Review of Respiratory Disease 131: 393–396

Rose HS, Balthazar EJ, Megibow AJ, Horowitz L, Laubenstein LJ 1982 Alimentary tract involvement in Kaposi's sarcoma: radiographic and endoscopic findings in 25 homosexual men. American Journal of Roentgenology 139: 661–666

Teixidor HS, Honig CL, Norsoph E, Albert S, Mouradian JA, Whalan JP 1987 Cytomegalovirus infection of the alimentary canal: radiologic findings with pathologic correlation. Radiology 163: 317–325

Wallace JM, Hannah J 1987 Cytomegalovirus pneumonitis in patients with AIDS. Chest 92: 198–203

# 6

# Injection drug use related HIV and AIDS

*R.P. Brettle P.J. Flegg L.R. MacCallum*

## INTRODUCTION

The importance of injection drug use (IDU) related human immunodeficiency virus (HIV) infection cannot be overstressed since it is recognised that this is the route by which HIV can and does spread into the general heterosexual population (Drucker 1986). It is therefore important that all practitioners dealing with HIV patients be conversant with the particular problems and management difficulties of IDU-related HIV infection.

The medical complications of IDU include the excessive or addictive effects of drugs, the withdrawal effects from drugs, and infections associated with drug use. Infections associated with IDU centre around the use of non-sterile equipment such as needles, syringes, spoons, cups etc. in the preparation and administration of drugs. The use of non-sterile equipment and solutions may then lead to bacterial infections.

The practice of sharing equipment between users allows the spread of a number of blood-borne viruses. Two particular practices are thought to favour this spread. Firstly washing the drug out of the syringe by repeatedly drawing back and injecting the user's own blood. This results in heavy contamination of the equipment with blood which can then be passed on to the next user. Secondly, there is the practice of washing the equipment in a communal glass or bowl of water which rapidly becomes contaminated with blood.

The best known blood-borne virus associated with needle drug abuse is hepatitis B virus but more recently another blood borne virus, the AIDS virus or HIV, has infected drug users.

## INJECTION DRUG USE AND AIDS

The first 9 cases of AIDS amongst injection drug users were diagnosed retrospectively in 1980 and 4 of these were also homosexuals (Des Jarlais et al 1985). The number of cases associated with IDU in the USA increased from 29 in 1981 to 148 in 1982, 324 in 1983, 4500 in 1986 and 26 321 by May 1989 accounting for at least 17% of AIDS cases in the USA (Centres for Disease Control 1989). In Europe in 1984 IDU-related AIDS accounted for only 2% of cases but this had risen to 26.8% by 1989 and it had been noted that in Europe IDU-related AIDS was the fastest growing risk group (Communicable Diseases Scotland 1987, World Health Organisation 1989).

IDU-related HIV and AIDS are noted for their geographical clustering. For instance some 75% of IDU-related AIDS in the USA has occurred in the New York City metropolitan area and in Europe 70% of the cases have been reported from Italy, Spain and France (Des Jarlais et al 1988, Brunet et al 1987). As yet explanations for this clustering are not forthcoming although there are suggestions that it is linked to the intense sharing of equipment in localised areas together with mobility of a small number of users (Bisset et al 1989).

IDU-related HIV was first noted from retrospective analysis of sera to have begun in New York in 1978, in Italy in 1979, in Germany in 1982, in Edinburgh, Dublin and Sweden in 1983, and in Copenhagen in 1984 (Novick et al 1986, Lazzarin et al 1986, Brunet et al 1987, Robertson et al 1986a, Shattock et al 1986, Blix & Grönbladh 1988). The extent of HIV seroposi-tivity in drug users is by and large related to the time of introduction of HIV into the community. For instance by 1984 in New York and 1985 in Edinburgh HIV seroprevalence of drug users had passed 50% (Spira et al 1984, Marmor et al 1987, Brettle et al 1987). The extent and variability of IDU-related HIV seroprevalence is demonstrated in Table 6.1.

In these differing communities the spread of IDU-related HIV seems to follow two broad patterns, a slow gradual spread and a rapid explosive spread. The reasons for the differing pattern is probably differing relationships between drug users. In some areas, drug users remain in tight knit communities often along racial lines. There may be little mixing between such groups other than the purchase of drugs. As such, spread is rapid within groups but not between groups. In other situations possibly where there is only one racial group there is more dynamic interchange between users and spread is very rapid.

The scattered pockets of IDU-related HIV around Europe may be explained by the movement of small numbers of very mobile users between areas of varying drug availability (Brettle et al 1987, Bisset et al 1989). In Italy relatively high seroprevalence amongst drug users around US Air Force bases has been suggested as one means of entry of the virus into Europe (Franceschi et al 1986). This pattern of the sudden appearance of pockets of HIV amongst drug users may well be set to continue into developing countries with the reports of HIV seroprevalence amongst drug users of 44% in Bangkok and 22–48% in Argentina (Vanichseni et al 1989, Weissenbacher et al 1988a,b).

The risk factors associated with HIV infection amongst drug users have not been well elucidated. The link with the frequency of equipment sharing is, however, now well established and in the USA there is also a link with injecting in 'shooting galleries' (Robertson et al 1986b, Brettle et al 1986, Brettle 1986, Esparza et al 1986, Chaisson et al 1986, Bouchard et al 1986, Ginzburg et al 1986, Pont el al 1986, Merino et al 1986, Marmor et al 1987). Less well recognised is the importance of the type of drug used. For instance,

**Table 6.1**   IDU-related HIV seroprevalence

| Location | Year | % | Total sample size | Reference |
|---|---|---|---|---|
| **UNITED KINGDOM** | | | | |
| *SCOTLAND* | | | | |
| Edinburgh | 1982 | 0.0 | 182 | Peutherer et al 1986 |
| | 1983 | 14.0 | 124 | Peutherer et al 1986 |
| | 1984 | 42.0 | 205 | Peutherer et al 1986 |
| | 1985 | 38.0 | 106 | Peutherer et al 1985 |
| | 1986 | 51.0 | 164 | Robertson et al 1986b |
| | 1986 | 52.0 | 191 | Brettle et al 1987 |
| | 1988 | 56.0 | 164 | Robertson et al 1988 |
| | 1988 | 64.0 | 203 | Skidmore & Robertson 1989 |
| Dundee | 1986 | 39.0 | 251 | Scottish Home & Health Department 1986 |
| Glasgow | 1986 | 4.5 | 600 | Follett et al 1986 |
| *ENGLAND* | | | | |
| Newcastle-Upon-Tyne | 1986 | 1.0 | 400 | Scottish Home & Health Department 1986 |
| Manchester | 1986 | 0.0 | 100 | Scottish Home & Health Department 1986 |
| Liverpool | 1986 | 0.0 | 200 | Scottish Home & Health Department 1986 |
| Southport | 1986 | 0.0 | 36 | Scottish Home & Health Department 1986 |
| South London | 1985 | 6.4 | 236 | Sutherland & McManus 1989 |
| | 1986 | 0.6 | 146 | Webb et al 1986 |
| | 1986 | 6.0 | 293 | Sutherland & McManus 1989 |
| | 1987 | 4.0 | 313 | Sutherland & McManus 1989 |
| | 1988 | 5.0 | 216 | Sutherland & McManus 1989 |
| *ENGLAND & WALES* | 1983 | 1.5 | 269 | Mortimer et al 1985 |
| | 1984 | 2.5 | 203 | Mortimer et al 1985 |
| | 1985 | 6.4 | 236 | Mortimer et al 1985 |
| | 1986 | 10.0 | 239 | Mortimer et al 1985 |
| | 1986–7 | 2.1 | 2712 | Miller & Kaye 1988 |
| *IRELAND* | | | | |
| Dublin | | | | |
|    healthy | 1985 | 27.0 | 451 | Shattock et al 1986 |
|    ill | 1985 | 37.0 | 152 | Shattock et al 1986 |
|    neonates | 1985 | 55.0 | 152 | Shattock et al 1986 |
| **EUROPE EXCLUDING UK** | | | | |
| *SWEDEN* | 1983 | 3.0 | 67 | Blix & Grönbladh 1988 |
| | 1984–6 | 16.0 | 32 | Blix & Grönbladh 1988 |
| | 1987 | 57.0 | 60 | Blix & Grönbladh 1988 |
| *GREECE* | | | | |
|    prisoners | 1987 | 2.1 | 288 | Romeliotou et al 1987/88 |
|    voluntary screening | 1987 | 2.8 | 434 | Romeliotou et al 1987/88 |
| *WEST GERMANY* | 1983 | 10.1 | 927 | Zoulek et al 1986 |
| | 1984 | 17.6 | | Zoulek et al 1986 |
| | 1985 | 23.9 | | Zoulek et al 1986 |
| Berlin | | | | |
|    autopsy | 1985 | 30.0 | | Zoulek et al 1986 |
| | 1986 | 49.0 | | Zoulek et al 1986 |
| | 1987 | 49.0 | | Zoulek et al 1986 |
| | 1988 | 38.0 | 362 | Bschor et al 1989 |

**Table 6.1** (*cont'd*)

| Location | Year | % | Total sample size | Reference |
|---|---|---|---|---|
| detox | 1988 | 13.0 | 362 | Bschor et al 1989 |
| prisoners | 1988 | 12.0 | 362 | Bschor et al 1989 |
| Hamburg | | | | |
| autopsy | 1985 | 0.0 | 362 | Bschor et al 1989 |
| | 1986 | 23.0 | 362 | Bschor et al 1989 |
| | 1987 | 16.0 | 362 | Bschor et al 1989 |
| | 1988 | 13.0 | 362 | Bschor et al 1989 |
| *PORTUGAL* | | | | |
| nationals | 1988 | 8.0 | 24 | Castroemelo et al 1988 |
| foreigners | 1988 | 67.0 | 86 | Castroemelo et al 1988 |
| *YUGOSLAVIA* | | | | |
| Belgrade | 1983 | 10.0 | 40 | Jankovic et al 1988 |
| | 1987 | 42.0 | 19 | Jankovic et al 1988 |
| | 1986–8 | 44.0 | 625 | Zenja et al 1988 |
| Zagreb | 1985 | 5.0 | 140 | Burek et al 1988 |
| | 1987 | 5.9 | 393 | Burek et al 1988 |
| *CZECHOSLOVAKIA* | 1987 | 0.0 | 228 | Bruckova et al 1988 |
| *POLAND* | 1986 | 0.0 | | Boron et al 1988 |
| North East | 1988 | 0.0 | 30 | Boron et al 1988 |
| Warsaw | 1988 | 2.9 | 718 | Staipinski et al 1989 |
| | 1989 | 8.0 | 718 | Staipinski et al 1989 |
| *SPAIN* | | | | |
| Valencia | 1983 | 11.0 | 58 | Rodrigo et al 1985 |
| North | 1983 | 35.0 | 478 | Carcaba et al 1988 |
| | 1983 | 71.0 | 478 | Carcaba et al 1988 |
| | 1984 | 40.0 | | Rodrigo et al 1985 |
| | 1985 | 48.0 | 174 | Rodrigo et al 1985 |
| Bilbao | 1984–5 | 50.0 | 75 | Esparza et al 1986 |
| | 1986 | 41.9 | 479 | Merino et al 1986 |
| Catalonia | 1985–8 | 40.7 | 313 | Casabona et al 1989 |
| Barceolona | 1985–8 | 70.0 | 55 | Tor et al 1989 |
| *FRANCE* | | | | |
| Paris | 1984 | 75.0 | 8 | Brun-Vezinet et al 1984 |
| | 1985 | 64.0 | 113 | Bouchard et al 1986 |
| Tours | 1982–3 | 0.0 | 52 | Goudeau et al 1986 |
| | 1984 | 15.0 | 40 | Goudeau et al 1986 |
| | 1985 | 17.0 | 125 | Goudeau et al 1986 |
| *HOLLAND* | | | | |
| Amsterdam | 1983 | 3.4 | 145 | Bunning et al 1986 |
| prostitutes | 1983 | 23.0 | 52 | Van Hastrecht et al 1989 |
| | 1986 | 33.3 | | Van Hastrecht et al 1989 |
| | 1987 | 28.3 | | Van Hastrecht et al 1989 |
| | 1988 | 27.8 | 560 | Van Hastrecht et al 1989 |
| *AUSTRIA* | | | | |
| Tyrol | 1985 | 44.0 | 34 | Fuchs et al 1985 |
| Vienna | 1985 | 8.5 | 82 | Pakesch et al 1987 |
| | 1986 | 14.4 | 159 | Pakesch et al 1987 |
| prisoners | 1986 | 17.0 | 71 | Pont et al 1986 |
| methadone | 1988 | 44.0 | 136 | Hutterer et al 1989 |

**Table 6.1** (*cont'd*)

| Location | Year | % | Total sample size | Reference |
|---|---|---|---|---|
| *SWITZERLAND* | | | | |
| Geneva | 1981 | 7.0 | 131 | Hirzchel et al 1986 |
| | 1985 | 52.0 | 131 | Hirzchel et al 1986 |
| Bern | 1979–81 | 0.0 | 93 | Hirzchel et al 1986 |
| | 1982 | 16.0 | 79 | Mortimer et al 1985 |
| | 1983 | 16.0 | 49 | Mortimer et al 1985 |
| | 1984 | 42.0 | 38 | Mortimer et al 1985 |
| | 1985 | 32.0 | 37 | Mortimer et al 1985 |
| Bern/Basel/Geneva/ | | | | |
| Louscree | 1983 | 36.0 | 103 | Schupbach et al 1985a |
| | 1984 | 53.0 | 55 | Schupbach et al 1985a |
| | 1985 | 36.0 | 103 | Schupbach et al 1985b |
| Lausanne | 1987 | 47.3 | 63 | Dolivo et al 1988 |
| *ITALY* | | | | |
| Milan | 1979 | 7.0 | | Lazzarin et al 1986 |
| | 1980 | 6.0 | | Lazzarin et al 1986 |
| | 1981 | 8.0 | | Lazzarin et al 1986 |
| | 1982 | 22.0 | | Lazzarin et al 1986 |
| | 1982 | 24.0 | 67 | Ferroni et al 1985 |
| | 1983 | 35.0 | | Lazzarin et al 1986 |
| | 1983 | 21.0 | | Ferroni et al 1985 |
| | 1984 | 45.0 | | Lazzarin et al 1986 |
| | 1985 | 60.0 | 716 | Lazzarin et al 1986 |
| | 1985 | 53.0 | 62 | Ferroni et al 1985 |
| | 1985 | 69.3 | | Titti et al 1987 |
| Bari | 1980 | 6.0 | 68 | Angarano et al 1985 |
| | 1981 | 10.0 | 58 | Angarano et al 1985 |
| | 1982 | 15.0 | 47 | Angarano et al 1985 |
| | 1983 | 31.0 | 49 | Angarano et al 1985 |
| | 1984 | 53.0 | 34 | Angarano et al 1985 |
| | 1985 | 76.0 | 59 | Angarano et al 1985 |
| Porderone/Udine | 1985 | 27.0 | 315 | Tirelli et al 1986 |
| | 1985–6 | 90.0 | 63 | Franceschi et al 1986 |
| Udine | 1985–6 | 10.0 | 134 | Franceschi et al 1986 |
| Rome | 1985 | 28.0 | 207 | Titti et al 1986 |
| | 1985 | 52.0 | 220 | Costigliola et al 1986 |
| | 1986 | 33.0 | 120 | Gradilone et al 1986 |
| Padua | 1985 | 43.0 | 460 | Bartolotti et al 1986 |
| Naples | 1986 | 14.0 | 164 | Gradilone et al 1986 |
| Sicily | 1987 | 68.4 | 684 | Accurso et al 1988 |
| **SOUTHERN CONTINENTS** | | | | |
| *SOUTH AMERICA* | | | | |
| (Buenos Aires) | | | | |
|     detoxification | 1987 | 22.0 | 268 | Weissenbacker et al 1988a |
|     hepatitis | 1987 | 48.0 | 97 | Weissenbacker et al 1988b |
| | 1988 | 63.9 | 36 | Boxaca et al 1989 |
| | 1988 | 60.3 | 338 | Cahn et al 1989 |
| *AUSTRALIA* | 1986 | 0.8 | 1905 | Dwyer et al 1988 |
| *THAILAND* | | | | |
| (Bangkok) | 1987 | 1.0 | | Thongcharoen et al 1988 |
|     March | 1988 | 16.0 | | Thongcharoen et al 1988 |
|     September | 1988 | 44.0 | 1811 | Vanichseni et al 1989 |

**Table 6.1** (*cont'd*)

| Location | Year | % | Total sample size | Reference |
|---|---|---|---|---|
| **NORTH AMERICAN CONTINENT** | | | | |
| *CANADA* | | | | |
| Manitoba | 1988 | 2.1 | 627 | Hammand et al 1989 |
| Montreal, Quebec | | | | |
|     hospitalised | 1985–8 | 4.4 | | Hammand et al 1989 |
|     detox unit | 1985 | 7.1 | | Hammand et al 1989 |
| | 1986 | 3.0 | 294 | Bruneau et al 1982 |
| | 1987 | 2.0 | | Bruneau et al 1982 |
| | 1988 | 6.6 | | Bruneau et al 1982 |
| *UNITED STATES* | | | | |
| San Francisco | 1985 | 10.0 | 281 | Chaission et al 1986 |
| Los Angeles | 1987 | 3.4 | 205 | Battjes and Pickers 1988 |
| Denver Colorado | 1985 | 2.0 | 76 | Scottish Home and |
| | | 5.0 | 262 | Health Department 1986 |
| Connecticut | 1981–3 | 30.0 | 283 | D'Aquila et al 1986 |
| Florida (Miami) | | | | |
|     In treatment | 1988 | 12.0 | | McCoy et al 1989 |
|     In street | 1988 | 33.0 | 500 | McCoy et al 1989 |
| Illinois (Chicago) | 1984–5 | 11.0 | 35 | Scottish Home and |
| | | | | Health Department 1986 |
| | 1986–7 | 33.0 | 200 | Sherer et al 1988 |
| Maryland (Baltimore) | 1988 | 24.7 | 441 | Nelson et al 1989 |
| Michigan (Detroit) | 1985–6 | 12.5 | 96 | Ognjan et al 1988 |
| | 1987–8 | 15.7 | 70 | Ognjan et al 1988 |
| | 1988–9 | 15.5 | 71 | Ognjan et al 1988 |
| Minnesota (Minneapolis) | 1987 | 1.3 | 231 | Thomas et al 1989 |
| | 1988 | 1.5 | 325 | Thomas et al 1989 |
| New York | 1978 | 9.0 | | Novick et al 1986 |
| | 1979 | 30.0 | | Novick et al 1986 |
| | 1980 | 40.0 | | Novick et al 1986 |
| | 1982 | 50.0 | | Novick et al 1986 |
|     drug treatment | 1983–4 | 33.0 | | Novick et al 1986 |
|     hospitalised | 1983–4 | 70.0 | | Maayan et al 1985 |
|     non-opportunistic infection | 1984 | 35.0 | 103 | Brown et al 1986 |
|     drug detox | 1984 | 58.0 | | Spira et al 1984 |
| | 1985 | 50.0 | | Spira et al 1984 |
|     methadone | 1985 | 32.0 | 445 | Selwyn et al 1988a |
|     methadone | 1987 | 59.5 | 222 | Battjes and Pickers 1988 |
| Texas | 1987 | 19.4 | 31 | Ognjan et al 1988 |
| Texas (San Antonio) | 1987 | 1.3 | 149 | Battjes and Pickers 1988 |

users inject cocaine intravenously often mixed with heroin and do so far more frequently than when they inject heroin alone (Drucker 1986). Recently a definite link between HIV seropositivity and the use of intravenous cocaine has been reported (Stark 1988a,b, Chaisson et al 1989).

Lastly, it is difficult to separate out the importance of the spread of HIV between drug users by sexual intercourse. However an estimate can be made by comparing the seroprevalence of injecting drug users and their non-drug using sexual partners. For instance in one Italian study the seroprevalence of double drug using couples was 45% compared to only 8% in non-drug using sexual partners (Tirelli et al 1986). In Edinburgh whilst the seroprevalence of injecting drug users was around 50% that in non-using partners was only 15% (France et al 1988). These studies suggest that needle sharing is between three to five times as efficient at spreading HIV as heterosexual intercourse.

## AIDS, HIV INFECTION AND INJECTION DRUG USE IN THE UNITED KINGDOM

Unlike the USA 82% of the patients with AIDS notified in the United Kingdom have involved homosexuality or bisexuality alone and only 2% of such reports have implicated IDU alone as a high risk activity (Anonymous 1989). Only 3.8% of the AIDS cases have come from Scotland and only 11 of these were drug users (Communicable Diseases Scotland 1989a,b,c). In the UK as a whole IDU represents only 16% of reports for those infected with HIV and this contrasts markedly with the position in Scotland in which 54% of those infected with HIV have implicated IDU and nearly 60% of those reports have come from Edinburgh (Communicable Diseases Scotland 1989a,b,c).

In 1985 and 1986 surveys found that between 38% and 52% of Edinburgh and 40% of Dundee drug users had been infected with HIV (Peutherer et al 1985, Robertson et al 1986, Brettle et al 1987, Urquhart et al 1987). However, at any one time, only about 30–40% of HIV seropositive patients were currently still injecting drugs. By comparison only 4.5% of drug users in Glasgow and 10% in England and Wales were infected with HIV (Follett et al 1986, Mortimer et al 1985). Whilst fewer IDU related HIV infections have occurred in England and Wales all areas have now reported cases. The known rate of HIV infection per head of population is 60 per 100 000 in the North West Thames Region of London and 110 per 100 000 or 0.1% in Edinburgh (Communicable Diseases Scotland 1988). By comparison, in the Bronx the HIV seroprevalence of women attending for termination was 2% and for patients attending hospitals in general it was 4.6% (Schoenbaum et al 1988).

The initial United Kingdom drug problem in the 1960's was centred around relatively affluent individuals in London with smaller numbers in other cities. In the late 1970s and early 1980s coincident with the arrival of relatively cheap brown heroin from Iran and then Pakistan different users appeared — unemployed individuals from large council estates (Pearson et al 1985). An epidemic of IDU occurred in Edinburgh starting around 1980 and peaking in 1983–84 (Brettle & Nelles 1988). There is also further supportive evidence of this epidemic of IDU from the increased number of IDU-related conditions admitted to hospital over this period (Table 6.2). This was unfortunately the time that HIV was introduced into this community (Robertson et al 1986a).

In 1985 drug users were generally unemployed, around 25 years of age, started their drug use around the age of 17–20 and at least one third were

**Table 6.2**  Injection drug use related illness — hospital discharges for Lothian 1976–86. Supplied by Information and Statistic Division of Common Services Agency (Scotland).

| Year | Endocarditis | Pneumonia | Skin infections (abscesses etc.) | Hepatitis B | Opiate overdoses |
|------|--------------|-----------|----------------------------------|-------------|------------------|
| 1976 | 0 | 0 | 0 | 0 | 0 |
| 1977 | 0 | 0 | 4 | 0 | 0 |
| 1978 | 0 | 2 | 3 | 0 | 0 |
| 1979 | 0 | 0 | 2 | 0 | 0 |
| 1980 | 1 | 2 | 5 | 2 | 36 |
| 1981 | 0 | 4 | 13 | 2 | 55 |
| 1982 | 2 | 0 | 23 | 3 | 53 |
| 1983 | 1 | 4 | 46 | 9 | 53 |
| 1984 | 7 | 8 | 66 | 19 | 83 |
| 1985 | 1 | 2 | 7 | 1 | 93 |
| 1986 | 1 | 0 | 9 | 3 | 69 |

female (Brettle et al 1986, Brettle 1986). These individuals often had no tradition of heroin use and knew little about how to avoid some of the complications. Comparisons of self-reported habits between Edinburgh and Glasgow or Edinburgh and London reveal considerably more sharing of needles and syringes in Edinburgh (Robertson et al 1986b, Brettle 1986). Further evidence for the epidemic of heroin use and the intense sharing of injecting equipment in Edinburgh users comes from the concurrent epidemic of injection-related medical conditions including hepatitis B amongst injection drug users between 1980–85 (Table 6.2 and Fig. 6.1).

Historically, drug users report that needles and syringes were in short supply in Edinburgh from around 1980/82 to 1985 when a surgical supplies shop ceased trading and pharmacists were generally unwilling to supply users. Users also report that equipment was commonly removed from them by the

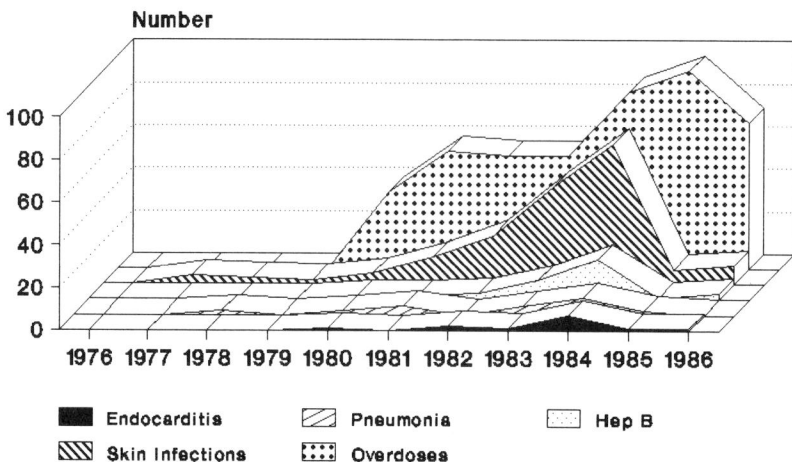

**Fig. 6.1**  Drug use and illness. Lothian hospital inpatients 1980–1986, supplied by Information and Statistics Division, CSA (Scotland).

police during searches and then destroyed. Possession of equipment contaminated with heroin may be used as evidence of illicit use and users might then give evidence against a supplier. This resulted in suppliers forcing users to use drugs on site so that on leaving the premises they were free of any incriminating evidence. Unfortunately, because of the limited supply of equipment considerable sharing occurred, with possibly only one or two sets of equipment being used for all the pushers' clients, which could number 20–40. There were also large gatherings of users, anything from 5 to 20, in the style of American 'shooting galleries' where one set of equipment was passed around the group.

## CONSEQUENCES OF AN HIV EPIDEMIC AMONGST INJECTION DRUG USERS

A number of studies in the USA and the United Kingdom have shown that between 60–100% of heterosexually acquired HIV is related to IDU (Centers for Disease Control 1987a, Evans et al 1988, France et al 1988). What is less well known is that at least 40% of injection drug users are in relationships with non-users (Drucker 1986). In addition approximately a third of injection drug users are female and as a consequence a further problem is one of vertical spread to newborn children (Drucker 1986, Robertson et al 1986a, Brettle 1986).

A subgroup of drug users are surprisingly mobile and this results in further geographical spread of HIV to other injection users (Robertson et al 1986a,b, Franceschi et al 1986, Brettle et al 1987, Bisset et al 1989).

A considerable proportion of drug users will spend periods in prison, and in view of the rising prevalence of drug use related HIV, prisoners constitute a group which is at high risk of HIV infection. Exact figures of HIV seroprevalence within United Kingdom prisons are unavailable as screening of individuals on entry to or inside prison is not performed. European figures are available however (Harding 1987) and give much cause for concern. In Italy, which screens all prison inmates, overall seroprevalence is 16.8% and in some reported studies is around 30% (Borroni 1986, Tirelli et al 1988). Small scales studies in other countries have revealed prevalence rates of 26% in Spain, 12.6% in France and 11% in Dutch and Swiss prisons (Harding 1987). It is not unreasonable to estimate a United Kingdom seroprevalence of a similar order. In one study of two Madrid prisons, an overall seroprevalence in males of 55% was found with the highest prevalence (77%) amongst drug users (Estebanez et al 1988). In the USA, seroprevalence rates of up to 15% have been reported (Centers for Disease Control 1987b).

One consequence of the high rates of HIV in drug using prisoners is that new infections with HIV are bound to occur because injection drug use continues within the prison environment. Owing to the lack of available injecting equipment, multiple sharing does occur and it has been anecdotally reported that as many as 30 inmates can regularly share a single set of injecting paraphernalia. This obviously puts HIV seronegative drug users at great risk of acquiring HIV. A recent study of prison inmates in one US prison suggested an annual rate of infection of 0.41% per person (Brewer et al 1988), and the incidence of seroconversion in Stockholm Central Prison has been estimated to be 1% per year (Olin & Käll 1988). Higher transmission rates are more likely in regions with high HIV seroprevalence in drug users.

Thus it is apparent that the key to the spread of HIV into the general population lies with the drug users. Improved services for drug users to prevent heterosexual spread must be viewed in the same light by the community as the use of confidential alternative testing sites to protect the blood supply.

## NATURAL HISTORY OF IDU RELATED HIV INFECTION

Several studies have assessed the rate of progression to AIDS amongst drug users. However, most of these reports relate the onset of symptoms of AIDS to the length of follow up, and not to the duration of HIV infection. Hence, these figures must be interpreted carefully as differing results may merely reflect differing intervals between infection and the start of the assessment period.

A study of 288 HIV positive drug users from the Bronx in New York showed that 16% had progressed to AIDS over 31 months, and in another series 25% of 25 drug users developed AIDS over a 3 year period (Selwyn et al 1989, Goedert et al 1986).

Results obtained in European studies show a slower rate of progression. In a large Spanish survey of 646 IDUs, the actuarial incidence of AIDS was 15% at 6 years, with a similar incidence being found amongst homosexuals (Gatell et al 1989). Other smaller scale studies show AIDS incidences of 6% after 14 months, 6.5% after 18 months, and 7.4% after 3 years follow up (Vaccher et al 1988, Zulaica et al 1988, Crovari et al 1988).

In one Italian study in which seroconversion dates were estimated, there was a 17.8% progression to AIDS after 4 years of HIV infection (Rezza et al 1989).

In Edinburgh, since October 1985, 289 patients known to be HIV seropositive have been medically examined and of these 245 (85%) acquired their infection between 1983–84 as a consequence of IDU. To date 8 (3.2%) of these 245 have died from either violence or apparent drug overdose. The Infectious Disease Unit of the City Hospital has cared for a total of 32 patients with the diagnosis of AIDS and 8 have died. Twelve (one of whom has died) of these 32 patients with AIDS were related to IDU either directly or via heterosexual transmission. One patient with AIDS acquired her HIV infection from her injection drug-using sexual partner.

In 1987 the Tayler Report predicted that in the South East of Scotland there would be 2 new cases of IDU-related AIDS (that is, users and heterosexual cases) in 1987, 9–10 in 1988 and between 111 and 182 by 1991 (Scottish Home and Health Department 1987). In fact there were 3 new cases in 1987 and 9 in 1988 very much in line with the predictions. The current doubling time, as for most early epidemics, is around 6 months (Flegg et al 1989a).

We have observed a rate of progression to AIDS of 1% after approximately 4 years and 3% after 5 years of infection. By comparison, of a cohort of homosexual men from San Francisco 5% had developed AIDS at 3 years, 10% at 4 years, 23% at 6 years and 37% at 8 years of infection (Hessol et al 1988). However, it is too soon to conclude that progression occurs at a slower rate in drug users. This will only be possible when studies are conducted in a standardised manner between centres, with data based on the duration of HIV infection, and with calculations of actuarial rates of progression to clearly defined end points.

There is increasing evidence that amongst drug users, data collected on AIDS cases greatly underrepresents serious IDU related HIV disease. In New York, Stoneburner has reported that there has been a rapid increase in both AIDS and non-AIDS narcotic related deaths (Stoneburner et al 1989). There were 276 narcotic related deaths in 1978, 1607 in 1985 and nearly 2000 in 1986. Thus by 1986, for every AIDS related death in a drug user, there was one other as a consequence of such conditions as tuberculosis, endocarditis and bacterial pneumonia. Similar data has been reported from Milan (Galli et al 1988).

Whilst it is generally assumed that the survival for drug users with AIDS is shorter a report on 5833 cases of AIDS from New York which adjusted for various factors found no difference between homosexuals and drug users in terms of survival. Injection drug use itself may be an adverse factor however, since the combination of IDU and homosexuality did lead to a shorter survival. Also a proportional hazards model showed a significant interaction between IDU and *Pneumocystis carinii* pneumonia (PCP) as factors shortening survival (Rothenberg et al 1987).

The apparent poor survival for drug users may be connected with the poor survival of women, possibly related to a delay in diagnosis as seen by the fact that 16.3% of women die at diagnosis of AIDS compared to 10.9% of men (Rothenberg et al 1987). A greater risk of respiratory failure was observed for women with PCP as well as a two fold increase in the mortality compared to a matched group of men (Verdegem et al 1988). In New Jersey amongst 345 women, 95% of whom were black and 63% drug users, the mean survival was only 14.5 weeks (Kloser et al 1988). By comparison one series of 24 women, all white from Rhode Island suggested improved survival since the mean length of survival was 19 months and only 5 had PCP (Carpenter et al 1988). Overall however, the prognosis seems to be poorer for women since in the New York series the cumulative probability of survival at 1 year was 75.4% for white males with Kaposi's sarcoma (KS) but only 37% for black female drug users with PCP (Rothenberg et al 1987).

Thus, it is necessary when considering progression of HIV amongst drug users to consider these additional factors, and until this is done it is probably inaccurate to consider that progression is slower or faster in drug users.

## CLINICAL FEATURES

Injection drug use-related AIDS or HIV infection has little to differentiate it clinically from that occurring in the other risk groups, and the range of opportunistic disease that occurs is similar. However, differences in lifestyle and environment have an influence over the organisms encountered and hence the prevalence of some diseases does vary between risk groups.

In the USA, figures are available on the 30 632 cases of AIDS notified to the Centers for Disease Control by the 9 February 1987 (Selik et al 1987). These show that conditions such as KS are unusual in the absence of homo/bisexuality. In drug users, KS, cytomegalovirus and chronic cryptosporidiosis are all significantly less common than for all other risk groups notified with AIDS; while PCP, tuberculosis, oesophageal candidiasis and extra-pulmonary cryptococcosis are more common.

Drug use has been identified as a risk factor for tuberculosis prior to the advent of AIDS (Reichman et al 1979), but nonetheless the incidence of tuberculosis is much higher in HIV infected drug users than in other risk groups outside the tropics or in HIV negative drug users. In the USA, most patients with AIDS and tuberculosis have been drug users (Sunderam et al 1986, Handwerger et al 1987). The latter of these studies showed a prevalence of 15.1% in drug users with AIDS but only 4.4% in other risk groups within a New York hospital. A similar pattern has been shown in San Francisco (Chaisson et al 1987). In New York the rate of tuberculosis was 4% amongst HIV positive drug users compared to 0% in HIV negative drug users and the 36% increase in reported cases of tuberculosis between 1984 and 1986 has been largely ascribed to infection amongst HIV positive drug users (Centers for Disease Control 1987c, Selwyn et al 1989).

Encapsulated bacteria such as *Streptococcus pneumonia* and *Haemophilus influenzae* are frequent respiratory pathogens and causes of bacteraemia in HIV seropositive individuals (Simberkoff et al 1984). IDU related HIV patients have a higher incidence of recurrent bacterial infections such as pneumonia, 12% with a mortality of 2.2% compared to 3% with a mortality of 0% in HIV negative drug users (Selwyn et al 1988a). The annual incidence of pneumonia was 9.7% for HIV seropositive drug users compared to under 2% for a population of mainly homosexual males with AIDS (Selwyn et al 1988b, Polsky et al 1986). There is a rising mortality from pneumonia in young adults in New York City primarily as a consequence of IDU related HIV and other cities in the USA are showing similar trends (Centers for Disease Control 1988).

The morbidity and mortality of bacterial endocarditis in HIV seropositive individuals is greater than for seronegative individuals. For instance the mortality was 24% in seropositives compared with 4% in the seronegatives. The poorer outcome was related to more frequent embolisation, a greater diversity of organisms, more prolonged fever, persistent bacteraemia and greater immunological dysfunction. It was not related to recognised opportunistic infections (Slim et al 1988, Ruggeri et al 1988).

The reasons for the increase in bacterial infections are not yet clear. Antibody production is impaired in HIV infected patients, and low levels of IgG$_2$ have been associated with bacterial infection (Parkin et al 1989). This is not specific for injection drug users however, and the fact that they make less use of medical services may be of importance. Additional factors may be that opiates themselves depress the cough reflex as well as the immune system and unsterile IDU exposes the individual to recurrent episodes of bacterial infection.

A common clinical problem is the combined effect of pneumonia and opiates. It is now our standard practice to consider the use of naloxone in patients presenting with pneumonia in order to overcome the effect of opiates on respiratory drive. It is also necessary to use controlled infusions of naloxone in order to produce a controlled withdrawal from opiates which not only improves oxygenation but can be tolerated by the patient. Acute withdrawal from opiates without an explanation of the need can result in the patients' self discharge.

One major concern when dealing with IDU related HIV is the fact that many conditions may be either HIV related or drug-use related (Table 6.3). For instance lymphadenopathy may be associated with injecting foreign materials or HIV infection, whilst the fatigue, lethargy and excessive sweating of HIV can all also be caused by mild withdrawal from opiates.

Diarrhoea is common with acute opiate withdrawal and as an outpatient there may be a history of diarrhoea for longer than 1 month. If not caused by any pathogens or other illness this would be suggestive of stage IVa of HIV but there is a need to search for specific pathogens seen in AIDS such as Cryptosporidium or *Isospora belli*. It is a common complaint first thing in the morning for those on methadone but in general diarrhoea is an uncommon problem for IDU related HIV.

The intermittent use of benzodiazepines can cause epileptic fits as can cerebral toxoplasmosis and other neurological conditions seen in AIDS. The excessive use of cannabis and benzodiazepines can interfere with memory and other cognitive functions as can HIV. Thus early dementia, which might be picked up in other risk groups by psychometric testing, is extremely difficult to be confident about in current users. Syncopal attacks in HIV infection or AIDS may be associated with an autonomic neuropathy or low levels of steroids from a failing adrenal cortex. This problem can also be caused however by the use or misuse of antidepressant tricyclic drugs such as amitriptyline.

Shortness of breath and a persistent cough are common early symptoms of PCP but can also occur with endocarditis, excessive smoking, recurrent bronchitis and obstructive airways disease. Weight loss and sweating are associated with heavy drug use, yet in the setting of HIV, infection with Mycobacteria must be considered. Thus it is often difficult to be sure with injection drug users, especially current users, whether the problem is real or spurious, drug or HIV related, and admission to hospital for a period of observation may be the only way to unravel this dilemma.

**Table 6.3**   Comparison of drug and IDU related HIV problems

| Problem | Drugs effects | Injection related | HIV related |
|---|---|---|---|
| Respiratory tract: shortness of breath/ cyanosis/cough | Excess amphetamines/ cocaine | Septic pulmonary embolism, bacterial pneumonia, endocarditis | PCP — note increased susceptibility to bacterial infections |
| | Heart failure 2° cocaine Myocardial infarction 2° cocaine | Aspiration pneumonia Chronic bronchitis | |
| | Excess opiates Pulmonary oedema 2° to excess opiates Methaemoglobin 2° Nitrites (poppers) | | PCP — note increased suceptibility to bacterial infections |
| Fever | Dirty fix/withdrawals from opiates/excess cocaine | Pneumonia/ endocarditis etc. | PCP, TB, etc. or CDC IVa |
| Rash: small blood spots | | Septicaemia, endocarditis | Immune thrombocytopenia/ failing bone marrow |
| Bruises | | Arterial injection | Immune thrombocytopenia/ failing bone marrow |
| Itchy spots | | Poor diet, infestation | Allergy/seborrhoeic dermatitis/papular urticaria |
| Abscess | | Missed hit (chemical damage) especially barbiturates, Diconal, temazepam | Note excess susceptibility to bacterial infections |
| Sores around mouth | | Poor diet | Chronic Herpes simplex |
| Sore mouth | | Poor diet | Herpes simplex, thrush, oral leukoplakia |
| Weight loss | Frequent injecting of cocaine/amphetamines | Poor diet | CDC IVA, TB, other infections |
| Vomiting/nausea | Withdrawal from benzodiazepines Withdrawal from opiates | Hepatitis, septicaemia, pneumonia, etc | Toxoplasmosis |
| Diarrhoea | Withdrawal from opiates, excess amphetamine/cocaine | | Cryptosporidiosis/ isosporiasis, CMV, etc |
| Constipation | Excess opiates | | ? Autonomic dysfunction |
| Flu-like symtoms | Withdrawal from opiates | Bad fix/septicaemia/ endocarditis, etc | CDC III, IVA |
| Sweating | Withdrawal from opiates | Bad fix/septicaemia/ endocarditis, etc | CDC III, IVA |
| Loss of vision | | Endocarditis, local injection damage, Candida ophthalmitis | CMV, choroidoretinitis |

| | | | |
|---|---|---|---|
| Confusion/coma/ delirium | Withdrawal from barbiturates, excess opiates/ benzodiazepines/ barbiturates, excess cocaine | Pneumonia/ endocarditis, etc. | Toxic confusional state, meningitis, toxoplasmosis, etc |
| Psychological disturbance, hallucinations/ paranoia | Excess amphetamines/ cocaine, cannabis/phencyclidine (angel dust) | | Toxoplasmosis, HIV encephalopathy |
| Slurred speech/ abnormal gait | Excess barbiturates, benzodiazepines | | Toxoplasmosis, HIV encephalopathy |
| Headache | Excess amphetamines/ cocaine | | Toxoplasmosis, HIV encephalopathy |
| Fits/episodic/ loss of consciousness/ postural syncope | Excess cocaine, withdrawal from benzodiazepines, barbiturates and alcohol | Meningitis | Toxoplasmosis etc |
| | Antidepressants  — excess methaqualone used to 'cut' heroin | | |
| Paralysis | | Arterial/nerve injection | Toxoplasmosis/HIV encephalopathy |

Hepatitis B is frequent amongst injection drug users. For instance in our population of HIV seropositives 91% have markers of infection as opposed to 51% in HIV seronegative drug users reflecting the frequency of drug use and the extent of equipment sharing (Burns et al 1987). A recently described event is the reactivation of hepatitis B infection amongst drug users during the course of HIV infection (Vento et al 1989) and we have also observed this phenomenon in IDU-related HIV infection.

## MANAGEMENT OF IDU RELATED HIV INFECTION

The management of IDU-related HIV infection is based upon:

1. The prevention of further spread of HIV,
2. The prevention of progression to AIDS once infected with HIV,
3. The treatment of opportunistic cancers and infections and
4. Specific anti-HIV therapy.

### Prevention of transmission of HIV

The particular measures which have been suggested to reduce transmission include:

1. A reduction in the number of sexual partners,
2. Avoidance of anal intercourse for homosexuals and heterosexuals,
3. Use of barrier contraceptives especially condoms or sheaths combined with spermicides,

4. Avoidance of needle and syringe sharing, and
5. Avoidance of pregnancy with the increased chance of infecting the child.

*Spread by needles and syringes*

The management of drug users at risk of, or infected with, HIV has a number of particular problems not often seen elsewhere. Abstinence has, until now, been the major goal of dealing with users but with the appearance of HIV these goals need to be adjusted to one of 'risk or harm reduction'. The *eventual* goal is still one of abstinence but initially it is important to start with a more realistic goal identified for each patient. Depending upon the individual, this may encompass substitution therapy on a long or short term basis in order to avoid needles drug abuse, or the provision of needles and syringes to reduce equipment sharing.

Recent work suggests that oral methadone reduces not only high risk injecting behaviour but also acquisition of HIV and the incidence of AIDS. For instance in a 3 year study of methadone maintenance treatment programme (MMTP) in New York, Philadelphia and Baltimore 715 clients who remained in MMTP for more than 1 year ceased IDU (Ball et al 1988). By comparison 82% of those who left the programme continued to inject. In addition only 10% of clients in MMTP shared equipment compared to 27% amongst dropouts. This latter figure increased to 48% once they had been out of treatment for longer than 1 year.

Another New York study looked at clients on the waiting list for MMTP (Yancovitz et al 1988). These clients were randomly divided into two groups to receive counselling, methadone and biweekly urine toxicology or counselling and biweekly urine toxicology only until they were admitted to the regular MMTP. Needle use was identical for each group at 95 injections per month but at entry into MMTP only 33% of those on methadone were injecting compared to 87% of those in the counselling group. In the Swedish MMTP the HIV seroprevalence of those admitted was 3% in those admitted in 1983, 16% in 1984–86 and 57% in 1987 suggesting a protective effect for the acquisition of HIV related to MMTP (Blix & Grönbladh 1988). Lastly the Montefiore group showed that the incidence of AIDS was lower (11.4 and 33.0/1000 person years) for entrants to their MMTP before and after 1983 (Hartel et al 1988).

The concept of harm reduction grew out of the Amsterdam approach to drug use which began in the late 1970's with the establishment of a mobile distribution vehicle, known as the Methadone Bus. The basic underlying principle was to dispense methadone to encourage contact, to provide information and wait for attitude and behaviour changes to occur in the user towards drug use. Whilst waiting for these changes it was thought necessary to reduce the harm that might befall the user via dangerous injection practices. There were few restrictions surrounding the methadone other than a need to collect it daily and drink it on the bus.

In 1984 as an extension to the principle of harm reduction the Amsterdam Junkie Union proposed and started a pilot needle exchange scheme which was taken up by the Municipal Health Authority and other voluntary organisations such that by 1987 there were 11 participating sites. In 1984 less than 50 000 syringes/needles were distributed with perhaps 30% being returned. By 1987 700 000 syringes/needles were distributed with 70% being returned and in 1988 650 000 syringes/needles were distributed with 95% being returned (Bunning 1989 Personal communication).

Scientific evaluation of the schemes only began recently. A group of exchangers were compared with users not using exchanges but recruited from other areas such as hospitals, police stations etc. When asked to compare their current IDU with that of 6 months previously only 29% of the exchangers were injecting more by comparison to 50% of the non-exchangers. Thus there was no suggestion that the exchanges promoted IDU. As far as equipment sharing was concerned only 10% of exchangers were sharing compared to 24% of non-exchangers and 74% of exchangers were using equipment only once by comparison to only 27% of non-exchangers. Perhaps of even more interest was the fact that 25% of the exchangers were outside the methadone system thus increasing even more the number of users the Municipal Health Authority were in contact with (Bunning 1989 Personal communication).

Partly as a consequence of the Amsterdam experience numerous United Kingdom practitioners began to exchange equipment and the United Kingdom Government, under pressure from the McClelland report which called for the availability of equipment in the management of IDU, set up 15 experimental exchanges throughout England and Scotland in early 1987 (Scottish Home and Health Department 1986). The evaluation was recently reported by the Monitoring Research Group of Goldsmith College London (Stimson et al 1988a,b, Donoghue et al 1989).

The final report on 2449 clients concluded that these schemes reached a considerable number of injection drug users, the majority living within 2 miles of the schemes. 40% had never been in a treatment programme and nearly 75% were not in a current treatment programme. The attenders were however older opiate users with a mean age of 27.8 years, mostly male (78%) and had an initial lower level of risk behaviour compared to injectors who did not attend. For instance only 36% had shared equipment within the previous 4 weeks and only 19% had shared with more than 2 individuals in the last 4 weeks. By comparison 62% of a group of non-attenders were injecting in the previous 4 weeks and 36% with more than 2 individuals. Thus non-attenders at exchange schemes had riskier injecting behaviour despite the fact that this sample was interviewed after the government's publicity campaign. The commonest reason for sharing was difficulty in obtaining equipment and this did not differ between attenders or non-attenders. The non-attenders however paid more attention to the cleaning of equipment than the attenders.

The major problems were the high turnover of clients which varied from a low of 25% to a high of 85% returning for a second visit. The average retention rate was 61% for the second visit falling to 17% for the tenth visit and only 1% returning for more than 40 visits. The exchange rate also varied from 23% to 100% with a mean of 62%. The number of syringes/needles issued per visit varied from 3 (the legal maximum per visit in Scotland) to 30, with a mean of 9 per visit.

Amongst clients who continued to attend there was evidence of self reported reduction in needle related risk behaviour. For instance sharing in the previous 4 weeks declined from 34% to 27% and the % sharing with 2 or more individuals declined from 17% to 11%. Over 70% of attenders and non-attenders reported that as a consequence of AIDS they had made some change in their drug use usually a reduction in sharing or an increase in using clean equipment.

Interestingly clients in Scotland, possibly because the schemes ran under stricter legal controls with fewer needles and syringes given out per visit and shorter opening hours, showed greater sharing risk behaviour compared to their English counterparts. For instance 76% of Scottish injectors had shared equipment in the previous 4 weeks compared to only 52% of English injectors. This is in keeping with previous reports of increased equipment sharing in Scotland. In Scotland injectors found equipment harder to obtain, were more likely to find the exchanges closed or to share in custody.

The changes in sexual behaviour were also small but in the right direction. The number of attenders who were sexually active declined from 77% to 69% and the number with multiple sexual partners in the previous 3 months declined from 26% to 21%. Marginally more attenders (48%) reported changes in sexual behaviour because of AIDS than non-attenders (42%). Only 25% of the sexually active non-attenders reported using a condom compared to 38% of the sexually active attenders.

In the United States as yet few needle exchange schemes have managed to open often because of political opposition. As a consequence voluntary organisations have begun campaigns to teach injection users to clean their equipment using commonly available disinfectants such as bleach, alcohol, detergent or peroxide. Such compounds are effective and available to the majority of injection drug users (Flynn et al 1988). Street based education, utilising outreach workers has successfully improved 'safe' needle hygiene (Watters et al 1988). As with needle exchanges it is difficult to collect scientific data to prove their effectiveness but they are popular with clients. Cleaning agents such as household detergent are effective in killing HIV in vitro provided cold water is used to reduce or slow blood clotting. It may be that such campaigns could be used effectively in the United Kingdom in areas such as prisons where needle exchange is unlikely to occur because of political dogma or security reasons.

Whilst for many the scientific case for needle exchange is still not yet proven the epidemic of injection drug associated illness and the spread of both HIV and hepatitis B that overtook Edinburgh from 1982 onwards serve as a demonstration of the effects of reducing the availability of injecting equipment for drug users.

Thus despite the pessimism it is possible for injection drug users to change their injecting behaviour and this is in keeping with other reports (Skidmore et al 1988). It appears however, that it is more difficult to change heterosexual behaviour.

Preventive strategies to decrease possible transmission of HIV within prisons should include measures in addition to the present policy of education and drug screening vigilance. Consideration should be given to the continuation of maintenance methadone for those who are on programmes prior to their conviction and education provided on safe methods of sterilising injection equipment. Unlimited provision of sterile needles is not viewed as a viable option since these can be used as weapons. Segregation or isolation of known HIV seropositives would be a retrograde step, denying rights to those infected and yet not identifying all those who are potentially infectious. Voluntary rather than mandatory testing of inmates would be most appropriate (Andrus et al 1988).

Much has been made of the risks of HIV transmission between normally heterosexual males by homosexual contacts in prison. It is not known to what extent such behaviour occurs but the provision of condoms is one possible means for reducing the risks of such activity.

*Pregnancy*

Pregnancy is important in HIV infection because of the risk of transmission to the child. The factors responsible for vertical transmission are as yet not well understood and the risk of transmission from mother to child may be as low as 0% if HIV infection occurs during the pregnancy (Stewart et al 1985). Reports which unfortunately rely upon the identification of a symptomatic child, will suggest high rates of perinatal transmission and these may not be widely applicable. Preliminary reports of prospective surveys suggest a risk of between 22% and 51% (Selwyn et al 1987, Mok et al 1987a,b, Willoughby et al 1987, Blanche et al 1987, Bradick et al 1987). Of more importance may be the immunological status of the mother. The risk of transmission from a haemophiliac to his spouse seems to depend upon low numbers of T4 helper lymphocytes, the presence of thrombocytopenia and HIV antigenaemia (Eyster et al 1987, Lange et al 1986). One report from Africa suggested a similar correlation between low numbers of T4 lymphocytes in the mother and transmission to the child (Nzila et al 1987). Because we do not understand the factors involved in transmission it is difficult at present to advise prospective HIV infected mothers of what they can do to reduce the risks of transmission.

In addition a recent study of 136 pregnant women, 61 HIV seropositive has shown that HIV has little effect on pregnancy itself early on in the course of HIV infection. A comparison of HIV seropositive and seronegative pregnancies revealed features of lifestyle and deprivation that would be expected to have an adverse effect on pregnancy but no evidence that HIV per se affected the outcome of pregnancy. The only significant difference was the fact that the spontaneous abortions rate was 18% for the HIV seropositives compared to 6.6% for the HIV seronegatives (Johnstone et al 1988).

## Progression of HIV infection

The particular measures which have been suggested to reduce the influence of cofactors for progression to AIDS once infected are:

1. Avoidance of needle sharing to reduce further HIV infection
2. Avoidance of needle drug use
3. Avoidance of pregnancy.

### Reduction in further HIV infection

It has been suggested that the drift in molecular composition demonstrated in different HIV isolates might result in the acquisition of differing strains of HIV (Hahn et al 1986). These additional doses of HIV, acquired as a consequence of persistent needle sharing, might be expected to hasten disease progression and emphasise the need for continued avoidance of needle sharing.

### Reduction in injection drug use

There is a continuing debate over the benefit of substitution therapy in the management of opiate IDU whether HIV seropositive or not (Stevenson 1986, Lipsedge & Cook 1987, Szasz 1987, MacNair 1986). Oral substitution therapy for drug use has been evaluated over a number of years but the majority of studies have concentrated upon retention rates, frequency and prevention of illicit drug use, reduction of criminal behaviour, the return to normal social activities and/or the possibility of curing drug use (Dole & Nyswander 1965, 1967, 1968, Newman 1976, 1987, Gossop 1978, Newman & Whitehill 1979). More recently methadone has been evaluated in the prevention of acquisition of HIV but there is little if anything concerning its possible effects on the progression of HIV once infected (Ball et al 1988, Yancovitz et al 1988, Blix & Grönbladh 1988, Hartel et al 1988).

In the United States of America MMTP are common place but in the United Kingdom maintenance regimens until recently were not favoured (Medical Working Group on Drug Dependence 1984). There is concern about the General Medical Council's current attitude towards maintenance methadone regimens and one proponent of such therapy has recently had his contract terminated (Brahams 1987, Anonymous 1987a).

Before the advent of HIV infection, drug use per se had a relatively low mortality with alternating periods of abstinence and use together with natural recovery (Ritson & Plant 1977, Robertson & Bucknall 1986, Waldorf & Biernachie 1979, Wille 1983). The advent of IDU related HIV infection has added a new dimension to the problem. For instance workers in New York have demonstrated a relationship between the frequency of IDU and the loss of T4 lymphocytes from the peripheral blood (Des Jarlais et al 1987). We have similarly seen an increased rate of loss of T4 lymphocytes amongst injectors compared to non-injectors (Flegg et al 1989b).

Opiates themselves depress the immune system. Morphine given to mice reduced the numbers of neutrophils and macrophages as well as their efficiency in phagocytosing and killing *Candida albicans*. Morphine treated mice succumbed more rapidly to *Klebsiella pneumonia* peritonitis and a depressed lymphoproliferative response to mitogens was noted in the presence of opiates (Tubaro et al 1983, Anonymous 1984). Morphine treated mice also develop marked atrophy of the spleen, thymus, lymph nodes and bone marrow as well as a reduced lymphocyte helper/suppressor ratio within 24 hours. The effects were maximal at 3 days but took 20 days to reverse completely (Arora et al 1988).

Thus even after HIV infection, for the individual rather than for the community as a whole, there are good reasons to discourage IDU. Methadone mixture DTF 1 mg per ml has been used for those unable or unwilling to become abstinent. This preparation, recommended in the Government's guidelines, is preferred because of the difficulty in its use as an injection unlike a number of other preparations, such as buprenorphine (Temgesic), dihydrocodeine, dipipanone (Diconal), etc. Attempts are made to establish a reducing regimen but if this fails patients may be maintained for long periods on regular doses.

In 1988 an assessment was made with regard to 107 injection drug users and their drug use classified as follows:

*Group 1.*   Those thought to be persistently using illicit injection drugs and who were not prescribed methadone.

*Group 2.*   Those considered to have ceased drug use and to have been prescribed methadone.

*Group 3.*   Those considered to be utilising both oral methadone and illicit injection drugs.

*Group 4.*   Those who were observed not to be using illicit drugs by injection and not in receipt of methadone either from ourselves or from general practitioners.

Significantly, more patients on methadone were noted to register a net gain in weight during the follow-up period. Overall, all methadone users were found to have a mean net weight increase of 2.5 kg versus 0.2 kg ($P = 0.02$) for those patients who received no methadone. There was no significant difference in the follow-up period for these patients (8.1 months versus 7.6 months). When the patients were divided into groups according to their drug use, a significant increase in weight of 3.7 kg was noted for Group 2 or methadone only users (Table 6.4). Over the short follow-up period there was no significant difference in the initial and final T4 counts, IgG, IgA, IgM levels between the groups.

We have been impressed by the physical improvement in those patients giving up injection drug use. This improvement is, however, difficult to measure and weight gain provides one objective measure of improvement in general health. The weight gain associated with methadone use is almost

**Table 6.4**   HIV and Methadone. *Key:* IDU, continued injection drug use;meth., use of oral drugs including methadone;meth. + IDU, use of oral drugs including methadone and injection drug use;Nil, use of oral drugs from general practitioners but *not* methadone or abstinence from drugs.

| Group | No. | Months of follow-up (range) | Net weight change in Kg (range) | Two sample, analysis with reference to group II P |
|---|---|---|---|---|
| I (IDU) | 19 | 6.5 (1–14) | – 0.4 ( – 9.3 to 8.0) | 0.005 |
| II (meth.) | 38 | 8.3 (2–19) | + 3.7 ( – 10.6 to 24.8) | |
| III (meth. + IDU) | 12 | 8.1 (2–20) | – 1.2 ( – 5.8 to 3.4) | 0.002 |
| IV (nil) | 38 | 8.1 (2–19) | + 0.6 ( – 10.5 to 21.5) | 0.01 |

certainly associated with the cessation of IDU and has been historically reported to us in those patients giving up IDU by other means. A general improvement in health is important in those infected with HIV and the regular attendance of those on oral methadone makes them available for other health education messages.

Although methadone mixture DTF is not the only oral substitute therapy available it does have a number of advantages. In modest doses of 40–60 ml, it prevents withdrawal symptoms but does not provide significant euphoria. It is thus suitable for those not willing to suffer withdrawal symptoms. Whilst the drug may enter the 'black market', its dilution and constituents discourage its use by injection. This is in contra-distinction to opiates in tablet form for which there is a ready 'black market' because of the ease with which tablets may be dissolved and then injected.

Guidelines from the Medical Working Group on Drug Dependence state that 'it is the responsibility of any doctor to provide care for general health means and drug related problems as they would for patients with other relapsing disorders' (Medical Working Group on Drug Dependence 1984). This message was reiterated by Dr John Strang, Advisor to the Department of Health and Social Security (Anonymous 1987b). Since over half of our drug use related HIV patients were still injecting when first seen, the management of their drug use is as important as the management of their HIV disease.

*Effect of pregnancy*

The prevention of pregnancy is important on the grounds of progression to AIDS in the mother as well as the prevention of transmission to the child.

In the United States only about 25% of HIV infected mothers were well 2.5 years after delivery (Scott et al 1985). In one series of 16 mothers identified by the birth of a child with AIDS only 4 remained asymptomatic at a mean follow up time of 2.5 years after delivery of the child. However, 11 of 16 women had a subsequent pregnancy during this time and we know nothing of their total parity. Additionally, in 5 of these 11 subsequent pregnancies the mothers developed AIDS or AIDS Related Complex (ARC) during that pregnancy. A second study in New York looked at 34 mothers, again identified by the birth of an affected child, after a mean of 27.8 months. Fifteen, or 44%, of the mothers had become symptomatic with AIDS or ARC. Fourteen mothers had gone on to have subsequent pregnancies (Minkoff et al 1987). The problem with both these studies was that the patients were identified by the ill health of a child and if there is a link between maternal and child ill health then it will be exaggerated by this form of selection. By comparison only 2 of 31 patients in Edinburgh had become symptomatic 2 years after delivery (MacCallum et al 1989).

In 88 non-pregnant and 7 pregnant females there was no association between parity and clinical or immunological deterioration (MacCallum et al 1988). Similar conclusions were reported by the Montefiore group but others have reported the fact that pregnancy seems to accelerate progression to AIDS although their studies are unable to control for length of infection (Schoenbaum et al 1989, Deschamps et al 1989). Despite what seemed to be adequate counselling, planned and unplanned pregnancies occur. Many mothers elect to continue with the pregnancy despite the possible risks to themselves and their future child. The Montefiore group reported that counselling with regard to the risks for mother and child had no influence on the rate of elective terminations in seropositive and seronegative women. The decision to continue pregnancy was more influenced by race, or a prior intention to become pregnant (Selwyn et al 1988c). We would recommend at present that consideration for termination be made on an individual basis rather than on any theoretical risk for the mother. However pregnancy with evidence of severe immunodeficiency and possible opportunistic infections is not without hazard and it is important to ensure that mother understands the risks to herself and the child.

**Specific treatment for opportunistic infections and HIV infection**

There are no particular differences with regard to IDU in the treatment of the opportunistic infections that occur in serious HIV infection. The most difficult area is the lack of adequate venous access and the use of indwelling intravenous catheters in current injection drug users with all the possible complications.

Specific anti-HIV chemotherapy is now becoming available. The most well known is azidothymidine (AZT) also known as Zidovudine or Retrovir. Zidovudine has been shown to increase survival and lessen the morbidity of patients with AIDS and ARC but because 60–70% of Zidovudine is metabolised via liver glucuronidation there is considerable potential for drug interactions. The early toxicity studies noted an association between neutropenia and concurrent paracetamol ingestion, utilised a 4 hourly dosage regime, closely monitored the subjects for toxicity and were conducted in highly motivated patient group (Fischl et al 1987, Richman et al 1987).

IDU is the fastest growing risk group for HIV infection in Europe and the second commonest risk group in both the USA and Europe yet little has been reported with regard to Zidovudine treatment. Since periods of abstinence may be interspersed with drug use it is necesary to establish the safety of Zidovudine in IDU related HIV infection under a variety of conditions.

Our experience of Zidovudine therapy with IDU related HIV was recently reported (Cowan et al 1989a). Forty patients were treated with Zidovudine, 30 males and 10 females. Thirteen patients acquired the virus homo/bisexually, while 26 patients became infected secondary to IDU related HIV and 1 patient from a blood transfusion. The average age of the homo/bisexual patients was 38 years (range 29–58 years), while those with intravenous drug related infection had an average age of 28.8 years (range 22–39 years).

Patients were started on Zidovudine when they developed AIDS or other CDC category IV problems. The mean absolute T4 counts of patients commencing on treatment with Zidovudine were as follows: IDU related HIV with AIDS (4 patients) $0.15 \times 10^9$/l (range 0.06–0.26); others with AIDS (11 patients) $0.11 \times 10^9$/l (range 0.05–0.2); IDU related HIV without AIDS (22 patients) $0.28 \times 10^9$/l (range 0.1–0.46); others without AIDS (3 patients) $0.12 \times 10^9$/l (range 0.09–0.16). Thirty-four of the 40 patients have had HIV antigen tests performed to date and 24 (70.5%) were found to be positive. There was no significant difference between the risk groups or CDC status as far as HIV antigenaemia was concerned.

Three (7.5%) patients who received Zidovudine had died. The one IDU related HIV with concomitant cirrhosis secondary to type B chronic active hepatitis died after 6 months of Zidovudine therapy of a massive variceal haemorrhage. His HIV related problems did not progress whilst he was taking Zidovudine.

Of the 26 IDU related HIV patients, 1 patient denied intravenous drug use and acquired her infection heterosexually from her drug using partner, 7 (28%) were no longer using oral or intravenous drugs (although 4 continue to smoke cannabis), 18 (72%) patients were on oral substitution therapy. In total 6 (24%) patients admitted to continued IDU whilst taking Zidovudine. The average length of follow up for the 26 IDU related HIV patients was 8.2 months (range 2–14 months) compared with 8.76 months (range 3–18 months) for the 13 homo/bisexual patients.

Of the 40 patients started on Zidovudine, 14 (35%) developed side effects severe enough to necessitate a reduction in the dose of Zidovudine. Eleven (27.5%) patients became anaemic, 10 (25%) severely enough to require transfusion and 1 was stabilised on a reduced dose of Zidovudine. As has been shown previously, the patients with full blown AIDS were more likely to become transfusion dependent than those with the ARC (Chi square = 10.98 with Yates' correction, $P < 0.001$). Continuing to use drugs orally or via injection did not have an adverse effect on the T4 count or make transfusion more likely. Three (7.5%) patients became neutropenic on Zidovudine (2 with AIDS).

Injection drug users are notorious for defaulting from outpatient appointments and for non-compliance with treatment due to their chaotic lifestyle. None of the homo/bisexual group missed any clinic appointments. Of the 26

IDU related HIV patients on Zidovudine 11 (42%) patients had no defaults, 12 (46%) missed 1–3 clinic visits and 3 (12%) missed 4–5 clinic visits. When the attendance of drug users was further assessed it was apparent that missed appointments were not related to continued IDU, current versus ex-IDU, AIDS versus non-AIDS or gender. The most reliable attenders were those receiving oral methadone from our clinic (Chi square = 3.72 with Yates' correction, $P = 0.05$).

If a rise in red blood cell mean corpuscular volume (MCV) is taken as an indication of Zidovudine compliance, our data suggests that compliance in the IDU related patients is comparable with those in the other groups (mean rise in MCV in IDU related HIV patients on Zidovudine is + 21.2 fl, in the other groups it is + 18.0 fl (the data from those patients who have received transfusions has not been included in this analysis).

In 12 (30%) patients the course of Zidovudine was interrupted and in 5 (12.5%) patients this was for medical reasons (anaemia, neutropenia, or gastrointestinal upset). One of these patients already mentioned had to discontinue Zidovudine permanently. Six patients, all IDU related HIV, discontinued the drug without consulting the clinic. In one patient whose lifestyle was particularly chaotic it was felt unsafe to continue with Zidovudine as its effects were being inadequately monitored. None of these patients suffered ill effects as a result of these stoppages. Two patients, 1 who had not used drugs for 4 years and 1 on oral methadone have defaulted for long periods (mean 5.5 months) and then returned to the clinic. None of the homo/bisexual patients have given up Zidovudine without medical indication.

It is not surprising perhaps that IDU related HIV as a group had a worse attendance record than homo/bisexual patients and this is probably more related to differing life style and background. A study of general practice in Muirhouse, Edinburgh, revealed a uniform default rate of two visits per patient per year irrespective of drug use (Bickler 1985).

Overall 58% of IDU related HIV patients missed one appointment but 75% of the ex- or non-IDU patients also missed at least one appointment. By comparison only 50% of those judged to be still injecting whilst on oral substitute therapy missed at least one appointment.

In two preliminary reports of IDU related HIV and Zidovudine, the populations studied were not exactly the same as our own since 14/60 or 23% of the IDU related HIV patients from New York were heterosexual contacts compared to our 4% (1 patient). Only 30% admitted to concurrent medication whereas at least 88% of our patients were using concurrent drugs and 24% admitted to current IDU (Spears et al 1988). Superficially however the results were surprisingly similar in that 81% from New York missed from 0–3 appointments compared to our 86%. However only 1% of the patients in New York had no defaults compared to our 42% and New York had 12/60 or 20% lost to follow up compared to our 2 (8%). Even these latter patients are still in contact with their general practitioners or our counselling clinic. As with ourselves other groups have not reported any excess toxicity (Spears et al 1988, Slim et al 1989, Cowan et al 1989b, Vella et al 1989). A further study concluded that: 'addicts stabilised on methadone or in drug free treatment regimes were as reliable as homosexual patients and seemed to become less sociopathic' with Zidovudine treatment (Kaplan et al 1988). Lastly, an inner city population, predominantly black and drug using, showed acceptable although not ideal compliance with Zidovudine (Williams et al 1989).

Thus the preliminary results of clinical monitoring of Zidovudine treated IDU related HIV suggest that it is safe in a variety of drug use situations including recent IDU. Caution and careful monitoring are required, however, in view of the preliminary report that opiates increase the plasma levels of Zidovudine (Brettle et al 1989).

## PRACTICAL ISSUES OF TREATING IDU-RELATED HIV

Without doubt there are a number of problems in managing IDU-related HIV. Current injection drug users are of course usually involved in an illegal activity, often tend to manipulate those with whom they are in contact and distrust official organisations such as social work and health care. This is often matched by a distrust of drug users by those same organisations and professions. Injection drug users often have a high default rate for appointments and consequently tend to utilise existing services at times of crisis.

The medical care of individuals engaged in IDU is difficult and is complicated by a lack of support in the community and often differing goals for doctors and users. Periods of IDU are interspersed with variable periods of abstinence such that therapy which demands abstinence would be fraught with dangers. Abstinence, or a particular form of drug use (eg. oral vs inhalation vs injection), would not be safe criteria on which to initiate treatment since their drug use state might alter during treatment.

In Edinburgh a number of seriously ill patients have been transferred to the Infectious Diseases Unit because of their HIV status, and there is a continuing reluctance to cope with seriously disturbed HIV patients on the grounds of infection risk.

Within the wards there are a number of difficulties which can arise. These include continued IDU, patients found unconscious as a consequence of alcohol or other drugs, the supply of drugs to each other by patients and visitors, disturbances by visitors, aggression both verbal and physical from both patients and visitors, in combination with the problems of managing seriously ill patients. In other areas such difficulties lead to discharge either by the patient or staff but this is more difficult when the patient has a condition that is life threatening or infectious. There is also the not unnatural concern by the staff over legal liability in such situations.

Within the outpatient setting there is the problem of aggression towards medical staff which might even culminate in the patient being removed horizontally from the clinic by four policemen as has happened in the past. This is obviously not very conducive to a continuing patient–doctor relationship. As far as the rest of the hospital is concerned all the disturbances and thefts are not surprisingly attributed, sometimes falsely, to such patients.

Whilst all of these problems are encountered elsewhere in the Health Service it is the relative concentration in one area which increases the difficulties.

A major problem for the patients is the apparent discrepancy between media information and local knowledge. The current relatively low rate of vertical transmission with little or no effect on the mothers in Edinburgh has encouraged further pregnancies. Similarly the low rate of transmission between heterosexual couples even after long periods of unprotected intercourse has made it difficult to encourage the use of condoms. Unfortunately seroconversions are now occurring in these couples and the rate of vertical transmission may well rise as the duration of HIV infection increases in the mothers.

There are a number of practical issues which are more specific to drug users. Since our patients are issued with a 1 month's supply of Zidovudine at each visit, intermittent treatment has occurred because of missed appointments, but this has not resulted in any harm to the patients. In addition, several treatment courses were interrupted on medical grounds and no deterioration was observed unlike recent reports (Helbert et al 1988). Currently because of the unknown effect of Zidovudine upon the fetus we recommend termination in the case of pregnancy although we would continue treatment if requested.

A commonly expressed fear is that IDU related HIV patients will sell their Zidovudine on a 'black market'. Whilst this may have happened the rise in MCV in our group suggests this is infrequent. It would also appear to be uncommon when a reasonable supply of an oral opiate substitute is given even if injecting does continue. Thus the MCV change is a convenient and a cheap method of assessing compliance. Thus only those patients who did not experience an MCV rise need be further investigated for malabsorption or lack of compliance. Interestingly, the MCV change also occurred with a far less rigorous regimen, usually two to four per day organised around meal times.

Venous access is a considerable problem in a few patients and because of the need for repeated venepuncture over many months or years we currently favour sampling from the external jugular in the head down tilt rather than the femoral vein. However current IDU does result in difficulties as far as outpatient intravenous therapy is concerned if indwelling lines need to be used, in view of their possible use by patients.

The improvement in health induced by Zidovudine has on a number of occasions resulted in individuals feeling well enough to return to IDU. Continued IDU does and will occur in patients on Zidovudine treatment. Thus, it is important to keep up the harm reduction message.

A number of our patients have started on Zidovudine whilst being in prison and others have spent time there after commencing treatment. It might be expected that this would result in difficulties with therapy but this has not occurred and prison authorities and their medical staff have provided the service for such patients to continue with their treatment and attend follow up appointments.

## CONCLUSIONS

As far as the future is concerned, until we better understand the natural history of IDU related HIV and the factors affecting progression, management strategies will be difficult to develop. For instance, it was initially thought that as far as female drug users were concerned pregnancy was detrimental to their health. However this is now far from proven since the initial reports were influenced by selection bias. Gender may well be something that must be taken into account in assessing progression since in New York females seem less susceptible, whilst in Scotland they seem more susceptible in the early stages. Gender may also affect presentation in view of the fact that other forms of immunosuppression in females result in an increased risk of cervical cancer (Alloub et al 1989).

Further work is needed into whether continued drug use by injection, by mouth or by inhalation has a dramatic influence on outcome. The importance of bacterial infections must not be overlooked. Since as many individuals with IDU related HIV die from a bacterial pneumonia as die from AIDS in New York, this susceptibility to bacterial infections needs to be considered in management strategies. It may be that immunoglobulin replacement therapy or active vaccination might be required.

Finally, treatment regimes for IDU related HIV must take into account continued drug use. For instance complex timings schedules, the need for frequent blood tests, a lack of venous access or drug interactions might all make a particular treatment impossible in certain situations.

The importance of IDU related HIV cannot be overstressed since this is the route by which the virus can and will spread into the general heterosexual population. The Presidential Commission on HIV in the USA recognised that 'the future course of the HIV epidemic depends greatly on the effectiveness of our nations ability to address IV drug use' (Watkins et al 1988). Thus it is not only important for us to develop drug therapies and care systems that address the problems of IDU related HIV but also to reconsider our approach to drug use in the light of HIV.

## ACKNOWLEDGEMENT

We would like to acknowledge Dr AG Bird, Dr PL Yap, Dr SM Burns and Dr JM Inglis for their continued laboratory support, and the Lothian Health Board for financial assistance. We thank Miss BA Hamilton for typing the manuscript and the nursing and clerical staff of the Infectious Diseases Unit Outpatient Department for their continued help without whom this work would not be possible. Dr LR MacCallum and Miss BA Hamilton are supported by the AIDS Virus Research and Education Research Trust (AVERT). Dr PJ Flegg is supported by the American Foundation for AIDS Research (AmFAR).

## REFERENCES

Accurso V, Mancuso S, Mitra ME, Caravello E, Cajozzo A 1988 The epidemiology of HIV infection in Sicily: our experience (Abstract). IV International Conference on AIDS: 13–16 June, Stockholm, Sweden: Abstract 4170

Alloub MI, Barr BBB, McLaren K M, Smith IW, Bunney MH, Smart GE 1989 Human papillomavirus infection and cervical intraepithelial neoplasia in women with renal allografts. British Medical Journal 298: 153–156

Andrus JK, Fleming D, Knox C, McAllister R, Skeels M, Foster L 1988 HIV antibody testing in prisons: assessment of voluntary vs mandatory (Abstract). IV International Conference on AIDS: 13–16 June, Stockholm, Sweden: Abstract 4201

Angarano G, Pastore G, Monno L, Santantonio T, Luchena N, Schiraldi O 1985 Rapid spread of HTLV-III infections among drug addicts in Italy. Lancet ii: 1302.

Anonymous 1984 Editorial: opiates, opioid peptides, and immunity Lancet i: 774–775

Anonymous 1987a Maintenance treatment of drug addicts — end of a short era. Lancet ii: 1103

Anonymous 1987b The scale of drug misuse. Lancet i: 640

Anonymous 1989 AIDS in the UK and worldwide. Lancet i:1151

Arora PK, Fride E, Petitto J, Waggie K, Skolnick P 1988 Morphine-induced modulation of the immune system: implications for AIDS (Abstract). IV International Conference on AIDS: 13–16 June, Stockholm, Sweden: Abstract 8021

Ball JC, Lange WR, Myers CP, Friedman SR 1988 The effectiveness of methadone maintenance treatment in reducing IV drug use and needle sharing among heroin addicts at risk for AIDS (Abstract). IV International Conference on AIDS: 13–16 June, Stockholm, Sweden: Abstract 8503

Battjes RJ, Pickens R 1988 HIV infection among intravenous drug abusers (IVDAs) in five U.S. cities (Abstract). IV International Conference on AIDS: 13–16 June, Stockholm, Sweden: Abstract 4523

Bickler CB 1985 Defaulted appointments in general practice. Journal of the Royal College of General Practitioners 35: 19–22

Bisset C, Jones G, Davidson J et al 1989 Mobility of injection drug users and transmission of HIV. Lancet ii: 44

Blanche S, Rouzioux C, Veber F et al 1987 Prospective study on newborns of HIV seropositive women (Abstract). In: Abstracts from the III International Conference on AIDS, 1–5 June, Washington DC, USA: Abstract 158

Blix O, Grönbladh L 1988 AIDS and IV heroin addicts: the preventative effect of methadone maintenance in Sweden (Abstract). IV International Conference on AIDS: 13–16 June, Stockholm, Sweden: Abstract 8548

Boron P, Bobrowska E, Kaczmarska, Rembergowa W, Grzeszczuk A 1988 Prophylactic and serological screening of anti-HIV-antibodies in selected potentially risk populations from Bialystok region/Poland (Abstract). IV International Conference on AIDS: 13–16 June, Stockholm, Sweden: Abstract 4177

Borroni G 1986 Seroepidemiologic case finding in HTLV III infection, lues and HBV in a prison. Bollittino Dell Istituto Sieroterapicoi Milanese, 65(6): 487–493

Bortolotti F, Cadrobbi P, Carretta M, Meneghetti F, De Rossi A, Chieco-Bianchi L 1986 HTLV-III infection in drug abusers with acute viral hepatitis (Abstract). II International Conference on AIDS: June, Paris, France: Abstract 172

Bouchard I, Espinoza P, Buffet C et al 1986 Prevalence of antibody to LAV in parenteral drug users (Abstract). II International Conference on AIDS: June, Paris, France, Abstract 175

Boxaca M, Belli L, Casco R et al 1989 HIV infection in heterosexuals from Buenos Aires City consulting for venereal disease (Abstract). V International Conference on AIDS: 5–9 June, Montreal, Canada: Abstract W.G.P.18

Bradick M, Kreiss JK, Quin T et al 1987 Congenital transmission of HIV in Nairobi, Kenya (Abstract). III International Conference on AIDS, 1–5 June Washington DC, USA, Abstract TH.7.5

Brahams D 1987 Private treatment for drug dependence: GMC ban upheld by Privy Council. Lancet ii: 696–697

Brettle RP 1986 Epidemic of AIDS related virus infection among intravenous drug abusers. British Medical Journal 292: 1671

Brettle RP, Nelles B 1988 Special problems of injecting drug misusers. British Medical Bulletin 44: 149–60

Brettle RP, Davidson J, Davidson SJ et al 1986 HTLV-III Antibodies in an Edinburgh clinic. Lancet i: 1099

Brettle RP, Bisset K, Burns S et al 1987 Human immunodeficiency virus and drug misuse — The Edinburgh experience. British Medical Journal 295: 421–424

Brettle RP, Jones GA, Bingham J, Spacey BEM, Weatherley B, Churchus R 1989 Pharmacokinetics of zidovudine in IDU related HIV infection (Abstract). V International Conference on AIDS: 5–9 June: Montreal, Canada: Abstract W.B.U.3.

Brewer TF, Vlahov D, Taylor E, Hall D, Munoz A, Polk BF 1988 Transmission of HIV-1 within a statewide prison system. AIDS 2:363–367

Brown DK, Gindi EJ, Gandhi RP, Grieco MH, Klein EB, Reddy MM 1986 Initial report of a prospective study of intravenous drug users enrolled in a methadone program (Abstract). II International conference on AIDS: June, Paris, France: Abstract 176

Bruneau J, Lamothe F, Soto J, Brabant M, Vincelette J, Fauvel M 1989 Sero-epidemiology of HIV-1 infection among injection drug users seeking medical help in Montreal 1985–1988 (Abstract). V International Conference on AIDS: 5–9 June, Montreal, Canada: Abstract T.A.P. 59

Brunet J-B, Des Jarlais DC, Koch MA 1987 Report on the European Workshop on Epidemiology of HIV Infections: spread among intravenous drug abusers and the heterosexual population. AIDS 1: 59–61

Brun-Vezinet F, Barre-Sinoussi F, Saimot AG et al 1984 Detection of IgG antibodies to lymphadenopathy-associated virus in patients with AIDS or lymphadenopathy syndrome. Lancet i: 1129

Bruockov M, Syrucek L, Sejda J, Kopeck D, Vojtechovsk K 1988 Prevalence of HIV-1 Antibodies in Czechoslovakia (Abstract). IV International Conference on AIDS, 13–16 June, Stockholm, Sweden: Abstract 4182

Bschor F, Bornemann R, Pueschel K, Rex R, Platz W, Lueth R 1989 Comparative monitoring of HIV spread in the IVDU population of Berlin and Hamburg (Abstract). V International Conference on AIDS: 5–9 June, Montreal, Canada: Abstract T.A.P. 60.

Bunning EC 1989 Personal communication

Bunning EC, Coutinho RA, van Brassel GHA, van Santen, Van Zadelhoff AW 1986 Preventing AIDS in drug addicts in Amsterdam. Lancet i:1435

Burek V, Maretio T, Zrinscak J, Soldo I 1988 Dynamics of HIV infection in the past two years in Yugoslavia (Abstract). IV International Conference on AIDS: 13–16 June, Stockholm, Sweden: Abstract 4180

Burns SM, Collacott IA, Hargreaves FD, Inglis JM 1987 Incidence of hepatitis B markers in HIV seropositive and seronegative drug misusers in the Edinburgh area. Communicable Diseases Scotland (Weekly Report) 87/08: 7–8

Cahn P, Perez H, Casiro A, Vallejo N, Wolk D, Muchnik G 1989 HIV infection among IV drug abusers in Buenos Aires, Argentina (Abstract). V International Conference on AIDS: 5–9 June, Montreal, Canada: Abstract Th.D.P. 46

Carcaba V, Carton J A, Asensi V, Fernandez-León A, Maradona J A , Anibas J M 1988 Epidemiological, clinical and immunological experience with HIV infection in different risk populations in the North of Spain (Abstract). IV International Conference on AIDS: 13–16 June, Stockholm, Sweden: Abstract 4164

Carpenter CCJ, Fisher A, Desai M, Durand L, Indacochea F, Mayer KM 1988 Clinical characteristics of AIDS in women in Southeastern New England (Abstract). IV International Conference on AIDS: 13–16 June, Stockholm, Sweden: Abstract 7274

Casabona J, Barba G, Segura A 1989 Demographic and epidemiological characteristics of HIV positive blood donors in Catalonia (Abstract). V International Conference on AIDS: 5–9 June, Montreal, Canada: Abstract M.B.P. 137

Castro e Melo J, Santos E, Campos M, Vasconcelos C 1988 Immunological studies of two populations at risk of HIV infection: drug addicts and hemofiliacs (Abstract). IV International Conference on AIDS: 13–16 June, Stockholm, Sweden: Abstract 4163

Centers for Disease Control 1985 Recommendations for assisting in the prevention of perinatal transmission of HTLV-III/LAV and AIDS. Morbidity and Mortality Weekly Report 34(48): 721–732

Centers for Disease Control 1987a Antibody to HIV in female prostitutes. Morbidity and Mortality Weekly Report 36, 157–161

Centers for Disease Control Editorial 1987b Human immunodeficiency virus infection in the

United States: a review of current knowledge. Morbidity and Mortality Weekly Report 36 (Suppl No. 6) 1–48

Centers for Disease Control Editorial 1987c Tuberculosis and acquired immunodeficiency syndrome — New York. Morbidity and Mortality Weekly Report 36(48): 785–790, 795

Centers for Disease Control Editorial 1988 Increase in pneumonia mortality among young adults and the HIV epidemic — New York City, United States. Morbidity and Mortality Weekly Report 37(38): 593–596

Centers for Disease Control 1989 Statistics from WHO and CDC. AIDS 3: 471

Chaisson RE, Onishi R, Moss AR, Osmond D, Carlson JR 1986 Risk of HTLV-III/LAV infection in heterosexual intravenous drug abusers (IVDAS) in San Francisco (SF) (Abstract) II International Conference on AIDS: June, Paris, France: Abstract 174

Chaisson RE, Schecter GF, Theuer CP, Rutherford GW, Echenberg DF, Hopewell PC 1987 Tuberculosis in patients with the acquired immunodeficiency syndrome. Clinical features, responses to therapy, and survival. American Review of Respiratory Diseases 136: 570–574

Chaisson RE, Bacchetti P, Osmond D, Brodie B, Sande MA, Moss AR 1989 Cocaine use and HIV infection in intravenous drug users in San Francisco. Journal American Medical Association 261: 561–565

Communicable Diseases (Scotland) 1987 AIDS Surveillance in Europe: update to 30th June 1987 (Part 2). Communicable Diseases (Scotland), Answer, 87/47:1

Communicable Diseases (Scotland) 1988 Human immunodeficiency virus infection in the United Kingdom: Quarterly Report No. 2. Communicable Diseases (Scotland), Answer, 88/16:1

Communicable Diseases (Scotland) 1989a Acquired immune deficiency syndrome (AIDS)-United Kingdom. Communicable diseases (Scotland), Answer, 89/09 (A92) 1–2

Communicable Diseases (Scotland) 1989b Human immunodeficiency virus (HIV) infection Scotland: Aug 1983–Dec 1988. Communicable Diseases (Scotland), Answer, 89/06 (A89) 1–3

Communicable Diseases (Scotland) 1989c HIV infection in the U.K. Communicable Diseases (Scotland), Answer, 89/17 (A99) 1–2

Costigliola P, Ricchi E, Verani P et al 1986 Time of appearance and rapid spread of LAV/HTLV-III infection among Italian drug addicts (Abstract). II International Conference on AIDS: June, Paris, France: Abstract 171

Cowan FM, Jones G, Bingham J et al 1989a Use of Zidovudine for drug misusers infected with human immunodeficiency virus. Journal of Infection 18: 1: 59–66

Cowan FM, Jones ME, Flegg PJ et al 1989b Use of Zidovudine (AZT) in injection drug use (IDU) related HIV infection — clinical outcome (Abstract). V International Conference on AIDS: 5–9 June: Montreal, Canada: Abstract W.B.P.371

Crovari P, Penco G, Valente A et al 1988 HIV infection in two cohorts of drug addicts prospectively studied. Association of serological markers with clinical progression (Abstract). IV International Conference on AIDS: 13–16 June, Stockholm, Sweden: Abstract 4527

D'Aquila R, Williams AB, Kleber HD 1986 Prevalence and natural history of HTLV-III/LAV infection among New Haven, Connecticut, USA intravenous drug abusers (Abstract). II International Conference on AIDS: June, Paris, France: Abstract 178

Deschamps MM, Pape JW, Madhavan S, Johnson WD 1989 Pregnancy and acceleration of HIV related illness (Abstract). V International Conference on AIDS: 5–9 June, Montreal, Canada: Abstract M.B.P.6.

Des Jarlais DC, Friedman S R, Hopkins W 1985 Risk reduction for the acquired immunodeficiency syndrome among intravenous drug users. Annals Internal Medicine 103: 755–759

Des Jarlais DC, Friedman S R, Marmor M et al 1987 Development of AIDS, HIV seroconversion, and potential co-factors for T4 cell loss in a cohort of intravenous drug users. AIDS 1: 105–111

Des Jarlais DC, Friedman S R, Stoneburner RL 1988 HIV infection and intravenous drug use: critical issues in transmission dynamics, infection outcomes, and prevention. Reviews of Infectious Diseases 10: 1:151–158

Dole VP, Nyswander M 1965 A medical treatment for Diacetylmorphine (heroin) addiction. Journal of American Medical Association 193: 646–50

Dole VP, Nyswander M 1967 Heroin addiction — a metabolic disease. Archives of Internal Medicine 120: 19–24

Dole VP, Nyswander M, Warner A 1968 Successful treatment of 750 criminal addicts. Journal of American Medical Association 206: 2708–2711

Dolivo N, Claeys M, Chave J, Peitrequin R, Frei PC 1988 Distribution of the different risk groups among newly found seropositive subjects (Abstract). IV International Conference on AIDS: 13–16 June, Stockholm, Sweden: Abstract 4168

Donoghue M, Stimson GV, Dolan K, Alldritt L 1989 Changes in HIV risk behaviour in clients of syringe exchange schemes in England and Scotland. AIDS 3: 267–272

Drucker E 1986 AIDS and addiction in New York City. American Journal Drug Alcohol Abuse 12(1 & 2): 165–181

Dwyer DE, Bell J, Batey R, Cunningham AL 1988 HIV in a Sydney methadone programme and in pregnant intravenous drug users (Abstract). IV International Conference on AIDS: 13–16 June, Stockholm, Sweden: Abstract 4536

Esparza B, Merino E, Aizpiri J, Fernandez J, Cogrral J, Carcia L 1986 HTLV-III/LAV infection in drug addicts in the Vasque country, Northern Spain (Abstract). II International Conference on AIDS: June, Paris, France: Abstract 164

Estebanez P, Colomo C, Zunzunegui MV, Rua M 1988 Prevalence and risk factors for HIV infection among inmates (Abstract). IV International Conference on AIDS: 13–16 June, Stockholm, Sweden: Abstract 4202

Evans BA, McCormack SM, Bond RA, MacRae KD, Thorp RW 1988 Human immunodeficiency virus infection, hepatitis B virus infection, and sexual behaviour of women attending a genito urinary medicine clinic. British Medical Journal 296: 473–475

Eyster ME, Gail MH, Ballard JO, Al-Mondhiry N, Goedert JJ 1987 Natural history of human immunodeficiency virus infection in haemophiliacs: effects of T-cell subsets, platelet counts and age. Annals Internal Medicine 107: 1–6

Federlin M, Smilovici W, Montalegre A, Watrigant MP, Ducos J, Armengaud M et al 1986 LAV/HTLV III Virus endemic among a population of 431 former drug users (Abstract). II International Conference on AIDS: June, Paris, France: Abstract 168

Ferroni P, Geroldi D, Galli C, Zanetti AR, Cargnel A 1985 HTLV-III Antibody among Italian drug addicts. Lancet 2: 52–53

Fischl MA, Richman DD, Grieco MH et al 1987 The efficacy of Azidothymidine (AZT) in the treatment of patients with AIDS and AIDS-related complex. New England Journal of Medicine 317: 185–191

Flegg PJ, Cowan FM, Jones ME, MacCallum LR, Whitelaw JM, Brettle RP 1989a Prospective evaluation of HIV progression in Edinburgh injection drug users (Abstract). V International Conference on AIDS: 4–9 June, Montreal, Canada: Abstract M.A.P. 105

Flegg PJ, Jones ME, MacCallum LR, Bird AG, Whitelaw JM, Brettle RP 1989b Continued injecting drug use as a cofactor for progression of HIV (Abstract). V International Conference on AIDS: 4–9 June, Montreal, Canada: Abstract M.A.P. 92

Flynn N, Jain S, Keddie E, Harper S, Carlson J, Bailey V 1988 Cleaning IV paraphernalia: bleach was just the beginning (Abstract). IV International Conference on AIDS: 13–16 June, Stockholm, Sweden: Abstract 8515

Follett EAC, McIntyre A, O'Donnell B, Clements GB, Desselberger U 1986 HTLV-III antibody in drug abusers in the West of Scotland: the Edinburgh connection. Lancet i: 446–447

France AJ, Skidmore CA, Robertson JR et al 1988 Heterosexual spread of human immunodeficiency virus in Edinburgh. British Medical Journal 296: 526–529

Franceschi S, Tirelli U, Vaccher et al, Serraino S 1986 Increased prevalence of HTLV-III antibody among drug addicts from Italian province with US Military Base. Lancet i:804

Fuchs D, Blecha HG, Deinhardt F et al 1985 High frequency of HTLV-III antibodies among heterosexual intravenous drug abusers in the Austrian Tyrol. Lancet i: 1506

Fuchs D, Wachter H, Wille R 1986 AIDS in haemophiliacs, parenteral drug abusers, and homosexuals. Lancet i: 324

Galli M, Carito M, Craccu V et al 1988 Cause of death in IV drug abusers — a retrospective survey on 4883 subjects (Abstract). IV International Conference on AIDS: 13–16 June, Stockholm, Sweden: Abstract 4520

Gatell JM, Podzamczer D, Clotet B, Ocana I, Estamy C et al Barcelona AIDS Study Group 1989 Incidence of AIDS in Spanish HIV infected patients (Abstract). V International Conference on AIDS: 5–9 June, Montreal, Canada: Abstract W.A.P. 55

Ginzburg HM, Weiss SH, Hubbard RL, French J, Hartsock PI, Blattner WA 1986 Needle and syringe sharing among parenteral drug users in high, moderate and low HTLV-III seroprevalence regions in the United States (Abstract). II International Conference on AIDS: June, Paris, France: Abstract 177

Goedert JJ, Biggar RJ, Weiss SH et al 1986 Three-year incidence of AIDS in five cohorts of HTLV-III-infected risk group members. Science 231: 992–995

Gossop M 1978 A review of the evidence for methadone maintenance as a treatment for narcotic addiction. Lancet i: 812–5

Goudeau A, Dubois F, Barin F, Choutet P, Jusseaume P, Royer JM 1986 Emergence of HTLV-III/LAV and delta agent in French intravenous drug abusers populations: retrospective study (1982–1985) (Abstract). II International Conference on AIDS: June, Paris, France: Abstract 169

Gradilone A, Zani M, Barillari G et al 1986 HTLV-I and HIV infection in drug addicts in Italy. Lancet ii: 753–754

Hahn BH, Shaw GM, Taylor ME et al 1986 Genetic variation in HTLV-III/LAV over time in patients with AIDS or at risk for AIDS. Science 232: 1548–1553

Hammond G, Buchanan D, Malazdrewicz R, Tate R, Sekla L, Bhayana V 1989 Seroprevalence and demographic results of intravenous drug users among individuals at risk for HIV infection in a community based study in Winnipeg, Manitoba Canada (Abstract). V International Conference on AIDS: 5–9 June, Montreal, Canada: Abstract Th.D.P. 56

Handwerger S, Mildvan D, Senie R, McKinley FW 1987 Tuberculosis and the acquired immunodeficiency syndrome at a New York City Hospital. Chest 91: 176–180

Harding TW 1987 Prison medicine: AIDS in prison. Lancet ii: 1260–1263

Hartel D, Selwyn PA, Schoenbaum EE, Klein RS, Friedland GH 1988 Methadone maintenance treatment (MMTP) and reduced risk of AIDS and AIDS-specific mortality in intravenous drug users (IVDUs) (Abstract). IV International Conference on AIDS: 13–16 June, Stockholm, Sweden: Abstract 8546

Helbert M, Robinson D, Peddle B et al 1988 Acute meningo-encephalitis on dose reduction of zidovudine. Lancet i: 1249–1252

Hessol NA, Rutherford GW, Lifson AR, et al 1988 The natural history of HIV infection in a cohort of homosexual and bisexual men; a decade of follow-up (Abstract 4096). In: Programs and abstracts of the Fourth International Conference on AIDS. Stockholm: Swedish Ministry of Health and Social Affairs.

Hirschel B, Carpentier N, Male P-J et al 1986 Lymphadenopathy virus (LAV/HTLV-III) Infection in Geneva heroin addicts: high prevalence of lymphadenopathy, low incidence of AIDS (Abstract). II International Conference on AIDS: June, Paris, France: Abstract 166

Hutterer J, Presslich G, Pfersmann D, Hollerer E, Pfersmann V 1989 Survey of the methadone treatment programme of the out patient clinic of the Vienna Psychiatric University Hospital (Abstract). V International Conference on AIDS: 5–9 June, Montreal, Canada: Abstract Th.D.P.71

Jankovic T, Suvakovic V, Svirtlih N, Zerjav S, Jevtovic DJ, Pelemis M, 1988 Drug abusers as a high risk group for contracting HIV infection (Abstract). IV International Conference on AIDS: 13–16 June, Stockholm, Sweden: Abstract 4181

Johnstone FD, MacCallum L, Brettle R et al 1988 Does infection with HIV affect the outcome of pregnancy. British Medical Journal 296: 467

Kaplan MH, Farber B, Smith M, Coronesi M 1988 An open trial of Zidovudine in 112 patients (Abstract). IV International Conference on AIDS: 13–16 June, Stockholm, Sweden: Abstract 3607

Kloser P, Grigoriu A, Kapila R 1988 Women with AIDS: a continuing study 1987 (Abstract). IV International Conference on AIDS: 13–16 June, Stockholm, Sweden: Abstract 4065

Lange JMAA, Paul DA, Huismaan HG et al 1986 Persistent HIV antigenaemia and decline of HIV core antibodies associated with transition to AIDS. British Medical Journal 293: 1459–1462

Lazzarin A, Crocchiolo P, Galli M et al 1986 Milan as possible starting point of LAV/HTLV III epidemic among Italian drug addicts. Bollettino Dell Instituto Sieroterapico Milanese 66(1): 9–13

Lipsedge MS, Cook CCH 1987 Prescribing for drug addicts. Lancet ii: 451–452

MacCallum LR, France AJ, Jones ME, Steel CM, Burns SM, Brettle RP 1988 The side effects of pregnancy on the progression of HIV infection (Abstract). IV International Conference on AIDS: 13–16 June, Stockholm, Sweden: Abstract 4032

MacCallum LR, Cowan FM, Whitelaw J, Burns SB, Brettle RP 1989 Disease progression following pregnancy in HIV seropositive women (Abstract). V International Conference on AIDS: 5–9 June, Montreal, Canada: Abstract M.B.P.3

McCoy CB, Chitwood DD, Page JB 1989 A comparative analysis of HIV infection among IV drug users in treatment and on the street (Abstract). V International Conference on AIDS: 5–9 June, Montreal, Canada: Abstract Th.D.P.82

MacNair A 1986 What to do about drug abuse. Lancet ii: 811

Maayan S, Backenroth R, Rieber E et al 1985 Antibody to lymphadenopathy associated virus/HTLVIII in various illicit drug abusers in New York City. Journal of Infectious Diseases 152(4): 843

Marmor M, Des Jarlais DC, Cohen H et al 1987 Risk factors for infection with human immunodeficiency virus among intravenous drug abusers in New York City. AIDS 1: 39–44

Medical Working Group on Drug Dependence Report 1984 Guidelines of good clinical practice in the treatment of drug misuse. Department of Health and Social Security, London

Merino F, Esparza B, Aizpiri J et al 1986 Antibodies to AIDS-associated retrovirus (HTLV-III/LAV) in drug addicts from Vizcaya, northern Spain. AIDS Research 2(2): 133–140

Miller E & Kaye PA 1988 HIB antibody prevalence by risk group in different parts of the UK (Abstract). IV International Conference on AIDS: 23–16 June, Stockholm, Sweden: Abstract 4158

Minkoff H, Nanda D, Menez R, Fikeig S 1987 Pregnancies resulting in infants with AIDS or AIDS related complex. Obstetrics and Gynecology, 69: 285–287

Mok J, Giaquinto C, Grosch-Wörner I, Ades A, Peckham C 1987a Perinatal HIV infection: preliminary report of prospective study on 71 infants (Abstract). III International Conference on AIDS: 1–5 June, Washington D.C., U.S.A.: Abstract MP 47

Mok JQ, Giaquinto C, de Rossi A, Grosch-Wörner I, Ades AE, Peckham CS 1987b Infants born to mothers seropositive for human immunodeficiency virus. Lancet i: 1164–1167

Morbidity and Mortality Weekly Report 1987a Epidemiologic notes and reports: tuberculosis and acquired immunodeficiency syndrome – New York City. 36(48): 785–790, 795

Morbidity and Mortality Weekly Report 1987b Human immunodeficiency virus infection in the United States: a review of current knowledge. 36(6) 1–48

Morbidity and Mortality Weekly Report 1988 Increase in pneumonia mortality among young adults and the HIV epidemic — New York City, United States. 37(38): 593–596

Mortimer PP, Vandervelde EM, Jesson WJ et al 1985 HTLV-III antibody in Swiss and English intravenous drug abusers. Lancet ii: 449–450

Mortimer PP, Jesson WJ, Vandervelde EM, Pereira MS, Burkhardt F 1986 Prevalence of antibody to human T lymphotropic virus type III by risk group and area, United Kingdom 1978–84. British Medical Journal 290:1176

Nelson K, Vishov D, Solomon L, Lindsay A, Chowdhury N 1989 Clinical symptoms and medical histories of a cohort of IV drug users: correlation with HIV seroprevalence (Abstract). V International Conference on AIDS: 5–9 June: Montreal, Canada: Abstract Th.D.P.79

Newman RG 1976 Methadone maintenance: it ain't what it used to be. British Journal of Addiction 71: 183–186

Newman RG 1987 Methadone treatment. New England Journal of Medicine, 317 (No. 7) 447–450

Newman RG, Whitehill WB 1979 Double blind comparison of methadone and placebo maintenance treatment of narcotic addicts in Hong Kong. Lancet ii: 485–488

Novick D, Kreek MJ, Des Jarlais DC et al 1986 Abstract of clinical research findings: therapeutic and historical aspects. In: Problems of drug dependence, 1985: (Proceedings of the 47th Annual Scientific Meeting, the Committee on Problems of Drug Dependence). NIDA research monograph 67. Washington DC: NIDA

Nzila N, Ryden RW, Behets F et al 1987 Perinatal HIV transmission in two African hospitals (Abstract). III International Conference on AIDS: Washington DC, USA: Abstract Th. 7.6. Quoted by Piot P, Kreiss JK, Ndinya-Achola JO et al 1987; Heterosexual transmission of HIV. AIDS 1: 199–206

Ognjan A, Burczak J, Markowitz N, Steaffens J, Mazurek C, Saravolatz L 1988 The emerging role of HTLV I and HIV among intravenous drug abusers (IVDA) in Detroit (Abstract). IV International Conference on AIDS: 13–16 June, Stockholm, Sweden: Abstract 4516

Ognjan A, Markowitz N, Pohlod D, Lee H, Belian B, Saravolatz L 1989 HIV-1 and HTLV-1 infections in intravenous drug users in Detroit 1985–89 (Abstract). V International Conference on AIDS: 5–9 June, Montreal, Canada: Abstract Th.A.P.10

Olin R, Käll K 1988 HIV status and risk behaviour among imprisoned intravenous drug abusers in Stockholm (Abstract). IV International Conference on AIDS: 13–16 June,

Stockholm, Sweden: Abstract 8036

Pakesch G, Presslich O, Willinger G et al 1987 Prevalence of HIV antibodies in intravenous drug dependent patients 1986 and 1987 in Vienna. Wiener Klinische Wochenschrift 99(22): 777–780

Parkin JM, Helbert M, Hughes CL, Pinching AJ 1989 Immunoglobulin G subclass deficiency and susceptibility to pyogenic infections in patients with AIDS-related complex and AIDS. AIDS 3: 37–39

Pearson G, Gilman M, McIver S 1985 Young people and heroin: an examination of heroin use in the North of England, Research Report No. 8, published by Health Education Council November 1985

Peutherer JF, Edmond E, Simmonds P, Dickson JD, Bath GE 1985 HTLV-III antibody in Edinburgh drug addicts. Lancet ii: 1129–30

Peutherer JF, Edmond E, Simmonds P, Dickson JD 1986 HTLVIII Infection in intravenous drug abusers in Edinburgh (Abstract). III International Conference on AIDS: 1–5 June, Washington D.C., USA: Abstract 173

Polsky B, Gold JW, Whimbey E et al 1986 Bacterial pneumonia in patients with the acquired immunodeficiency syndrome. Annals of Internal Medicine 104(1): 38–41

Pont J, Neuwald C, Kunz C, Werdenich W 1986 HTLV-III serology, epidemiology and clinical aspects of imprisoned i.v. drug-dependent males in Austria. Wiener Klinische Wochenschrift 98(14): 454–457

Reichman LB, Felton CP, Edsall JR 1979 Drug dependence, a possible new risk factor for tuberculosis disease. Archives of Internal Medicine 139: 337–339

Rezza G, Lassarin A, Angarano G et al 1989 The natural history of HIV infection in intravenous drug users: risk of disease progression in a cohort of seroconverters. AIDS 3: 87–90

Richman DD, Fischl MA, Grieco MH et al 1987 The toxicity of Azidothymidine (AZT) in the treatment of patients with AIDS and AIDS-related complex. New England Journal Medicine 317: 192–197

Ritson AB, Plant MA 1977 Drugs and young people in Scotland. Edinburgh: Scottish Health Education Unit

Robertson JR, Bucknall AB 1986 Heroin users in a Scottish city — Edinburgh drug addiction study, West Granton Medical Group, 1 Muirhouse Avenue, Edinburgh, EH4 4PL

Robertson JR, Skidmore CA, France AJ, Welsby PD, Rhein H, Galloway WBF 1988 1985 epidemic of HIV infection in Edinburgh IVDA: 3 years on (Abstract). IV International Conference on AIDS: 13–16 June, Stockholm, Sweden: Abstract 4528

Robertson JR, Bucknall ABV, Wiggins P 1986a Regional variations in HIV antibody seropositivity in British intravenous drug users. Lancet i: 1435–1436

Robertson JR, Bucknall ABV, Welsby PD et al 1986b An Epidemic of AIDS-related virus (HTLV-III/LAV) infection amongst intravenous drug abusers in a Scottish general practice. British Medical Journal 292: 527–530

Rodrigo JM, Serra MA, Aguilar E, Del Olmo JA, Gimeno V, Aparisi L 1985 HTLV-III antibodies in drug addicts in Spain. Lancet ii: 156–157

Rothenberg R, Woelfel M, Stoneburner R, Milberg J, Parker R, Truman B 1987 Survival with the acquired immunodeficiency syndrome. New England Journal of Medicine 317 (21): 1297–1302

Roumeliotou-Karayannis A, Tassopoulos N, Karpodini E, Trichopoulou E, Kotsianopoulou M, Papaevangelou G 1987 Prevalence of HBV, HDV and HIV infections among intravenous drug addicts in Greece. European Journal of Epidemiology 3(2): 143–146

Roumeliotou A, Nestoridou A, Kotsianopoulou M, Sapounas Th, Papaevangelou G 1988 Epidemiology of HIV infection in Greek IV drug addicts (Abstract). IV International Conference on AIDS: 13–16 June, Stockholm, Sweden: Abstract 4522

Ruggeri P, Sathe SS, Kapila R 1988 Changing patterns of infectious endocarditis (IE) in parenteral drug abusers (PDA) with Human Immunodeficiency Virus (HIV) Infections (Abstract). IV International Conference on AIDS: 13–16 June, Stockholm, Sweden: Abstract 8028

Schoenbaum EE, Webber M, Ernst J, Davenny K, Gayle H 1988 High prevalence of HIV antibody in heterogenous populations of the Bronx, New York City (Abstract). IV International Conference on AIDS: 13–16 June, Stockholm, Sweden: Abstract 4189

Schoenbaum EE, Davenny K, Selwyn PA, Hartel D, Rogers M 1989 The effect of pregnancy on progression of HIV-related disease (Abstract). V International Conference on AIDS: 5–9

June, Montreal, Canada: Abstract M.B.P.8

Schupbach J, Vogt M, Bhuschan R et al 1985a Prevalence of antibodies against HTLV-III in various regions in Switzerland. Schweizerische medizinische Wochenschrift Journal Suisse de Medecine 115(30): 1048–1054

Schupbach J, Haller O, Vogt M et al 1985b Antibodies to HTLV-III in Swiss patients with AIDS and pre-AIDS and in groups at risk for AIDS. New England Journal of Medicine 312(5): 265–270

Scott GB, Fischl MA, Klimas N et al 1985 Mother of infants with the acquired immune deficiency syndrome. Journal American Medical Association 253: 363–66

Scottish Home and Health Department 1986 HIV Infection in Scotland. Report of the Scottish Committee on HIV Infection and Intravenous Drug Misuse. Scottish Home and Health Department, Edinburgh

Scottish Home and Health Department 1987 Report of the National Working Party on Health Service Implications of HIV Infection. Scottish Home and Health Department, Edinburgh

Selik RM, Starcher ET, Curran JW 1987 Opportunistic diseases reported in AIDS patients: frequencies, associations, and trends. AIDS 1: 175–182

Selwyn PA, Schoenbaum EE, Mayers MM et al 1986 HTLV III/LAV infection and pregnancy outcomes in intravenous drug abusers (Abstract). III International Conference on AIDS: 1–5 June: Washington DC, USA: Abstract 200

Selwyn PA, Feingold AR, Schoenbaum EE, Davenny K, Robertson V, Shulman J 1987 Pregnancy outcome and HIV infection in intravenous drug abusers (Abstract). III International Conference on AIDS: 1–5 June, Washington DC, USA: Abstract MP.156

Selwyn PA, Schoenbaum EE, Hartel D et al 1988a AIDS and HIV-related mortality in intravenous drug users (IVDUs) (Abstract). IV International Conference on AIDS: 13–16 June, Stockholm, Sweden: Abstract 4526

Selwyn PA, Feingold AR, Hartel D, Schoenbaum EE et al 1988b Increased risk of bacterial pneumonia in HIV-infected intravenous drug users without AIDS. AIDS 2:267–272

Selwyn PA, Carter RJ, Hartel D et al 1988c Elective termination of pregnancy (TOP) among HIV seropositive (SP) and seronegative (SN) intravenous drug users (IVDU's) (Abstract). IV International Conference on AIDS: 13–16 June, Stockholm, Sweden: Abstract 9511

Selwyn PA, Schoenbaum EE, Hartel D et al 1988d AIDS and HIV-related mortality in intravenous drug user [abstract 4526] In: Programs and abstracts of the Fourth International Conference on AIDS. Stockholm, Sweden: Swedish Ministry of Health and Social Affairs

Selwyn PA, Hartel D, Lewis VA et al 1989 A prospective study of the risk of tuberculosis among intravenous drug users with human immunodeficiency virus infection. New England Journal of Medicine 320(9): 545–550

Shattock AG, Kaminski GZ, Hillary IB 1986 HTLV III serology, AIDS and ARC cases in Ireland (Abstract) II International Conference on AIDS: June, Paris, France: Abstract 143

Sherer R, Seibert D, Cadena R et al 1988 HIV seroprevalence at Cook County Hospital, Chicago (Abstract). IV International Conference on AIDS: 13–16 June, Stockholm, Sweden: Abstract 4190

Simberkoff MS, El-Sadr W, Schiffman G, Rahal JJ Jr 1984 Streptococcus pneumoniae infections and bacteremia in patients with acquired immune deficiency syndrome, with report of a pneumococcal vaccine failure. American Review of Respiratory Disease 130(6): 1174–1176

Skidmore C, Robertson JR 1989 Long term follow up and assessment of HIV serostatus and risk taking in a cohort of 203 intravenous drug users (Abstract). V International Conference on AIDS: 5–9 June: Montreal, Canada: Abstract T.A.P.31

Skidmore CA, Robertson JR, Roberts JJK, Foster K, Smith JH, Rhein H 1988 HIV infection in IVDA: a follow-up study indicating changes in risk taking behaviour (Abstract). IV International Conference on AIDS: 13–16 June, Stockholm, Sweden: Abstract 8510

Slim J, Boghossian J, Perez G, Johnson E 1988 Comparative analysis of bacterial endocarditis in HIV( + ) and HIV(-) intravenous drug users (Abstract). IV International Conference on AIDS: 13–16 June, Stockholm, Sweden: Abstract 8027

Slim J, Perez G, Forrester C, Tonnesen G, Johnson ES 1989 Zidovudine use in intravenous drug users (Abstract). V International Conference on AIDS: 5–9 June: Montreal, Canada: Abstract W.B.P. 336

Spears A, Berge P, Cancellieri, Druckman D, Landesman S 1988 Efficacy of Zidovudine in intravenous drug users and women (Abstract). IV International Conference on AIDS: 13–16 June, Stockholm, Sweden: Abstract 3680

Spira TJ, Des Jarlais DC, Marmor M et al 1984 Prevalence of antibody to lymphadenopathy associated virus among drug detoxification patients in New York. New England Journal of Medicine 313: 467–468

Stapinski A, Mazurkiewicz W, Ochelska B, Gzwska T, Seliborska Z 1989 HIV infection in intravenous drug addicts (Abstract). V International Conference on AIDS: 5–9 June: Montreal, Canada: Abstract Th.D.P.4

Stark C 1988a Cocaine and HIV seropositivity. Lancet i: 1052

Stark C 1988b Cocaine and HIV seropositivity. Lancet ii: 965

Stevenson RC 1986 The benefits of legalising heroin. Lancet ii: 1269–1270

Stewart GJ, Tyler JPP, Cunningham AL et al 1985 Transmission of HTLV-III by artificial insemination by donor. Lancet ii: 581–585

Stimson GV, Alldritt L, Dolan K, Donoghue M 1988a HIV and the injecting drug user: clients of syringe exchange schemes in England and Scotland (Abstract). IV International Conference on AIDS, 13–16 June, Stockholm, Sweden: Abstract 8511

Stimson GV, Alldritt LJ, Dolan KA, Donoghue MC, Lart RA 1988b Injecting equipment exchange schemes final report for Department of Health and Social Security and Scottish Home and Health Department. Sociology Department, Goldsmith College, New Cross, London SE14 6NW

Stoneburner RL, Des Jarlais DC, Benezra D et al 1989 A larger spectrum of severe HIV-1 related disease in intravenous drug users in New York City. Science 242: 916–918

Sunderam G, McDonald J, Maniatis T, Oleske J, Kapila R, Reichman LB 1986 Tuberculosis as a manifestation of the acquired immune deficiency syndrome (AIDS). Journal of the American Medical Association 256: 362–366

Sutherland S, McManus TJ 1989 HIV Seroprevalence in injecting drug users in South London 1985–1988 (Abstract). V International Conference on AIDS: 5–9 June: Montreal, Canada: Abstract T.A.P.55

Szasz TS 1987 Aids and drugs: balancing risk and benefits. Lancet ii: 450

Thomas J, Danila R, Osterholm M, Shultz J, Falkowski C, MacDonald K 1989 A comparison of HIV-1 infection rate in Minnesota IV drug users between 1987 and 1988 (Abstract). V International Conference on AIDS: 5–9 June: Montreal, Canada: Abstract T.A.P. 43

Thongcharoen P, Wasi C, Wangroongsarb Y 1988 HIV infection in Thailand (Abstract). IV International Conference on AIDS: 13–16 June, Stockholm, Sweden: Abstract 5523

Tirelli U, Vaccher E, Carbone A et al 1986 HTLV-III Infection among 315 intravenous drug abusers: seroepidemiological, clinical and pathological findings. AIDS Research: 2: Number 4

Tirelli U, Vaccher E, Diodato S et al 1987 HIV infection among female and male prostitutes (Abstract). III International Conference on AIDS: 1–5 June, Washington DC, USA: Abstract WP.95

Tirelli U, Serraino D, Vaccher E, Tamburlini R, Saracchini S, Modolo L 1988 Human immunodeficiency virus (HIV) infection among prisoners in North-Eastern Italy (Abstract). IV International Conference on AIDS Abstract 4217

Titti F, Verani P, Rossi GB et al 1986 HTLV-III/LAV antibodies in intravenous drug abusers: a follow-up study of methadone maintenance outpatients (Abstract). II International Conference on AIDS: June, Paris, France: Abstract 170

Titti F, Lazzarin A, Costigliola P et al 1987 Human immunodeficiency virus (HIV) seropositivity in intravenous (i.v.) drug abusers in three cities of Italy: possible natural history of HIV infection in I.V. drug addicts in Italy. Journal of Medical Virology 23(3): 241–248

Tor J, Soviano V, Muga R, Ribera A, Clotet V, Foz M 1989 HTLV1 and HIV1 infection in intravenous drug abusers of Barcelona (Abstract). V International Conference on AIDS: 5–9 June, Montreal, Canada: Abstract Th.A.P.19

Tubaro E, Borelli G, Croce C, Cavallo G, Santiangeli C 1983 Effect of morphine on resistance to infection. Journal of Infectious Diseases 148: 656–666

Urquhart GED, Scott SS, Wooldridge E et al 1987 Human immunodeficiency virus (HIV) in intravenous drug abusers in Tayside. Communicable Diseases Scotland 87/09: 5–10

Vaccher E, Saracchini S, Errante D et al 1988 Progression of HIV disease among intravenous drug abusers (IVDA): a three-year prospective study (Abstract). IV International Conference on AIDS: 13–16 June, Stockholm, Sweden: Abstract 4529

Van Haastrecht H, Van den Hock JAR, Coutinho RA 1989 No trend in yearly HIV-seroprevalence rates among IVDU in Amsterdam: 1986–1988 (Abstract). V International Conference on AIDS: 5–9 June: Montreal, Canada: Abstract T.A.P.36

Vanichseni S, Sonchai W, Plangsringarm K, Akarasewi P, Wright N, Choopanya K 1989 Second seroprevalence survey among Bangkok's intravenous drug addicts (IVDA) (Abstract). V International Conference on AIDS: 5–9 June: Montreal, Canada: Abstract T.G.O.23

Vella S, Menniti Ippolito F, Agresti MG 1989 Long term safety and efficacy of Zidovudine in large cohorts on IV drug abusers: 20 month experience with 200 asymptomatic, 500 ARC and 400 AIDS patients (Abstract). V International Conference on AIDS: 5–9 June: Montreal, Canada: Abstract W.B.P.370

Vento S, Di Perri G, Luzzati R et al 1989 Clinical reactivation of hepatitis in anti-HBs-positive patients with AIDS. Lancet i: 332–333

Verdegem TD, Sattler FR, Boylen CT 1988 Increased fatality from Pneumocystis carinii pneumonia (PCP) in women with AIDS (Abstract). IV International Conference on AIDS; 13–16 June, Stockholm, Sweden: Abstract 7271

Waldorf D, Biernachie PJ 1979 Natural recovery from heroin addiction: a review of the incidence literature. Journal of Drug Issues 9: 281–289

Watkins JD, Conway-Welch C, Creedon JJ et al 1988 Interim report of the Presidential Commission on the HIV Epidemic: Chairman's Recommendations — Part 1. Journal of AIDS 1: 69–103

Watters JK, Case P, Huang K, Cheng Y-T, Lorvick J, carlson J 1988 HIV seroepidemiology and behaviour change in intravenous drug users: progress report on the effectiveness of street-based prevention (Abstract). IV International Conference on AIDS: 13–16 June, Stockholm, Sweden: Abstract 8523

Webb G, Wells B, Morgan JR, McManus TJ 1986 Epidemic of AIDS related virus infection among intravenous drug abusers. British Medical Journal 292: 1202

Weissenbacker M, Libonatti O, Gertiser R et al 1988a Prevalence of HIV and HBV markers in a group of drug addicts in Argentina (Abstract). IV International Conference on AIDS: 13–16 June, Stockholm, Sweden: Abstract 4513

Weissenbacker M, Diaz Lestrem M, Fainboim H et al 1988b HIV infection in IV drug addicts with clinical manifestations of hepatitis in a hospital of Buenos Aires City (Abstract). IV International Conference on AIDS: 13–16 June, Stockholm, Sweden: Abstract 4539

Wille R 1983 Processes of recovery from heroin dependence: relationship to treatment social change and dry use. Journal of Drug Issues 13: 333–342

Williams IY, Noel-Connor J, El-Sadar W 1989 Compliance with Zidovudine (AZT) therapy in an inner city HIV infected population (Abstract). V International Conference on AIDS: 5–9 June: Montreal, Canada: Abstract W.B.P.373

Willoughby A, Mendez H, Minkoff H et al 1987 HIV in pregnant women and their offspring (Abstract). III International Conference on AIDS: 1–5 June, Washington DC, USA: Abstract Th.7.3

World Health Organisation 1989 WHO Collaborating Centre, Paris AIDS: 3: 474

Yancovitz S, Des Jarlais D, Peyser N et al 1988 Innovative AIDS risk re-education project: interim methadone clinic (Abstract). IV International Conference on AIDS: 13–16 June, Stockholm, Sweden: Abstract 8547

Zerjav S, Jevtovic DJ, Fridman V, Suvakovic V, Jankovic T 1988 Two years of experience with HIV infection in Belgrade (Yugoslavia) (Abstract). 4th International Conference on AIDS: 13–16 June, Stockholm, Sweden: Abstract 4179

Zoulek G, Gurtler L, Eberle J, Lorbeer B, Deinhardt F 1986 Increase in the prevalence of antibodies against LAV/HTLV III in drug addicts in West Germany. Deutsche Medizinische Wochenschrift 111 (15) 567–570

Zulaica D, Arrizabalaga J, Iribarren JA, Perex-Trallero E, Rodriguez- Arrondo F, Garde C 1988 Follow-up of 100 HIV infected intravenous drug abusers (Abstract). IV International Conference on AIDS: 13–16 June, Stockholm, Sweden: Abstract 4532

# 7

# Prostatitis

*A. Doble*

Any discussion on recent advances in prostatitis, particularly the chronic form, starts from a disadvantaged position clothed in pessimism. In their textbook of genitourinary diseases, White & Wood (1898) remarked that 'chronic prostatitis is relatively more frequent than is the acute form of the disease, but much less understood', and more recently Stamey (1981) concluded that 'little more is known about prostatitis than was reported by Hugh H. Young and associates in 1906'. However, advances have been made in the classification and diagnosis of prostatitis but a satisfactory treatment and, in the case of chronic abacterial prostatitis, knowledge of aetiological factors, have yet to be found.

## INTRODUCTION

In his treatise on venereal diseases Hunter (1786) described prostatic inflammation as arising from distension and irritation of the urethra secondary to a stricture, instillations or violent gonorrhoea. The first formal description of chronic prostatitis appeared in Sir Henry Thompson's Diseases of the Prostate (1857) and since that time a steady supply of articles on the subject has appeared in the literature. The gonococcus was undoubtedly the most common causative organism (Martin 1899) until the work of Notthaft (1904) noted increasing difficulty in isolating *Neisseria gonorrhoeae* with increasing chronicity of the disease. The gonococcus now only accounts for the rare case. Researchers were aware at an early stage of the difficulty in the collection and interpretation of specimens from the prostate and the perennial problem of urethral contamination of prostatic secretions. A variety of sampling techniques were employed, including irrigation of the urethra with antiseptics (Hitchens & Brown 1913, Culver 1916) and the use of elaborate endoscopes (Player et al 1923), and as a result more interest was taken in the role of aerobic and anaerobic bacteria such as the staphylococci, streptococci and coliforms (Culver 1916, Baker 1925, Von Lackum 1927, Herrold 1928, Nicol 1930).

A great break through was made by Stamey et al (1965) by indicating the value of segmenting the voided bladder urine into three aliquots namely, first void (VB1), mid stream (VB2) and post-prostatic massage urine (VB3), enabling differentiation between urethral and prostatic infection in the presence of sterile mid-stream urine. This work confirmed and highlighted the role of Gram negative organisms and enterococci in the aetiology of chronic prostatitis. However, the debate did not end there as some workers still hold Gram positive organisms (excluding enterococci) responsible for chronic infection (Drach 1975) though their view is far from universal (Meares & Stamey 1968, Jimenez Cruz et al 1982, Pfau 1986).

On the basis of these localisation techniques, the various forms of prostatitis have been categorised into a practical classification (Drach et al 1978) which broadly separates patients in terms of their aetiology. However, confusion still exists and prostatitis continues to have a bad reputation primarily due to imprecise methods of diagnosis. Unfortunately the situation will not improve until clinicians pursue meticulous diagnostic techniques and subsequent research of those bona fide cases.

## ANATOMY

A knowledge of the anatomy of the prostate is an important prerequisite for understanding the pathophysiology of prostatitis. The original descriptions of the prostate (Lowsley 1912) subdivided the organ into lobes based on their embryological origin. However, these areas become distorted by disease and are unidentifiable as separate entities in the adult. A more logical description arose from the work of McNeal (1965), who divided the prostate into a central zone and peripheral zone (Fig. 7.1). This scheme achieves greater credibility

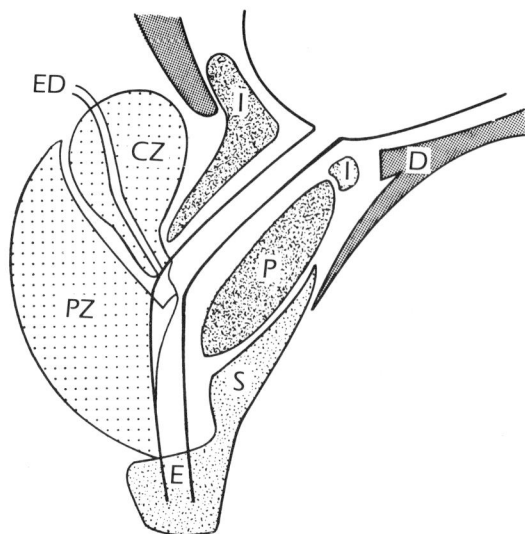

Fig. 7.1 The zonal anatomy of the prostate. Saggital section of human prostate. *Key :* D, detrusor; I, internal sphincter; P, preprostatic sphincter; CZ, central zone; PZ, peripheral zone; ED, ejaculatory duct; S, prostatic sphincter; E, external sphincter (After McNeal.)

in that the peripheral zone is the site of prostatitis and prostatic carcinoma (McNeal 1968), the central zone being involved much less frequently.

The glands of the peripheral zone drain the urethra by long tortuous ducts and at an angle to the prostatic urethra that is either horizontal or obliquely against the flow of urine (Blacklock 1974). In contrast the central zone glands have shorter ducts and these are orientated obliquely in the direction of urine flow. It has thus been postulated that any infection within the peripheral zone glands would not drain dependently and therefore may not respond fully to therapy. Also the ductal anatomy may promote retention of any substances that may reflux into the prostatic ducts during micturition.

## CLASSIFICATION

On the basis of localisation studies patients with prostatitis separate into four groups: acute bacterial prostatitis (ABP), chronic bacterial prostatitis (CBP), chronic abacterial prostatitis (CAP) and prostatodynia (Pd). The patients are categorised according to the cytological and microbiological findings in both the urine and expressed prostatic secretion (Drach et al 1978, Table 7.1).

The acute bacterial and chronic bacterial forms are distinguished readily despite similar findings in the urine and expressed prostatic secretion (EPS), by the patients in the former group being systemically unwell and having an exquisitely tender prostate on palpation; prostatic massage is inadvisable in ABP as it may induce bacteraemia. Of greatest importance in the classification of the chronic forms is the differentiation of those patients with an infective aetiology (CBP), those with an inflammatory reaction but no obvious infective aetiology (CAP), and those who, although symptomatic, do not appear to have an inflammatory disease of their prostate (Pd). It is impossible on clinical grounds alone to differentiate between these three groups as their symptoms of perigenital pain, irritative voiding and voiding dysfunction, are broadly similar.

Another variant of chronic prostatitis is the granulomatous form: a histological diagnosis characterised by foci of generally non-caseating granulomata with nodular aggregates of histiocytes and multinucleated giant cells. In a recent review (Stillwell et al 1987), the majority of cases (71%) were associated with a recent urinary tract infection, though it may develop

**Table 7.1**   The classification of prostatitis based on prostatic localisation studies. Key: ABP acute bacterial prostatitis; CBP chronic bacterial prostatitis; CAP chronic abacterial prostatitis; PD prostatadynia; WC white cells.

| Category | Mid-stream urine (VB2) | | Expressed prostatic secretion (EPS) | | Organisms |
|---|---|---|---|---|---|
| | WC | Culture | WC | Culture | |
| ABP | + + | + | + + | + | Enterobacteraciae |
| CBP | + | + | + | + | Enterobacteraciae |
| CAP | – | – | + | – | Nil |
| PD | – | – | – | – | Nil |

following previous trans-urethral resection (17%) or a needle biopsy (7.5%) of the prostate. However, half of these latter groups also had a recent urinary infection. Occasionally the granulomatous response may reflect tuberculous infection (3%) or systemic granulomatous disease (3%).

## AETIOLOGY

### Bacterial prostatitis

The aetiological organisms in acute (ABP) and chronic bacterial (CBP) prostatitis are well established and identical, consisting of the Gram negative *Enterobacteriacae* family or *Streptococcus faecalis* in the majority of cases (Meares 1987). More rarely isolated organisms are *Staphylococcus aureus* (Giamarellou et al 1982), *Neisseria gonorrhoeae* and *Mycobacterium tuberculosis*. Atypical bacteria and fungi are more likely to be causative in immunocompromised hosts (Lief & Sarfarazi 1986, Clairmont et al 1987). Protozoal infection by *Trichomonas vaginalis* within the prostate has also been described but is uncommon (van Laarhoven 1987). Although mixed infections may occur, a single aetiological organism is isolated in approximately 80% of cases, being most commonly *Escherichia coli,* followed by *Klebsiella spp., Pseudomonas aeruginosa* and *Proteus spp.* in order of prevalence (Meares 1987). The debate regarding the role of Gram positive organisms in prostatitis has raged from the early part of this century (Young et al 1906) and continues no less vociferously to the present day. There is little doubt *Streptococcus faecalis* has an aetiological role and not uncommonly (in approximately half the cases in which it is isolated), in partnership with another organism (Meares 1987). The main problem arises with Gram positive organisms such as *Staphylococcus epidermidis,* micrococci, non-group D streptococci and diphtheroids. These organisms are skin and urethral commensals, and unless scrupulous attention to detail is observed in the collection of samples during the Stamey localisation procedure, they may cloud the diagnostic picture. Although the consensus of opinion is that these organisms are contaminants and commensals (Meares & Stamey 1968, Meares 1973, Stamey 1981, Jimenez-Cruz et al 1982, Thin & Simmons 1983, Pfau 1986, Meares 1987), some authors (Drach 1975, 1986, Greenberg et al 1985) still feel that the Gram positive organisms cited above are pathogenic. The reason for this diversity of opinion may be the level at which a bacterial colony count is regarded as significant. Meares & Stamey (1968, Stamey 1981), feel there must be a tenfold increase in the bacterial colony count obtained from VB3 (post-massage urine aliquot) and/or expressed prostatic secretion (EPS) compared to the colony count obtained from VB1 (urethral urine) when VB2 (midstream urine) is sterile. Drach (1975) however, is prepared to accept pure numbers of bacteria, namely 5000 organisms/ml in EPS or VB3 provided the count is less than 3000 organisms/ml in VB1 and VB2; these values leave little margin for error. In addition this latter group of authors failed to perform leucocyte counts on their specimens, which provide circumstantial evidence that the organism isolated is actually responsible for the inflammatory process.


## Abacterial prostatitis

As the aetiological organisms involved in chronic bacterial prostatitis are the subject of debate, so the factors and organisms contributing to chronic abacterial prostatitis are confused, contradictory and poorly defined.

The possibility that *Chlamydia trachomatis* organisms (chlamydiae) might be involved was first raised on the basis of serological analysis (Mårdh et al 1972). Later work by the same group of investigators (Mårdh et al 1978) using culture and more subtle serological techniques, cast doubt on their original findings. The role of chlamydiae was given further support by the isolation of organisms from the prostate of 33% of patients after blind transrectal prostatic aspiration biopsy (Poletti et al 1985). However, all the patients in this study had *Chlamydia trachomatis* detected in their urethrae which raises doubt as to whether this group was a homogeneous sample with chronic abacterial prostatitis, or whether some in fact had acute urethritis. Subsequent studies (Berger et al 1987, 1989, Doble et al 1989a) have been unable to corroborate the conclusions of Poletti et al (1985), though support has been forthcoming from Weidner et al (1988) who felt *Chlamydia trachomatis* and *Ureaplasma urealyticum* must be considered as aetiological agents in chronic abacterial prostatitis.

In an attempt to overcome the problems of urethral contamination and blind prostatic biopsy, we used ultrasound guided biopsy to ascertain the role of chlamydiae in chronic abacterial prostatitis (Doble et al 1989a). All patients were diagnosed as having prostatitis by means of the Stamey localisation procedure and underwent transrectal prostatic ultrasound followed by subsequent transperineal biopsy of the abnormal areas under ultrasound control. A chronic inflammatory reaction was confirmed on histological analysis in 86% of the biopsies, but chlamydiae were not recovered in McCoy cell culture or detected by a direct immunofluorescence technique from the prostatic tissue of any of the patients, although they were detected in the urethra in 2% by the immunofluorescence technique. It was concluded that there was no evidence that *Chlamydia trachomatis* was directly implicated in chronic abacterial prostatitis, although the possibility that a chlamydial infection, evidence for which had disappeared, may have initiated the process, could not be excluded. Indeed using a monoclonal antibody against *Chlamydia trachomatis*, chlamydial antigen has been detected in the prostatic tissue of 31% of patients with histologically proven prostatitis (Shurbaji et al 1988), but not in a group of controls; there were no morphological characteristics of active chlamydial infection. This study not only was retrospective, but also based on tissue obtained from patients with acute or chronic prostatitis, and thus appeared to reflect a heterogeneous group. However, it does add further weight to the possibility of *Chlamydia trachomatis* being an initiator of the inflammatory response in chronic abacterial prostatitis.

The debate concerning *Chlamydia trachomatis* in chronic prostatitis is relatively recent, when compared to discussions on the infective aetiology of this condition. Earliest descriptions of chronic prostatitis (Christian 1899), commonly referred to as chronic catarrhal or non-specific prostatitis, laid blame for the condition on a variety of causes, namely posterior urethritis, excessive sexual activity and bicycle riding! Later work considered the possibility of ascending infection from the urethra, but also felt foci of sepsis, such as infected teeth and sinuses were contributory (Frederick 1940, Ill 1951). During the last 30 years or so the debate has been as keen as ever, but searches for consistent aetiological organisms have failed to find any real contenders (O'Shaughnessy et al 1956, Meares 1973, Mårdh & Colleen 1975). The lattermost study (Mårdh & Colleen 1975) attempted to isolate aerobes, anaerobes, mycoplasmas, fungi and viruses from the EPS and was unable to detect differences between the study and control groups, supporting the earlier findings of Meares (1973) in his search for *Neisseria gonorrhoeae*, ureaplasmas, aerobic and anaerobic bacteria.

At the same time as chlamydiae, *Ureaplasma spp.* and *Mycoplasma spp.* entered the fray and as noted above, were disregarded (Meares 1973, Mårdh & Colleen 1975) until Brunner et al (1983) found evidence of *Ureaplasma urealyticum* postatitis from localisation studies in 13.7% of a group of over 500 patients with chronic abacterial prostatitis. More recent studies of EPS (Berger et al 1989, Doble et al 1989b) and ultrasound guided biopsy (Doble et al 1989b), have failed to support Brunner's claims. In this last study, a search for anaerobes was also fruitless in support of earlier work (Meares 1973, Nielsen & Justesen 1974, Mårdh & Colleen 1975).

A viral aetiology has been sought (Gordon et al 1972, Nielsen & Vestergaard 1973), but like so many studies in chronic abacterial prostatitis, failed to implicate these organisms.

A major problem in assigning aetiology to an organism in prostatitis is urethral contamination of EPS. The localisation techniques of Meares & Stamey (1968) go a long way to eliminating this problem, but the viscid nature of prostatic secretions and their resultant slow passage along the urethra may 'recruit' significant numbers of misleading urethral contaminants (Stamey 1981). In an attempt to overcome this problem a number of researchers have employed prostatic biopsy in their search for aetiological organisms (Schmidt & Patterson 1966, Meares 1973, Nielsen & Justesen 1974, Poletti et al 1985, Doble et al 1989a,b). The first four studies all employed 'blind' biopsy techniques and as prostatitis is a focal disease (McNeal 1968) it is perhaps not surprising that the consensus of two of these studies (Schmidt & Patterson 1966, Nielsen & Justesen 1974) was that prostatic biopsy was of no consistent value in chronic prostatitis. Drach (1975) used cold-punch biopsies taken from an endoscope in the prostatic urethra and found an organism identical to that recovered from the prostatic fluid in 84% of patients. However, this serves to confirm that contamination is likely to account for the prostatic fluid bacteriology in this study as contamination would be very difficult to avoid by this method. The work of McNeal (1968) suggested that the peripheral zone is the site of the inflammatory reaction in chronic prostatitis and transurethral biopsy would be unlikely to include tissue from this zone.

The study of Poletti et al (1985) raises serious doubt as to their original diagnosis. In a recent pilot study (Doble et al, unpublished data) 7 patients with acute non-gonococcal urethritis due to *Chlamydia trachomatis*, underwent ultrasound guided aspiration of their prostate and in all patients *Chlamydia trachomatis* could not be detected using an immunofluorescence technique.

The role of ultrasound guided biopsy however requires further elucidation. We found a chronic inflammatory infiltrate in over 86% of our cases of chronic abacterial prostatitis who underwent biopsy and felt this was a clear vindication of the technique (Doble et al 1989a,b).

## DIAGNOSIS

### Microbiology

In order to make a diagnosis of prostatitis, prostatic localisation studies (Meares & Stamey 1968) are mandatory. Any attempt to cut corners and rely on expressed prostatic secretion (EPS) alone or worse still solely symptoms, will result in incorrect diagnosis and spurious data.

The diagnosis of prostatitis rests on finding excessive numbers of white cells in the EPS and/or post-prostatic massage (VB3) urine over and above that found in urethral (VB1) and bladder (VB2) urine. As with much in prostatitis, there is disagreement over the level at which the EPS leucocyte count is deemed pathological. Normal individuals possess leucocytes in their EPS and the range of the upper limit of normal varies between 2 cells per high power field (Andersen & Weller 1979) and 20 cells per high power field (Drach et al 1978), with other authors suggesting values within this range (Blacklock & Beavis 1974, Pfau et al 1978, Stamey 1980, Schaeffer et al 1981). However, a compromise has been struck: by means of a Fuchs-Rosenthal chamber the total white cell count in the EPS in normal controls was estimated (Andersen & Weller 1979) and felt to be 10 white blood cells per high power field. This value is the generally accepted level for a diagnosis of prostatitis, although with some reservation as the white cell count can vary between estimations in both normal individuals and prostatitis patients (O'Shaughnessy et al 1956, Colleen & Mårdh 1975). In addition recent ejaculation can raise the prostatic fluid leucocyte count (Jameson 1967) and thus it is prudent to ensure sexual abstinence for 5 days prior to prostatic fluid collection.

All too commonly EPS cannot be obtained and the diagnosis rests on finding excessive numbers of leucocytes in VB3, over and above that found in

VB1 and VB2. In centrifuged urine, a leucocyte count of greater than or equal to 4 cells per high power field ( × 400), in excess of the count in VB1 and VB2 is highly suggestive of prostatitis, whereas greater than 10 cells per high power field is pathognomic (Weidner & Ebner 1985).

In cases of a dry expressate, one can substitute EPS with semen provided the semen sample is collected as part of a localisation study (Mobley 1975). The drawbacks of this method, however, are that semen is an admixture of secretions and only approximately 20% of its volume arises from the prostate, and secondly cytological interpretation is hampered by immature spermatozoa mimicking leucocytes (Ulstein et al 1976).

## Ultrasound

There is a desperate need for an aid to diagnosis in prostatitis, in order to reduce the numbers of those patients wrongly labelled as prostatitic as a result of shoddy diagnostic methods. Clinical interest in prostatic ultrasound has grown since the first reproducible and interpretable images were obtained (Watanabe et al 1974). Unfortunately, the ultrasound features of chronic prostatitis are far from clear cut and with the early bistable scanners were indistinguishable from those of prostatic cancer (Watanabe et al 1971). Despite technological improvements certain features of inflammatory prostatic disease and cancer remain similar (Harada et al 1980, Brooman et al

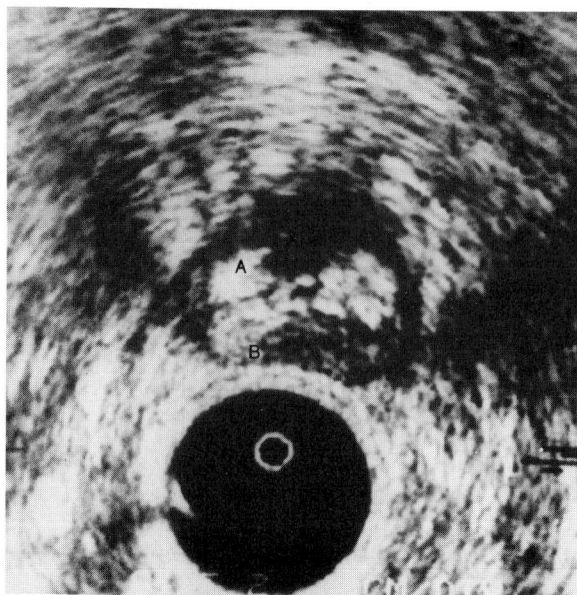

Fig. 7.2 Prostatic ultrasound scan with high density (A) and mid-range (B) echoes.

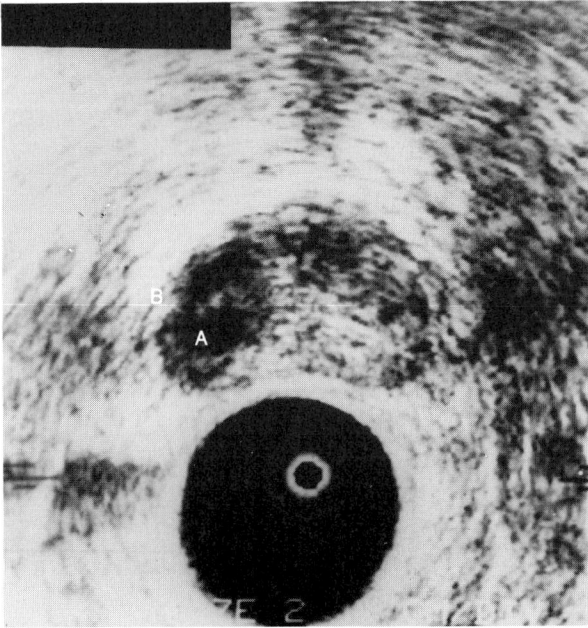

**Fig. 7.3** An echo-lucent zone (A) with adjacent capsular irregularity (B) in a prostatic ultrasound scan.

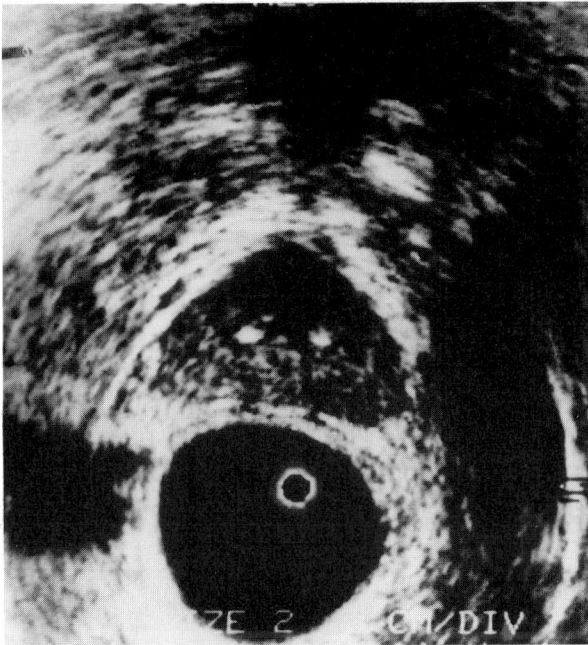

**Fig. 7.4** Bilateral ejaculatory duct echoes in a prostatic ultrasonagraph.

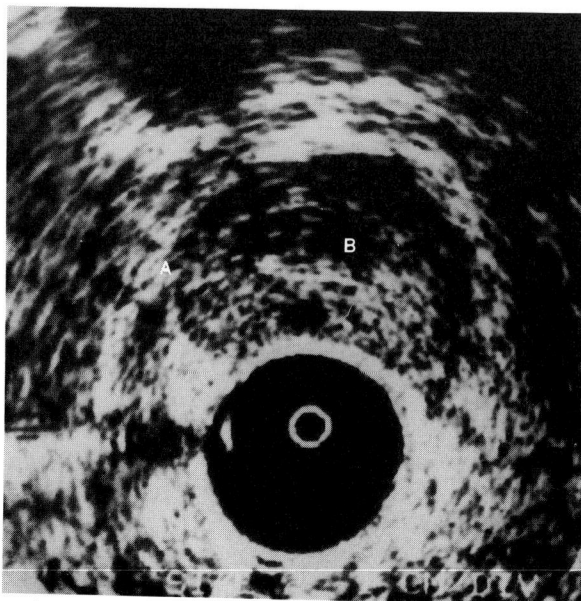

**Fig. 7.5** A prostatic ultrasound indicating capsular irregularity (A) and periurethral zone irregularity (B).

1981, Rifkin 1987), though the patient's age and clinical presentation may help differentiation of the two conditions.

The first study to specifically address the ultrasound features of chronic prostatitis (Griffiths et al 1984), investigated a group of patients diagnosed by the Stamey localisation procedure or examination of expressed prostatic secretion, and noted three ultrasound signs: a low-amplitude 'halo' around a slightly echogenic central area in the periurethral zone (100% of patients), multiple low amplitude echoes in the peripheral zone of the prostate with an ill-defined capsule (80%), and curvilinear, tubular, echo-free structures, immediately adjacent to the anterolateral aspect of the prostate (20%). The peripheral zone findings were felt to represent infection and the tubular signs adjacent to the capsule prominent peri-prostatic veins. The 'halo' sign is harder to explain and is felt by some workers to be non-specific (Harada et al 1980, Doble & Carter 1989) and by others significantly associated with chronic prostatitis (Wiegand & Weidner 1986). This latter group of research-ers compared the ultrasound findings of patients with chronic prostatitis and prostatodynia and detected four significant features: heterogeneous echo patterns, in 62.9% of prostatitis patients versus 16.5% of the prostatodynia cohort (P<0.001), solitary prostatic calculi (type A) 29% versus 15% (P< 0.05), diffuse prostatic calculi (type B) 43.6% versus 7.5% (P<0.001) and the 'halo' sign in 54.9% versus 24.5% (P <0.05).

A recent series of studies (Doble & Carter 1989) investigated patients with chronic prostatitis and prostatodynia, along with a normal control group, in

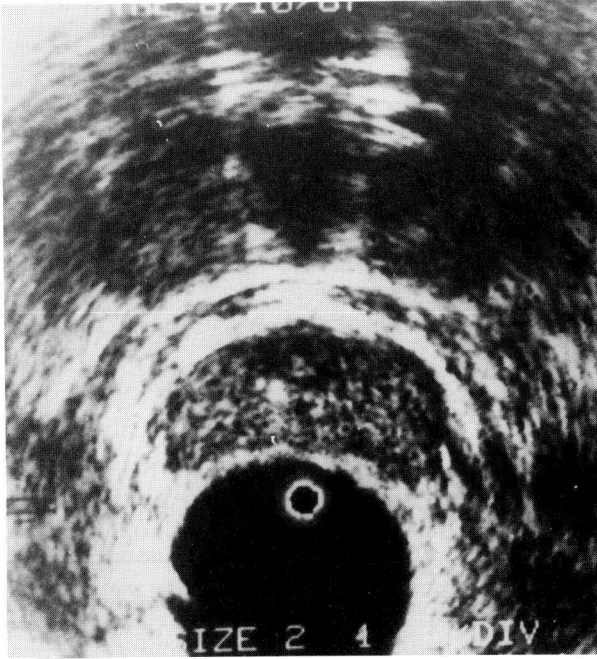

**Fig. 7.6** Capsular thickening in a prostatic ultrasound scan.

an attempt to correlate transrectal ultrasound abnormalities with the findings of the Stamey localisation procedure and histology.

Eight ultrasound abnormalities were identified for study (Table 7.2). Two hundred patients with a clinical diagnosis of chronic prostatitis comprising 105 with chronic prostatitis, 41 with borderline prostatitis and 54 with prostatodynia, as defined by the Stamey localisation procedure (Table 7.3), were studied. In addition, 35 patients with no evidence of lower genital tract disease were studied as controls. Seven of these ultrasound abnormalities, the exception being the 'halo' sign, were significantly associated (chi-square test) with the presence of symptoms of prostatitis compared with asymptomatic normal controls. Also within the group of patients with symptoms of chronic

**Table 7.2**   Ultrasound signs in chronic inflammatory prostatic disease

| Sign | Illustration |
|---|---|
| High density echoes | Fig. 7.2 |
| Mid-range echoes | Fig. 7.2 |
| Echo-lucent zones | Fig. 7.3 |
| Ejaculatory duct calcification | Fig. 7.4 |
| Capsular irregularity | Fig. 7.3, 7.5 |
| Capsular thickening | Fig. 7.6 |
| Periurethral-zone irregularity | Fig. 7.5 |
| 'Halo' sign | — |

**Table 7.3**    Scoring system for prostatitis based on the leucocyte count in the post massage urine (VB3) in cell mm$^3$

| Stamey score | Leucocyte count VB3 cells mm$^3$ | Diagnosis |
|---|---|---|
| 0 | 0 | Prostatodynia |
| 1 | <50 | Prostatodynia |
| 2 | 50–99 | Borderline prostatitis |
| 3 | 100–200 | Prostatitis |
| 4 | >200 | Prostatitis |
| 5 | 0 but documented past history of prostatitis | Prostatitis |

prostatitis there was a similar significant correlation (chi-square test) between each sign, save the 'halo' sign, and a leucocyte count in VB3 of greater than 50 white cells per cubic millimetre (Table 7.4). The borderline prostatitis group had a significant number of ultrasound abnormalities suggesting that these patients may have inflammatory changes within the prostate that are underestimated in the localisation studies. The same may be said of some patients labelled as having prostatodynia as shown by the latter group having a greater number of ultrasound abnormalities than normal controls.

Sensitivity and specificity values calculated from the data agree with a confidence level for the diagnosis of prostatitis of greater than 50 white cells per cubic millimetre in VB3 (Table 7.5). In making this judgement however, a compromise has to be struck. In order to achieve an acceptable specificity for the features of echo-lucent zones, capsular irregularity, capsular thickening and periurethral zone irregularity, a low sensitivity, ranging from 30.8% to 63.3% has to be accepted, with the resultant possibility of false-negative interpretations. The finding of high-density and mid-range echoes is predictive for the diagnosis of prostatitis (with sensitivities of 92.5% and 86.3%), but the relatively low specificity of these signs (51.9% and 40.7% respectively), make false positive interpretations a risk. With the possible exception of echo-lucent zones there is no single ultrasound sign indicative of chronic prostatitis and thus the diagnosis rests on finding a combination of signs; multivarate analysis was unable to provide more detailed information on this score in view of insufficient numbers studied.

**Table 7.4**   Significance of ultrasound abnormalities in symptomatic and chronic prostatitis patients

| Ultrasound signs | Correlation assessed by $x^2$ | |
|---|---|---|
| | Normal controls vs all others | Stamey score <2 vs Stamey score 2 + |
| High density echoes (HDE) | P<0.05 | P<0.001 |
| Mid-range echoes (MRE) | P<0.001 | P<0.001 |
| Echo-lucent zones (ELZ) | P<0.001 | P<0.001 |
| Capsular irregularity (CI) | P<0.001 | P<0.001 |
| Capsular thickening (CT) | P<0.001 | P<0.001 |
| Ejaculatory duct calcification (EDC) | P<0.001 | P<0.001 |
| Periurethral zone irregularity (PZI) | P<0.02 | P<0.001 |
| Halo | NS | NS |

**Table 7.5** Specificity and sensitivity values for the ultrasound signs assuming a diagnostic level for prostatitis at various Stamey scores. Key 5: HDE, high density echoes; MRE, mid-range echoes; ELZ, echo-lucent zones; CI, capsular irregularity; CT, capsular thickening; EDC, ejaculatory duct calcification; PZI, periurethral zone irregularity

| Stamey score | | HDE | MRE | ELZ | CI | CT | EDC | PZI |
|---|---|---|---|---|---|---|---|---|
| 1 + | Sensitivity | 83.7 | 90.6 | 57.5 | 58.7 | 41.9 | 54.4 | 30.0 |
| | Specificity | 40.0 | 60.0 | 100.0 | 87.5 | 90.0 | 70.0 | 87.5 |
| 2 + | Sensitivity | 86.3 | 92.5 | 61.0 | 62.3 | 44.5 | 56.2 | 30.8 |
| | Specificity | 40.7 | 57.9 | 94.4 | 85.2 | 88.9 | 68.5 | 85.2 |
| 3 + | Sensitivity | 83.8 | 96.2 | 57.1 | 67.6 | 48.6 | 57.1 | 29.5 |
| | Specificity | 26.3 | 36.8 | 66.3 | 70.5 | 78.9 | 58.9 | 76.8 |
| 4 + | Sensitivity | 89.5 | 100.0 | 54.4 | 66.7 | 47.4 | 56.1 | 26.3 |
| | Specificity | 25.2 | 27.3 | 57.3 | 57.3 | 69.2 | 53.1 | 73.4 |
| 5 | Sensitivity | 92.3 | 100.0 | 26.9 | 57.7 | 50.0 | 53.8 | 15.4 |
| | Specificity | 23.0 | 22.4 | 57.1 | 51.7 | 66.7 | 57.1 | 71.8 |

There was no ultrasound sign associated with long symptom duration and no difference in the features between patients with chronic bacterial prostatitis and abacterial prostatitis. The follow up data indicated that the development of new signs was more frequent than resolution of existing ones in patients with borderline and proven chronic prostatitis. There were minimal changes in the signs of patients with prostatodynia and therefore repeat scanning over a period of time may increase diagnostic accuracy.

Sixty of the larger group of patients discussed above underwent ultrasound guided biopsy (Holm & Gammelgaard 1981) of abnormal areas of echogenicity within the parenchyma, namely high density and mid-range echoes and echo-lucent zones. Routine histology revealed a chronic inflammatory infiltrate in 86% of cases and fibrosis in 30%. The relationship between ultrasound and histology showed a close correlation of high density echoes with corpora amylacea, of mid-range echoes with fibrosis or inflammation and of echo-lucent zones with inflammation. These pathological findings support the follow up ultrasound data which suggested that inflammation, indicated by echo-lucent zones, heals by fibrosis as manifest by mid-range echoes. High density echoes representing corpora amylacea tended to persist as would be expected.

The volume of the prostate can be calculated from the sonographs and a decrease in prostatic volume has been observed in patients whose chronic prostatitis showed clinical improvement after treatment but not in those whose symptoms remained the same (Griffiths et al 1984). However, the pre and post-treatment prostatic secretion cytology and microbiology was not detailed in this study and thus some doubt must exist as to the importance of this observation.

Few imaging studies have assessed seminal vesicular size and configuration in chronic prostatitis, though enlargement and septal thickening have been noted (Di Trapani et al 1988). The size of the seminal vesicles varies greatly in normal individuals and thus would be difficult to assess objectively.

Chronic prostatitis at present, cannot be diagnosed by transrectal prostatic ultrasound alone, though a normal ultrasound precludes the diagnosis and thus helps select patients who require further investigation. This imaging modality provides detail of intraprostatic pathology previously unsuspected and provides an objective assessment of the inflammatory process as well as enabling accurate biopsy in order for further research to be pursued. In time improved technology (Kimura et al 1986, Baran et al 1987), may enable more accurate diagnosis, but for the present transrectal ultrasound must remain a research tool in an attempt to further elucidate the pathology and natural history of chronic prostatitis.

Although readily diagnosed clinically, the ultrasonographic features of acute prostatitis are well documented (Harada et al 1980, Peeling & Griffiths 1984, Spirnak & Resnick 1984, Weidner 1985). The gland's capsule appears enlarged, rounded and symmetrical with a decreased echogenicity and sound transmission within the gland parenchyma, thought to represent oedema, is increased. After successful treatment the gland may return to a normal configuration.

A rare sequel of bacterial prostatitis is prostatic abscess formation. These lesions are readily visualised by transrectal ultrasound, appearing as irregular hypoechoic masses containing diffuse mid-range echoes within an enlarged gland (Rifkin 1985, Sugao et al 1986). It is possible to aspirate the abscess transperineally under ultrasound control and also monitor response to treatment by serial scanning.

In view of the focal nature of prostatitis (McNeal 1968), it is not surprising that blind biopsy techniques either proved to be of no consistent value (Schmidt & Patterson 1986, Nielsen & Justesen 1974), or perhaps provided misleading data (Poletti et al 1985). Also, the site of inflammatory changes in prostatitis generally reside in the peripheral zone of the gland (McNeal 1968) and thus endoscopic transurethral prostatic biopsy (Drach 1975) is liable to sample the wrong zone of prostate. However, by means of ultrasound guided biopsy (Holm & Gammelgaard 1981), the microbiology of chronic abacterial prostatitis has been studied (Doble et al 1989a, b) obviating the possibility of urethral contamination of samples. In these studies 86% of biopsies displayed a chronic inflammatory infiltrate, which was felt to be a clear vindication of the technique. However, prostatic biopsy should be regarded not as a routine clinical investigation but rather more as a research tool.

## Immunology

Immunoglobulins within the expressed prostatic secretion (EPS) were first noted, in normal subjects, in 1963 (Chodirker & Tomasi 1963). Since the finding of antibody coated bacteria in the urine of patients with chronic bacterial prostatitis, there has been great interest in the immunoglobulins within prostatic fluid (Jones 1974). A group of patients with a diagnosis of prostatitis, though no details of localisation studies were given, were found to have significantly increased levels of IgG, IgM and IgA within the EPS compared to controls (Gray et al 1974). Later studies in patients with both chronic bacterial and abacterial prostatitis, diagnosed by the Stamey localisation procedure, have noted elevated levels of IgG and IgA in prostatic fluid, the levels being greater in chronic bacterial than chronic abacterial prostatitis (Fowler & Mariano 1984, Shortliffe & Wehner 1986). Also, a satisfactory resolution of the inflammatory response was accompanied by a return of the immunoglobulins to normal levels albeit over a long period (6 to 24 months). In another study of chronic bacterial prostatitis (Shimamura 1979) IgM levels in addition to IgG, in the EPS, were found to follow a similar pattern.

The total and organism-specific immunoglobulin levels in EPS have now been measured by several investigators (Shortliffe et al 1981, Wishnow et al 1982, Fowler et al 1982, Fowler & Mariano 1984, Shortliffe & Wehner 1986) and the general consensus is that the levels of IgG and IgA in prostatitis are elevated compared to those in controls. The IgA response is most prominent and felt to represent local antibody production within the prostate rather than transudation from the serum. The immunoglobulin levels in chronic abacterial prostatitis are lower than those in chronic bacterial prostatitis and not organism specific for the Enterobacteriaceae (Shortliffe & Wehner 1986). It appears, therefore, that chronic abacterial prostatitis is not an occult infection by these organisms, that has escaped detection. Recently, Shortliffe and colleagues (Shortliffe et al 1989) have reported the use of an enzyme-linked immunosorbent assay (ELISA) to measure total urinary immunoglobulin and specific antibodies to common Gram-negative organisms, in pre and post-prostatic massage urine samples. In patients with chronic bacterial prostatitis elevated levels of IgA and IgG were detected in the post-massage urine. This method provides a simple test for diagnosing bacterial prostatitis and enables the diagnosis to be made in those cases who have an active urinary tract infection or in whom free EPS cannot be obtained.

In acute bacterial prostatitis antigen specific immunoglobulins of the IgA and IgG classes have been detected in the serum as well as the EPS, in contrast to chronic bacterial prostatitis where they are only detected in the EPS (Meares 1987). IgG is elevated in both compartments at the onset of infection and declines slowly over a period of 6 to 12 months with adequate treatment. In contrast, with IgA, the levels of immunoglobulin in the serum follow the pattern of IgG, but in the EPS this decline does not occur until approximately 12 months after successful treatment.

Tissue antibodies within the prostate have been noted in normal cadaveric and benign hyperplastic prostatic tissue (Ablin et al 1971). The immunoglobulins were found in granules within the ductal lumen (IgG and IgA), in the basal portion of the prostatic acini (IgG) and in the stroma (IgA); it was concluded these antibodies were part of the normal prostatic secretion. Frozen sections of prostatic tissue from a group of patients with chronic prostatitis detected a diffuse extracellular presence of IgA, IgG and IgM, and in some areas immunoglobulin containing cells (Vinje et al 1983). The authors were loath to make firm conclusions, save that the immunoglobulins had probably diffused passively from the serum. However, the patients were not diagnosed by standard localisation studies, a blind biopsy technique was adopted and there was no control group, making interpretation of the findings difficult.

Prostatic tissue obtained by ultrasound guided biopsy from patients with chronic abacterial prostatitis, diagnosed by standard techniques (Meares & Stamey 1968), has been studied for the presence of antibodies using a direct immunofluorescence technique (Doble et al 1990). Antibody deposition was detected in 57% of patients compared to 5% of controls (P <0.001), suggesting that the antibodies were directed against extrinsic proteins rather than being part of the normal secretions of the gland. In the patients with chronic abacterial prostatitis, positive immunofluorescence staining for IgM was found in 85%, for complement (C3) in 44%, for IgA in 35% and for fibrinogen in 24%. The site of antibody deposition was most commonly periglandular, but glandular and vessel wall sites were also prominent. Poor urinary flow, irritative voiding and urgency were significantly associated with IgM and C3 deposition and the link between symptomatology and these immunofluorescence findings may rest with functional outflow obstruction causing intraprostatic reflux of urine which in turn excites an inflammatory response (vide infra).

Recently, panels of monoclonal antibodies have become available to analyse tissue for the presence of lymphoid and non-lymphoid cells (Janossy et al 1980), in particular macrophages and antigen presenting cells (Poulter et al 1984). Prostatic biopsy specimens from 21 patients with chronic abacterial prostatitis, 2 patients with chronic bacterial prostatitis and 1 with granulomatous disease, along with samples from 10 control patients with no evidence of prostatitis, were analysed.

In normal prostate tissue a faint HLA-DR expression was observed in the basal epithelial cells, endothelial cells and mononuclear, non-macrophage cells in the periglandular region. Scanty T-lymphocytes, comprising roughly equal proportions of the helper/inducer (CD4) and suppressor/cytotoxic (CD8) subsets were noted, along with occasional mature tissue macrophages (RF D7). However, other members of the monocyte/macrophage series and B-lymphocytes were not detected in normal prostatic tissue.

The findings in the biopsy material from patients with prostatitis summarised in Table 7.6, were notably different. HLA-DR expression, strongest

**Table 7.6**   Distribution of inflammatory cells in chronic a prostatitis of different inflammatory grade. Key : +/-, less than 5 cells/high powered field (hpf); +, 5–10 cells/hpf; + +, 11–15 cells/hpf; + + +, greater than 15 cells/hpf.

| Antibody | Cells identified | | | | |
|---|---|---|---|---|---|
| | | 1 | 2 | 3 | Granulomatous |
| HLA-DR | MHC class II antigen | + | + + | + + + | + + + |
| T-mix | T-lymphocytes | + | + + | + + + | + + + |
| B-mix | B-lymphocytes | – | – | – | – |
| RF-D1 | Antigen presenting cells | +/– | +/– | + + | + |
| RF-D7 | Mature tissue macrophages | +/– | +/+ + | + + + | + + + |
| UCHM1 | Monocytes | – | +/– | + | + + |

in the glandular structures, increased with the more severe inflammation. The progressive increase in the number of T-cells with the degree of inflammation, was most marked in the CD8 subset. An increasing proportion of these T-lymphocytes also expressed the activation marker (CD7); a situation not seen in the CD4 subset. In the monocyte/macrophage series there was a progressive increase in the antigen-presenting cells (RFD1) and mature tissue macrophages (RFD7), whereas monocytes were found in only 50% of the biopsies with more severe inflammatory reactions. The RFD1/RFD7 relationship was in keeping with a type IV hypersensitivity reaction.

The consistent HLD-DR expression and presence of large numbers of T-cells and antigen-presenting cells (RFD1), along with the absence of B-cells, point to the inflammatory reaction in chronic prostatitis being cell-mediated. In contrast to rheumatoid arthritis, where the CD4 T-lymphocyte subset and the antigen-presenting cells (RFD1) predominate (Poulter et al 1983), and the pathological defect appears to be primarily one of immunoregulatory dysfunction (Poulter et al 1984), the pattern seen in chronic prostatitis is more in keeping with a persistent antigenic presence.

The nature of the inducing antigen in chronic abacterial prostatitis remains obscure, yet the predominance of the CD8 subset raises the possibility of a viral agent, though the same pattern was observed in chronic bacterial prostatitis. This data along with that of the immunofluorescence studies, cited earlier, raises the possibility of exogenous antigen entering the prostate along with urine which refluxes into the gland at the time of micturition. Our inability to implicate any micro-organisms in chronic abacterial prostatitis along with this immunological data suggests that treatment directed towards immunomodulation rather than antibiotics should be seriously contemplated in this condition.

A selected leucocyte defect, with resultant ineffective phagocytosis and killing of homologous isolates of Gram-positive bacteria obtained from patient's EPS, has been described (Wedren et al 1987). Although of limited value to the complex spectrum of prostatitis this study does add weight to the pursuance of immunological lines of research.

**Urodynamic studies**

It has been proposed that urine refluxes into the prostate during micturition and may be an aetiological factor in chronic abacterial prostatitis (Kirby et al 1982). The area of the prostate gland most commonly affected by chronic inflammatory disease is the peripheral zone (McNeal 1968) and the perpendicular orientation of the ducts draining this zone into the urethra makes urinary reflux an anatomical possibility. There is indirect evidence of intra-prostatic urinary reflux in that 50% of prostatic stones contain constituents derived from the urine (Sutor & Wooley 1974, Kim 1982). Furthermore, although distributed throughout the gland, prostatic calculi are most commonly located in the peripheral zone (Huggins & Bear 1944).

The prostatic urethra is bounded by two sphincters, the bladder neck and the distal sphincter complex. Incomplete relaxation of the distal sphincter during micturition leads to a high prostatic urethral pressure and a likelihood of urinary reflux into the prostatic ducts (Buck 1975, Hellstrom et al 1987). The reasons for the inappropriate distal sphincter relaxation may be local inflammation, abdominal straining with reflex enhanced distal sphincter tone, and psychological factors. In this way a vicious circle of urinary reflux leading to inflammation, which in turn perpetuates distal sphincter spasm with increased prostatic urethral pressure and subsequent further urinary reflux, may ensue (Hellstrom et al 1987). Persistence of the inflammatory process results in fibrosis of the prostatic ducts which may become patulous (Mitty 1971) and become prone to further reflux.

If urinary reflux does occur, as seems likely, it remains to be discovered whether this is a normal event. However, in chronic prostatitis, if urine containing pathogenic organisms refluxes into the prostate infection could ensue, but if sterile, the urine may act simply as a chemical irritant and initiate or perpetuate a non-bacterial inflammatory response.

## PSYCHOLOGICAL FACTORS

The psychological component of chronic prostatitis is well recognised (Bagge 1970, Mendlewicz et al 1971, Nilsson et al 1975), but difficult to assess objectively. Experimental studies in the rat, exposing the animals to standardised stress stimuli, have shown decreased blood flow and inflammatory changes within the prostates of the stressed animals compared to non-stressed controls (Gatenbeck et al 1987). The voicing of psychoneurotic complaints was shown in one study (Brähler et al 1986) to be more common in patients with chronic prostatitis than those with prostatodynia. The separation of psychological factors from physical ones in any chronic disease is difficult, prostatitis being no exception, and further studies are needed to clarify the situation.

## TREATMENT

The most appropriate therapeutic remedy for prostatitis has yet to be discovered, though many patients with acute and chronic bacterial prostatitis will gain relief from their symptoms, although in the case of the latter group, relapse is commonplace. The greatest problem lies in the management of chronic abacterial prostatitis, mainly due to the limited knowledge of its aetiology.

### Acute bacterial prostatitis

Fortunately, the acutely inflamed prostate provides no barrier to the diffusion of antimicrobial agents and therefore any antibiotic to which the offending organism is sensitive, is suitable in the treatment of this condition. As a general rule, treatment should initially be via the parenteral route in the form of either aminoglycosides or co-trimoxazole (Pfau 1986, Meares 1987) and thereafter antibiotics should be continued orally for 4 to 6 weeks. It is debatable as to whether acute bacterial prostatitis progresses to the chronic form if inadequately treated (Pfau 1986, Meares 1987), but the rationale for prolonged treatment is to prevent this sequel. Failure to respond to appropriate antimicrobial therapy may herald prostatic abscess formation, which can be imaged by transrectal ultrasound or CT scanning, and then drained by the transperineal route (Kadmon et al 1986, Sugao et al 1986, Vaccaro et al 1986).

The rare cases of acute prostatitis caused by unusual organisms are treated in standard fashion, namely *Salmonella* with co-trimoxazole or chloramphenicol, *Mycobacterium tuberculosis* with triple antituberculous therapy (Gorse & Belshe 1985) and mycotic infections with amphotericin B alone or in combination with 5-fluorocytosine (Bissada et al 1977, Sing et al 1979).

Occasionally the inflammatory process in acute bacterial prostatitis is so marked as to cause acute urinary retention. This should be managed by suprapubic catheterisation and on no account should urethral instrumentation be performed.

## Chronic bacterial prostatitis

The factors that require consideration in the medical treatment of chronic bacterial prostatitis are the choice of antibiotics, duration of therapy, route of administration and the definition of cure. The lack of consensus and the search for yet more potent antimicrobial agents indicate that an effective treatment is still awaited.

Much of the data on the pharmacokinetics of antibiotic diffusion into the prostate were obtained from experiments on dogs (Winningham et al 1968, Stamey et al 1970, Baumueller & Madsen 1977a,b). It was concluded that in order for a substance to cross the lipid membrane, the prostatic barrier, it had to be lipid-soluble, unbound to plasma proteins and have a suitable dissociation constant (pKa) such that at plasma pH there were large numbers of unionised molecules free to cross the prostatic epithelial barrier and thus enter the prostatic fluid. The ideal substance would be a lipid-soluble, non-bound, weak base which would dissociate once within the prostate and by means of ion-trapping, be concentrated in the prostate. Trimethoprim appeared to fit the bill achieving concentrations in the prostatic fluid in excess of those within the plasma both in the dog (Reeves & Gilchik 1970, Granato et al 1973), and the human gland (Oosterlinck et al 1975, Wright et al 1982). Unlike in the dog, the basic pH of prostatic fluid in the inflamed human gland (Blacklock & Beavis 1974, Pfau et al 1978), calls into question the validity of the above conclusions on the antibiotic pharmacokinetics in chronic prostatitis.

The early trials on treatment of chronic bacterial prostatitis studied the use of co-trimoxazole and found that short term treatment had little benefit, but long term therapy affected a permanent bacteriological cure in 33% to 55% of cases over a follow up period of 6 to 30 months (Meares 1973, McGuire & Lytton 1976, Pfau & Sacks 1976). Trimethoprim alone has been shown, in a small series (Pfau 1986), to be as effective with a 50% cure rate overall to 4 year follow up. In a larger series, the same author (Pfau 1986) reported a 44% cure rate using either co-trimoxazole for 4 to 8 months or trimethoprim for 4 to 6 months in a group of patients with *E. coli* or *Pseudomonas* chronic bacterial prostatitis, with a follow up period of 1 to 13 years. A similar cure rate was achieved in patients treated for 3 months with co-trimoxazole, but follow up was shorter (Meares 1982).

In view of the rather disappointing results achieved with co-trimoxazole and trimethoprim, other agents have been sought. Aminoglycosides first described as effective in 1968 (Meares & Stamey 1968) using kanamycin, have subsequently proved useful (Pfau & Sachs 1976, Pfau 1986) though cure rates are still in the order of 44%. Studies involving the tetracyclines, minocycline and doxycycline, have produced conflicting results: relapse rates range from 15% to 30% (Brannan 1975, Paulson & White 1978, Paulson et al 1986) but cure rates (clinical and bacteriological) in the order of 35% to 55%. Thus, it appears that the tetracyclines confer no benefit over co-trimoxazole or trimethoprim. Carbenicillin has been investigated and received favourable reports (Oliveri et al 1979, Nielsen et al 1980, Goldfarb 1984), but accurate bacteriological localisation studies and adequate follow up were lacking in these studies. Cephalosporins in particular cephalexin have proved inferior to the standard regimes (Mobley 1981, Paulson et al 1986). Rifampicin, theoretically a suitable antimicrobial on pharmacokinetic criteria, has proved effective in the treatment of prostatitis caused mainly by *Staphylococcus aureus* (Giamarellou et al 1982).

The antimicrobial agent receiving most press at present is ciprofloxacin, a quinolone derivative, which has been shown to reach high concentrations in prostatic secretions, semen (Dalhoff & Weidner 1984) and prostatic tissue (Dan et al 1986). Clinical studies have demonstrated that this antibiotic is effective in the short term (Weidner et al 1986) and in long term follow up (1 year), cure rates of 64% for *E. coli* prostatitis have been achieved (Weidner et al 1987). However, in this report chronic prostatitis due to *Streptococcus faecalis* and *Pseudomonas aeruginosa* relapsed between 6 weeks and 6 months after treatment. In another study, although symtomatic cure was achieved in 60% of cases, only 40% of those 'cured' had an accompanying bacteriological cure (Langemeyer et al 1987). All these studies lack standardisation of the definition of a cure and thus comparison is invalid. Pfau (1986) regards a 12 month period with repeated negative urine and prostatic fluid cultures as sufficient evidence of a cure, but in view of the chronic nature of the disease this may be too short a period of assessment.

The disappointing cure rates achieved with either oral or parenteral antibiotics in chronic prostatitis has led to a resurgence of the technique of intraprostatic injection of antibiotics, first described by Ritter & Lippow (1938). Initial results of this approach were encouraging with cure rates in the order of 66% (Plomp et al 1980, Baert et al 1983). This enthusiasm has been sustained on long term follow up (Baert & Leonard 1988), with remission periods of up to 6 months in 71% of patients after one to two instillations, and in a further 25% after repeated instillations. However, 30% of patients relapsed between 1 and 7 years after treatment. A criticism of this latter study was the blind passage of the needle into the prostate and in view of the focal nature of chronic prostatitis, administration of antibiotic to the infected foci was left very much to chance. The advent of transrectal prostatic ultrasound and methods to guide needle placement within the gland (Holm & Gammelgaard 1981) has enabled accurate delivery of antibiotic to diseased areas of the prostate. Intraprostatic antibiotic injections using aminoglycosides, in a group of patients with chronic prostatitis due to Gram-negative organisms, has resulted in a 'cure' in 70% of cases at 3 months and in 59% at 6 months after injection (Jimenez-Cruz et al 1988). The delivery of antibiotics by this method is well directed and provides high local concentrations of antimicrobial, but only for a short period, as within 27 hours it has been cleared from the gland (Schulteis et al 1986). In an attempt to provide a depot injection, an alcoholic emulsion of prolamine has been added to the antibiotic which has been shown to persist in the tissue for greater than 7 days (Schulteis et al 1986). These data provide some hope for the future if accurate delivery and persistence of antibiotics can be achieved, as side effects appear minimal.

An alternative approach to injection therapy has been administration of antibiotic via the prostatic ducts using a two ballon-four channel catheter which isolates the prostatic urethra. An 80% symptomatic and microbiological cure was achieved, though in 68% of cases *Staphylococcus epidermidis* was the causative organism and details of long term follow up were lacking (Jin & Guagi 1987).

The final medical option for chronic prostatitis is continuous suppressive therapy of low dose antibiotic, either co-trimoxazole or nitrofurantoin. Although relapse is common on stopping medication, patient's symptoms are controlled and their prostatic fluid remains sterile whilst on treatment (Meares 1982, Pfau 1986).

## Surgery

Although as a general rule surgery is not indicated in the treatment of chronic bacterial prostatitis, there are advocates of this approach. Smart et al (1976) achieved a cure in 50% and improvement in 30% of cases of chronic prostatitis, a mixture of bacterial and abacterial, with a follow up of 18 months to 3 years. However, other authors feel surgery should be reserved for recalcitrant cases of chronic bacterial prostatitis with evidence of marked prostatic calculus formation (Meares & Stamey 1968, Meares 1974, Stamey 1980, Pfau 1986). It would appear the best results are achieved in those patients who have concomitant bladder outflow obstruction which is undoubtedly relieved by surgery.

### Chronic abacterial prostatitis

In view of the uncertain aetiology of chronic abacterial prostatitis, there is no specific therapy available. The majority of patients have received antibiotics, the rationale being the possibility of an occult infection, or a past history of non-specific urethritis, or the misconception that chlamydiae or mycoplasmas are to blame.

A double-blind prospective trial comparing minocycline and diazepam produced symptomatic relief in 58% and 73% of cases respectively, and a fall in the EPS leucocyte count in 35% and 8% respectively (Simmons & Thin 1985). However, 56% of the minocycline group and 57% of the diazepam group still had elevated leucocyte counts in the EPS, diagnostic of prostatitis, following treatment. These results suggest, that although minocycline has greater efficacy than diazepam, the aetiology of the inflammatory response is unlikely to be an occult infection and neither treatment appears to be directed at the underlying cause.

A study comparing high-fluid intake versus dietary fibre, produced symptomatic improvement in 60% of the former group compared to 33% of the latter, but there was no corroborative microbiological data (Thin 1986). A pilot project using non-steroid anti-inflammatory agents produced symptomatic improvement in 75% of cases whilst on treatment, but all relapsed on stopping their medication; however a fall in EPS leucocyte account occured in only one case (Thin 1986). Sodium pentosanpolysulphate, a negatively charged polysaccharide with a number of properties including enzyme and complement inhibition, has been used to good effect in interstitial cystitis. It was employed in a double blind trial with a placebo in a group of patients with chronic abacterial prostatitis and statistical differences were observed in relief of musculoskeletal symptoms, functional bladder volume and mean urinary flow rate (Wedren 1987). No data was available on the effect on the EPS leucocyte count during treatment.

Attempts to reduce intraprostatic urinary reflux, thought to be an aetiological factor in chronic abacterial prostatitis, have included pharmacological manipulation with alpha-blockers to relax the distal sphincter mechanism and sacral-root electrostimulation to fatigue this sphincter (Hellstrom et al 1987). There is little objective data to support these regimes but the logic is sound and thus further study of these options is required.

Local hyperthermia applied transrectally by microwaves has claimed marked subjective and objective improvement in patients with chronic prostatitis (Servadio et al 1987), though details of the assessment criteria were lacking.

A number of less conventional approaches to treatment including acupuncture have been investigated. 46% of patients studied were cured on the basis of symptoms and cytology of prostatic fluid, and a further 20% were improved (Ge et al 1988). The belief that chronic abacterial prostatitis is related to stress has led to a number of studies where treatment of this element alone has brought favourable results (Mimoun 1987, Miller 1988). In an attempt to relieve distal urethral sphincter spasm, a proposed aetiological factor in chronic abacterial prostatitis, biofeedback has been proposed (Hellstrom et al 1987). Again, these studies lack objective data and rely on subjective criteria only.

It is clear from the preceding paragraphs that chronic abacterial prostatitis represents a therapeutic challenge as the nature of the enemy is unknown. At present simple reassurance that the disease is not life threatening and is likely to 'burn out' with time, along with sympathy for the symptoms, has acceptable results. Very often however the patient loses faith and seeks yet another opinion.

## CONCLUSIONS

Although our knowledge of prostatitis, particularly the chronic forms, has broadened over the past 50 years, there are some pressing problems: the reasons for failure in chronic bacterial prostatitis even when the aetiological organisms have been identified, the aetiological factors involved in chronic abacterial prostatitis and their treatment. So many studies into prostatitis have been poorly constructed, uncontrolled and relied on perfunctory methods of diagnosis and have only served to provide misleading information. Strict adherence to precise methods of diagnosis must be practised if any comparative data is to be accumulated and any valid conclusions drawn.

With the advent of improved technology such as transrectal prostatic ultrasound and immunological probing techniques, there is the opportunity to investigate in depth those bona fide cases of prostatitis and answer some of the outstanding questions. It is clear that the problem of prostatitis will not disappear. Thus, the options are to dismiss it as an insoluble problem or to attempt to unravel its complex and multifactorial pathophysiology. In view of the advances made in the last decade it would seem worth pursuing the latter option.

REFERENCES
Ablin R J, Gonder M J, Soanes W A 1971 Localisation of immunoglobulin in human prostatic tissue. Journal of Immunology 107: 603–604
Anderson R U, Weller C 1979 Prostatic leukocyte secretion studies in nonbacterial prostatitis (prostatosis). Journal of Urology 121: 292–294
Baert L, Leonard A 1988 Chronic bacterial prostatitis: 10 years of experience with local antibiotics. Journal of Urology 140: 755–757
Baert L, Mattelaer J, Nottlin P de 1983 Treatment of chronic bacterial prostatitis by local injection of antibiotic into prostate. Urology 21: 370–375
Bagge L 1970 Psychiatric aspects of chronic prostatitis. Nordisk Medicin 6: 786–789
Baker T 1925 Chronic prostatitis of non-venereal origin. Journal of the American Medical Association 85: 1606–1608

Baran G W, Golin A, Bergsma C et al 1987 Standardized endosonographic evaluation of prostatic cancer: receiver-operator-characteristic analysis. American Journal of Roentgenology 149: 975–980

Baumueller A, Madsen P O 1977a Experimental bacterial prostatitis in dogs. Urological Research 5: 211–213

Baumueller A, Madsen P O 1977b Secretion of various antimicrobial substances in dogs with experimental bacterial prostatitis. Urological Research 5: 215–218

Berger R E, Krieger J N, Paulsen C A et al 1987 Case control study of prostatic localisation cultures in men with chronic prostatitis. Journal of Urology 137: 136A

Berger R E, Krieger J N, Kessler D et al 1989 Case control study of men with suspected chronic idiopathic prostatitis. Journal of Urology 141: 328–331

Bissada N K, Finkbeiner A E, Redman J F 1977 Prostatic mycosis: non-surgical diagnosis and management. Urology 9: 327–328

Blacklock N J 1974 Anatomical factors in prostatitis. British Journal of Urology 46: 47–54

Blacklock N J, Beavis J P 1974 The response of prostatic fluid pH in inflammation. British Journal of Urology 46: 537–542

Brähler E, Brunner A, Girshausen C et al 1986 Psychosomatic and somatophysical aspects of chronic prostatitis. In: Weidner W, Brunner H, Krause W, Rothauge C F (eds) Therapy of prostatitis. Zuckswerdt Verlag, Munchen, pp 165–167

Brannan W 1975 Treatment of chronic prostatitis: comparison of minocycline and doxycycline. Urology 5: 626–631

Brooman P J, Griffiths G J, Roberts E et al 1981 Per rectal ultrasound in the investigation of prostatic disease. Clinical Radiology 32: 669–676

Brunner H, Weidner W, Schiefer H G 1983 Studies on the role of *Ureaplasma urealyticum* and *Mycoplasma hominis* in prostatitis. Journal of Infectious Diseases 147: 807–813

Buck A C 1975 Disorders of micturition in bacterial prostatitis. Proceedings of the Royal Society of Medicine 68: 508–511

Chodirker W B, Tomasi T B (jr) 1963 Gammaglobulins: quantitative relationships in the human serum and non-vascular fluids. Science 142: 1080–1081

Christian M D 1899 Chronic catarrhal prostatitis. Journal of Cutaneous and Genito-Urinary Diseases, New York 17: 18–22

Clairmont G J, Zon L I, Groopman J E 1987 Haemophilus parainfluenzae prostatitis in a homosexual man with chronic lymphadenopathy syndrome and HTLV-III infection. American Journal of Medicine 82: 175–178

Colleen S, Mardh P-A 1975 Studies on nonacute prostatitis: clinical and laboratory findings in patients with symptoms of nonacute prostatitis. In: Danielsson D, Juhlin L, Mardh P-A (eds) Genital infections and their complications. Almquist and Wiksell International, Stockholm, pp 121–132

Culver HB 1916 A study of bacteriology of chronic prostatitis and spermatocystitis. Journal of the American Medical Association 66: 553–557

Dalhoff A, Weidner W 1984 Diffusion of ciprofloxacin into prostatic fluid. European Journal of Clinical Microbiology 3: 360–362

Dan M, Golomb J, Gorea A et al 1986 Concentration of ciprofloxacin in human prostatic tissue after oral administration. Antimicrobial Agents & Chemotherapy 30: 88–89

Di Trapani D, Pavone C, Serretta V et al 1988 Chronic prostatitis and prostatodynia: ultrasonographic alterations of the prostate, bladder neck, seminal vesicles and periprostatic venous plexus. European Urology 15: 230–234

Doble A, Carter S St C 1989 Ultrasonographic findings in prostatitis. Urologic Clinics of North America 16: 763–772

Doble A, Thomas B J, Walker M M et al 1989a The role of *Chlamydia trachomatis* in chronic abacterial prostatitis: a study using ultrasound guided biopsy. Journal of Urology 141: 332–333

Doble A, Thomas B J, Furr P M et al 1989b A search for infectious agents in chronic abacterial prostatitis utilising ultrasound guided biopsy. British Journal of Urology 64: 297–301

Doble A, Walker M M, Harris J R W et al 1990 Intraprostatic antibody deposition in chronic abacterial prostatitis. British Journal of Urology 65: 598–605

Doble A, Thomas B J, Taylor-Robinson D Can chlamydiae be recovered from the prostate in patients with acute urethritis due to *Chlamydia trachomatis*. Unpublished data

Drach G W 1975 Prostatitis: man's hidden infection. Urologic Clinics of North America 2: 499–520

Drach G W 1986 Chronic bacterial prostatitis: problems in diagnosis and therapy. Urology 27 (Suppl.): 26–30

Drach G W, Fair W R, Meares E M et al 1978 Classification of benign diseases associated with prostatic pain: prostatitis or prostatodynia? Journal of Urology 120: 226

Fowler J E, Mariano M 1984 Longitudinal studies of prostatic fluid immunoglobulin in men with bacterial prostatitis. Journal of Urology 131: 363–369

Fowler J E, Kaiser D L, Mariano M 1982 Immunologic response of the prostate to bacteriuria and bacterial prostatitis. Immunoglobulin concentrations in prostatic fluid. Journal of Urology 128: 158–164

Frederick C O 1940 Management of chronic prostatitis. New Orleans Medical and Surgical Journal 93: 115–121

Gatenbeck L, Aronsson A, Dahlgren S et al 1987 Stress stimuli-induced histopathological changes in the prostate: an experimental study in the rat. Prostate 11: 69–76

Ge S H, Meng F Y, Xu B R 1988 Acupuncture treatment in 102 cases of chronic prostatitis. Journal of Traditional Chinese Medicine 8: 99–100

Giamarellou N, Kosmidis M, Leonidas M et al 1982 A study of the effectiveness of rifaprim in chronic prostatitis caused mainly by *Staphylococcus aureus*. Journal of Urology 128: 321–324

Goldfarb M 1984 Clinical efficacy of antibiotics in treatment of prostatitis. Urology 24 (Suppl.): 12–13

Gordon H L, Miller D H, Rawls W E 1972 Viral studies in patients with non-specific prostato-urethritis. Journal of Urology 108: 299–300

Gorse G J, Belshe R B 1985 Male genital tuberculosis: a review of the literature with instructive case reports. Reviews of Infectious Diseases 7: 511–524

Granato J J, Gross D M, Stamey T A 1973 Trimethoprim diffusion into prostatic and salivary secretion of the dog. Investigative Urology 11: 205–210

Gray S P, Billings J Blacklock N J 1974 Distribution of the immunoglobulins G, A and M in the prostatic fluid of patients with prostatitis. Clinica Chimica Acta 57: 163–169

Greenberg R N, Reilly P M, Luppen K L et al 1985 Chronic prostatitis: comments on infectious etiologies and antimicrobial treatment. Prostate 6: 445–448

Griffiths G J, Crooks A J R, Roberts E E et al 1984 Ultrasonic appearances associated with prostatic inflammation: a preliminary study. Clinical Radiology 35: 343–345

Harada K, Tanahashi Y, Igari D et al 1980 Clinical evaluation of inside echo patterns in gray scale prostatic echography. Journal of Urology 124: 216–220

Hellstrom W J G, Schmidt R A, Lue T F et al 1987 Neuromuscular dysfunction in nonbacterial prostatitis. Urology 30: 183–188

Herrold R D 1928 Interpretation of chronic infections of the prostate and seminal vesicles. Journal of the American Medical Association 91: 557–560

Hitchens A P, Brown C P 1913 Bacteriology of chronic prostatitis. American Journal of Public Health 3: 884–891

Holm H H, Gammelgaard J 1981 Ultrasonically guided precise needle placement in the prostate and seminal vesicles. Journal of Urology 125: 385–387

Huggins C, Bear R S 1944 The course of the prostatic ducts and the anatomy, chemical and x-ray diffraction analysis of prostatic calculi. Journal of Urology 51: 37–47

Hunter J 1786 A treatise on the venereal disease. London

Ill H M 1951 Chronic non-specific prostatitis. Journal of the Medical Society of New Jersey 48: 426–429

Jameson R M 1967 Sexual activity and the variations of the white cell content of the prostatic secretion. Investigative Urology 5: 297–302

Janossy G, Tidman N, Selby W S et al 1980 Human T-lymphocytes of inducer and suppressor type occupy different microenvironments. Nature 288: 81–84

Jimenez-Cruz J F, Ferrer M M, Almagro A A et al 1984 Prostatitis: are the gram-positive organisms pathogenic? European Urology 10: 311–314

Jimenez-Cruz J F, Tormo F B, Gomez J G 1988 Treatment of chronic prostatitis: intraprostatic antibiotic injections under echography control. Journal of Urology 139: 967–970

Jin C H, Guagi H 1987 Two-balloon and four-channel silicone rubber catheter for drug injection in the treatment of chronic bacterial prostatitis. European Urology 13: 116–117

Jones S R 1974 Prostatitis as a cause of antibody coated bacteria in the urine. New England Journal of Medicine 291: 365 (letter)

Kadmon D, Ling D, Lee J K T 1986 Percutaneous drainage of prostatic abscesses. Journal of Urology 135: 1259–1260

Kim K M 1982 The stones. Scanning Electron Microscopy 1982 (4): 1635–1660

Kimura A, Nakamura S, Niizuma M et al 1986 Quantitative analysis of ultrasonogram of the prostate. Journal of Clinical Ultrasound 14: 501–507

Kirby R S, Lowe D, Bultitude M I et al 1982 Intraprostatic urinary reflux: an aetiological factor in abacterial prostatitis. British Journal of Urology 54: 729–731

Langemeyer T N M, Ferwerda W H H, Hoogkamp-Korstanje J A A et al 1987 Treatment of chronic bacterial prostatitis with ciprofloxacin. Pharmaceutisch Weekblad Scientific Edition (suppl) 9: S 78–81

Lief M, Sarfarazi F 1986 Prostatic cryptococcosis in acquired immunodeficiency syndrome. Urology 28: 318–319

Lowsley O S 1912 The development of the human prostate gland with reference to the development of other structures at the neck of the urinary bladder. American Journal of Anatomy 13: 299–349

McGuire E J, Lytton B 1976 Bacterial prostatitis: treatment with trimethoprim-sulfamethoxazole. Urology 7: 499–500

McNeal J E 1965 Morphogenesis of prostatic carcinoma. Cancer 18: 1659–1666

McNeal J E 1968 Regional morphology and pathology of the prostate. American Journal of Clinical Pathology 49: 347–357

Mardh P-A, Colleen S 1975 Search for uro-genital tract infections in patients with symptoms of prostatitis. Scandinavian Journal of Urology and Nephrology 9: 8–16

Mardh P-A, Colleen S, Holmquist B 1972 Chlamydia in chronic prostatitis (letter). British Medical Journal 4: 361

Mardh P-A, Ripa K T, Colleen S et al 1978 Role of *Chlamydia trachomatis* in non-acute prostatitis. British Journal of Venereal Diseases 54: 330–334

Martin S C 1899 Acute and chronic prostatitis. American Journal of Dermatology and Genito-Urinary Diseases 3: 27–28

Meares E M 1973 Bacterial prostatitis versus prostatosis. A clinical and bacteriological study. Journal of the American Medical Association 224: 1372–1375

Meares E M 1973 Observations on activity of trimethoprim-sulfamethoxazole in the prostate. Journal of Infectious Diseases (suppl) 128: S679–685

Meares E M 1974 Infection stones of the prostate gland: laboratory diagnosis and clinical management. Urology 4: 560–566

Meares E M 1982 Prostatitis: review of pharmacokinetics and therapy. Reviews of Infectious Diseases 4: 475–483

Meares E M 1987 Acute and chronic prostatitis: diagnosis and treatment. Infectious Diseases Clinics of North America 1: 855–873

Meares E M, Stamey T A 1968 Bacteriologic localisation patterns in bacterial prostatitis and urethritis. Investigative Urology 5: 492–518

Mendlewicz J, Shulman C, de Schutte B et al 1971 Chronic prostatitis: psychosomatic incidence. Psychosomatic Medicine 19: 118–125

Miller H C 1988 Stress prostatitis. Urology 32: 507–510

Mimoun S 1987 L'approche psychosomatique des prostatitis chroniques. Contraception Fertilité-sexualité 15: 301–305

Mitty H A 1971 Roentgen features of reflux into the prostate, seminal vesicles and vasa deferentia. American Journal of Roentgenology 112: 603–606

Mobley D F 1975 Semen cultures in the diagnosis of bacterial prostatitis. Journal of Urology 114: 83–85

Mobley D F 1981 Bacterial prostatitis: treatment with carbenicillin indanyl sodium. Investigative Urology 19: 31–33

Nickel A C 1930 The bacteriology of chronic prostatitis and seminal vesiculitis and elective localisation of the bacteria isolated. Journal of Urology 24: 343–357

Nielsen M L, Justesen T 1974 Studies on the pathology of prostatitis. A search for prostatic infections with obligate anaerobes in patients with chronic prostatitis and chronic urethritis. Scandinavian Journal of Urology and Nephrology 8: 1-6

Nielsen M L, Vestergaard B F 1973 Virological investigations in chronic prostatitis. Journal of Urology 109: 1023–1025

Nielsen O S, Frimodt-Moeller N, Maigaard S et al 1980 Penicillanic acid derivatives in the canine prostate. Prostate 1: 79–85

Nilsson I-K, Colleen S, Mardh P-A 1975 Relationship between psychological and laboratory findings in patients with symptoms of non-acute prostatitis. In: Danielsson D, Juhlin L, Mardh P-A (eds) Genital infections and their complications. Almquist and Wiskell International, Stockholm, pp 133–144

Notthaft A 1904 Ubrer scheinbar mit der Prostat nicht zu sammenhängender aber dennoch durch Prostatitis bedingte Schmerzen. Archives fur Dermatologie und Syphilis 70: 277–312

Oliveri R A, Sachs R M, Caste P G 1979 Clinical experience with geocillin in the treatment of bacterial prostatitis. Current Therapeutic Research 25: 415–421

Oosterlinck W, Defoort R, Renders G 1975 The concentration of sulphamethoxazole and trimethoprim in human prostate gland. British Journal of Urology 47: 301–304

O'Shaughnessy E J, Parrino P S, White J D 1956 Chronic prostatitis — fact or fiction? Journal of the American Medical Association 160: 540–542

Paulson D F, White R D 1978 Trimethoprim-sulfamethoxazole and minocycline hydrochloride in the treatment of culture-proved bacterial prostatitis. Journal of Urology 120: 184–185

Paulson D F, Zinner N R, Resnick M I et al 1986 Treatment of bacterial prostatitis: comparision of cephalexin and minocycline. Urology 27: 379–387

Peeling W B, Griffiths G J 1984 Imaging of the prostate by ultrasound. Journal of Urology 132: 217–224

Pfau A 1986 Prostatitis: a continuing enigma. Urologic Clinics of North America 13: 695–715

Pfau A, Sacks T 1976 Chronic bacterial prostatitis: new therapeutic aspects. British Journal of Urology 48: 245–253

Pfau A, Perlberg S, Shapiro A 1978 The pH of the prostatic fluid in health and disease: implications of treatment in chronic bacterial prostatitis. Journal of Urology 119: 384–387

Player L P, Lee-Brown R K, Mathé C P 1923 The causative organisms and the effect of autogenous vaccines in cases of chronic prostatitis. Journal of Urology 10: 377–385

Plomp T, Baert L, Maes R A 1980 Treatment of recurrent chronic bacterial prostatitis by local injection of thiamphenicol into prostate. Urology 15: 542–547

Poletti F, Medici M C, Alinovi A et al 1985 Isolation of *Chlamydia trachomatis* from the prostatic cells in patients affected by non-acute abacterial prostatitis. Journal of Urology 134: 691–693

Poulter L W, Duke O, Hobbs S et al 1983 The involvement of interdigitating cells in the pathogenesis of rheumatoid arthritis. Clinical and Experimental Immunology 51: 247–254

Poulter L W, Duke O, Janossy G et al 1984 Immunoregulatory aspects of rheumatoid arthritis. Inflammation Research 7: 123–128

Poulter L W, Campbell D A, Munro C et al 1986 Discrimination of macrophages and dendritic cells of man using monoclonal antibodies. Scandinavian Journal of Immunology 24: 351–357

Reeves D S, Gilchik M 1970 Secretion of the antibacterial substance trimethoprim in the prostatic fluid of dogs. British Journal of Urology 42: 66–72

Rifkin M D 1985 Imaging of the lower genito-urinary tract. Raven Press, New York

Rifkin M D 1987 Endorectal sonography of the prostate: clinical implications. American Journal of Roentgenology 148: 1137–1142

Ritter S J, Lippow C 1938 Pathological and bacteriological processes present in prostatitis and tissue reaction to therapy. Journal of Urology 39: 111–117

Schaeffer A J, Wendel EF, Dunn J K et al 1981 Prevalence and significance of prostatic inflammation. Journal of Urology 125: 215–219

Schmidt J D, Patterson M C 1966 Needle biopsy of chronic prostatitis. Journal of Urology 96: 519–533

Schulteis K H, Schiefer H G, Alles J et al 1986 Intraprostatic injection of a tobramycin-prolamine compound. In: Weidner W, Brunner H, Krause W, Rothauge C F (eds) Therapy of prostatitis. Zuckschwerdt Verlag, Munchen, pp 73–75

Servadio C, Leib Z, Lev A 1987 Diseases of prostate treated by local microwave hyperthermia. Urology 30: 97–99

Shimamura M 1979 Immunological studies on bacterial prostatitis. Japanese Journal of Urology 70: 267–285

Shortliffe L M D, Wehner N 1986 The characterisation of bacterial and non-bacterial prostatitis by prostatic immunoglobulins. Medicine 65: 399–414

Shortliffe L M D, Wehner N, Stamey T A 1981 The detection of a local prostatic immunologic response to bacterial prostatitis. Journal of Urology 125: 509–515

Shortliffe L M, Elliot K, Sellers R G 1989 Measurement of urinary antibodies to crude bacterial antigen in patients with chronic bacterial prostatitis. Journal of Urology 141: 632–636

Shurbaji M S, Gupta P K, Myers J 1988 Immunohistochemical demonstration of chlamydial antigens in association with prostatitis. Modern Pathology 1: 348–351

Simmons P D, Thin R N 1985 Minocycline in chronic abacterial prostatitis: a double-blind prospective trial. British Journal of Urology 57: 43–45

Sing P, Sun S S Y, Crutchlow P F 1979 Coccidioido-mycosis of the prostate gland and its therapy. Journal of Urology 121: 127–128

Smart C J, Jenkins J D, Lloyd R S 1976 The painful prostate. British Journal of Urology 47: 861–869

Spirnak J P, Resnick M I 1984 Transrectal ultrasonography. Urology 23: 461–467

Stamey T A 1980 Urinary infections in males. In: Stamey T A (ed) Pathogenesis and treatment of urinary tract infections. Williams and Wilkins, Baltimore

Stamey T A 1981 Prostatitis. Journal of the Royal Society of Medicine 74: 22–40

Stamey T A, Govan D E, Palmer J M 1965 The localisation and treatment of urinary tract infections: the role of bactericidal urine levels as opposed to serum levels. Medicine 44: 1–36

Stamey T A, Meares E M, Winningham D G 1970 Chronic bacterial prostatitis and diffusion of drugs into prostatic fluid. Journal of Urology 103: 187–194

Stillwell T J, Engen D E, Farrow G M 1987 The clinical spectrum of granulomatous prostatitis: a report of 200 cases. Journal of Urology 138: 320–323

Sugao H, Takiuchi H, Sakurai T 1986 Transrectal longitudinal ultrasonography of prostatic abscess. Journal of Urology 136: 1316–1317

Sutor D J, Wooley S E 1974 The crystalline composition of prostatic calculi. British Journal of Urology 46: 533–535

Thin R N 1986 Treatment of non-bacterial prostatitis. In: Weidner W, Brunner H, Krause W, Rothauge C F (eds) Therapy of prostatitis. Zuckschwerdt Verlag, Munchen, pp 145–148

Thin N, Simmons P D 1983 Chronic bacterial and non-bacterial prostatitis. British Journal of Urology 55: 513–518

Thompson Sir H 1861 The diseases of the prostate, their pathology and treatment, 2nd ed, London

Ulstein M, Capell P, Holmes K K et al 1976 Non-symptomatic genital tract infection and male infertility. In: Hafez E S E (ed) Human semen and fertility regulation in man. Mosbe, St Louis, pp 355–362

Vaccaro J A, Belville W D, Kiesling V J et al 1986 Prostatic abscess: computerized tomography scanning as an aid to diagnosis and treatment. Journal of Urology 136: 1318–1319

Van Laarhoven P H 1987 Trichomonas vaginalis, a pathogen of prostatitis. Netherlands Journal of Surgery 19: 263–273

Vinje O, Fryjordet A, Brun A-L et al 1983 Laboratory findings in chronic prostatitis with special reference to immunological and microbiological aspects. Scandinavian Journal of Urology and Nephrology 17: 291–297

Von Lackum W H 1927 Clinical and experimental data on prostatic infection. Journal of Urology 18: 293–306

Watanabe H, Kaiho H, Tanaka M et al 1971 Ultrasonotomographic diagnosis of the prostate II. Sagittal tomography of the prostate by means of B mode scanning. Medical Ultrasonics 9: 26–35

Watanabe H, Igari D, Tanahashi Y et al 1974 Development and application of new equipment for transrectal ultrasonography. Journal of Clinical Ultrasound 2: 91–98

Wedren H 1987 Effects of sodium pentosanpolysulphate on symptoms related to chronic non-bacterial prostatitis. Scandinavian Journal of Urology and Nephrology 21: 81–88

Wedren H, Holm S E, Bergman B 1987 Can decreased phagocytosis and killing of autologous Gram-positive bacteria explain the findings of Gram-positive bacteria in 'non-bacterial' prostatitis Acta Pathologica Microbiologica et Immunologica Scandinavica section B 95: 75–78

Weidner W 1985 Use of transrectal ultrasonography of the prostate and seminal vesicles in andrology: 3 years experience. Acta Europaea Fertilitatis 16: 117–123

Weidner W, Ebner H 1985 Cytological analysis of urine after prostatic massage (VB₃) — a new technique for a discriminating diagnosis of prostatitis. In: Brunner H, Krause W, Rothauge C F, Weidner W (eds) Chronic prostatitis. Schattauer, Stuttgart, pp 141–151

Weidner W, Schiefer H G, Becker H C et al 1986 Clinical efficacy of ciprofloxacin in chronic bacterial prostatitis. In: Weidner W, Brunner H, Krause W, Rothauge C F (eds) Therapy of prostatitis. Zuckschwerdt Verlag, München pp 54–58

Weidner W, Schiefer H G, Dalhoff A 1987 Treatment of chronic bacterial prostatitis with ciprofloxacin. American Journal of Medicine 82 (supplement 4A): 280–283

Weidner W, Schiefer H G, Krauss H 1988 Role of *Chlamydia trachomatis* and mycoplasmas in chronic prostatitis. A review. Urologie Internationalis 43: 167–173

White J W, Wood A C 1898 Diseases of the prostate. In: American textbook of genitourinary diseases. Bags & Hardway, Philadelphia, pp 255–336

Wiegand S, Weidner W 1986 Per rectal ultrasonography of the prostate in the diagnosis of chronic prostatitis and prostatodynia. In: Weidner W, Brunner H, Krause W, Rothauge C F (eds) Therapy of prostatitis. Zuckschwerdt, Verlag, München, pp 177–180

Winningham D G, Nemoy N J, Stamey T A 1968 Diffusion of antibiotics from plasma into prostatic fluid. Nature 219: 139–143

Wishnow K I, Wehner N, Stamey T A 1982 The diagnostic value of the immunoglobulin response in bacterial and non-bacterial prostatitis. Journal of Urology 127: 689–694

Wright W L, Larking P, Lovell-Smith C J 1982 Concentrations of trimethoprim and sulphamethoxazole in the human prostate gland after intramuscular injection. British Journal of Urology 54: 550–551

Young D V, Portez D M 1978 Treatment of Salmonella prostatitis with trimethoprim-sulfamethoxazole. Southern Medical Journal 71: 742–743

Young H H, Geraghty J T, Stevens A R 1906 Bacteriology of chronic prostatitis. Johns Hopkins Hospital Report 13: 271–284

# 8

# Current trends in the diagnosis and treatment of gonorrhoea

*C.S.F. Easmon C.A. Ison*

## INTRODUCTION

Despite the increasing importance of other pathogens such as human immunodeficiency virus (HIV) and *Chlamydia trachomatis*, gonorrhoea continues to be one of the major sexually transmitted infections. Over the past 15 years there has been much basic research into the biology of the pathogenic neisseriae and since the last volume in this series diagnostic laboratories have begun to benefit from these advances. In that volume the two chapters on *Neisseria gonorrhoeae* were concerned with basic biology and the management of infections caused by penicillinase producing *N.gonorrhoeae* (PPNG). In this chapter we describe first the ways in which basic biology has been applied to the practical issues of diagnosis and sensitivity testing and secondly how the pattern of gonococcal resistance of antibiotics has developed and the implications of this for therapy.

## DIAGNOSIS AND SUSCEPTIBILITY TESTING

### Detection

A rapid preliminary diagnosis of gonorrhoea is needed to ensure adequate therapy and prevent further spread of the disease. The Gram stain is used routinely for this purpose and culture of the causative organism, *N.gonorrhoeae*, is used for confirmation. In urethral specimens from symptomatic men the Gram stain has a sensitivity of 98% but in women and asymptomatic males it falls to 40–50% (Handsfield et al 1974, Goodhart et al 1982). There have been many attempts to develop an alternative to the Gram stain using techniques such as ELISA, immunofluorescence and DNA probes.

An ELISA using a polyvalent antiserum to *N.gonorrhoeae* (Gonozyme, Abbott Laboratories) has been evaluated widely as an alternative. This method has been shown to have a good sensitivity and specificity in high-risk populations of symptomatic men (Danielsson et al 1983, Granato & Roefaro 1985) but is more time consuming and expensive and offers no advantage over the Gram stain. In women the test has been shown to have a lower sensitivity and specificity than in men (Manis et al 1984, Nachamkin et al 1984). The lower specificity is of particular concern in the diagnosis of a sexually transmitted disease because of the special problems that may arise from a wrong diagnosis or a request for further specimens. This has limited the use of Gonozyme even in populations of high-risk women. In low prevalence populations the predictive value has been found to be unacceptable and this test has rarely been used to screen these patients (Schachter et al 1984, Lieberman & Wheelock 1987, Thomason et al 1989).

Antibody linked to fluorscein has also been used to detect gonococci in direct smears (Ison et al 1985). It showed similar results to the ELISA, being useful in men but less so in women. DNA probes with either a radioactive (Totten et al 1983, Perine et al 1985) or chromogenic (Sprott et al 1989) label have been described but have not been used extensively as yet.

In women a number of factors influence the efficiency of any detection system, the lower numbers of gonococci, the presence of cervical mucus, of large numbers of other bacteria and of asymptomatic infection. Culture for *N.gonorrhoeae* still remains the most sensitive method of overcoming these problems and detecting gonorrhoea in women.

## Identification

The diagnosis of gonorrhoea by the laboratory isolation and identification of the infecting organism, *N.gonorrhoeae*, may have social and medicolegal consequences. It is, therefore, important that accurate and reliable tests are used for identification.

*N.gonorrhoeae* is a member of the genus *Neisseria*. This has many species of which only *N.gonorrhoeae* and *N.meningitidis* are considered primary pathogens. The remaining species are usually found on mucosal surfaces as commensals. Hence, any identification scheme must differentiate *N.gonor-rhoeae* from both *N.meningitidis* and the non-pathogenic *Neisseria*.

In many high risk populations, such as those attending sexually transmitted disease clinics, a presumptive identification of colonies growing on selective media as gonococci, on the basis of their being both oxidase positive and Gram negative cocci, has been considered sufficient. This assumption can be unreliable because non-pathogenic neisseria are not totally suppressed on the selective media used to isolate gonococci. In most laboratories, however, it is the practice to confirm the identification of *N.gonorrhoeae* and eliminate other non-pathogenic *Neisseria* without attempting full speciation. In situations where the likelihood of gonorrhoea is lower or there is a medicolegal issue, for example child abuse or rape cases, full speciation should always be attempted and it is often advisable to use more than one approach to avoid the possibility of misidentification of a non-pathogenic species as *N.gonorrhoeae*.

Historically carbohydrate utilisation tests have been considered the defin-itive means of identifying *N. gonorrhoeae*. However, the evolution of identification kits and the use of newer technologies such as monoclonal antibodies and DNA probes has broadened the spectrum of tests available for the identification of *Neisseria* spp. Many of the tests are aimed at producing a rapid identification for *N.gonorrhoeae* alone and should not be confused with, or used for, the full speciation of the genus, *Neisseria*. The tests available can be categorised as follows (1) detection of acid production from carbohydrates, (2) detection of preformed enzymes, (3) use of specific antibodies and (4) use of DNA probes.

## 1. Carbohydrate utilisation tests

Conventional carbohydrate utilisation tests originally used a serum agar medium with added carbohydrate. This has been largely replaced by the use of serum free medium such as cystine tryptic digest agar (CTA) base medium or a GC agar base with added supplements and carbohydrates (Flynn & Waitkins 1972) which are more efficient at supporting the growth of Neisseria. These media, whether used as slopes or as agar plates, require a pure growth for inoculation and 24 hours incubation before the result can be obtained. Identification therefore takes at least 48 hours from first isolation of suspect colonies. The reactions can also be difficult to interpret because of inadequate inoculum, mixed cultures or contamination of the maltose with glucose. Subsequent modifications of this technique using liquid media allowed identification within 1 to 4 hours of inoculation (Brown 1974, Lairsey & Kelly 1985) but many of the problems were not overcome.

A number of carbohydrate test kits are now available commercially (Neisseria-Kwik, RIM-N, Gonobio-Test, Minitek and Quad-FERM). For the identification of *N.gonorrhoeae* these tests have a sensitivity of 98–100% (Janda et al 1985, 1987, Dillon et al 1988). The specificity is also high, >90%, occasional isolates of *N.meningitidis, N.subflava* and *B.catarrhalis* have been wrongly identified as *N.gonorrhoeae* (Dillon et al 1988). Although these kits give a rapid result (between 1–4 hours), a heavy inoculum of the organism is required and consequently identification is always delayed for 24 hours after isolation. The advantage of such kits is that they remove the technical problems of preparing the carbohydrate media but at an increase in cost of 10–30 fold over CTA sugars (Dillon et al 1988).

## 2. Preformed enzymes

Rapid identification using enzyme profiles is mainly based on the work of D'Amato et al (1978). Chromogenic substrates are used to detect the presence of beta-galactosidase, gamma-glutamylaminopeptidase or hydroxyprolylaminopeptidase. A heavy pure growth of the test organism is usually required as an inoculum and a positive reaction produces a colour change. This approach is very useful both for distinguishing *N. lactamica* from *N.gonorrhoeae* by its ability to produce beta-D-galactosidase, and for the identification of *N.meningitidis*, particularly those strains which do not utilise maltose, by the production of gamma-glutamyl-aminopeptidase, an enzyme never produced by strains of *N.gonorrhoeae* (D'Amato et al 1978). In the United Kingdom the commercial kit most commonly used is Gonochek II. This has a high specificity for the identification of *N.gonorrhoeae* (Brown & Thomas 1985, Janda et al 1985, Dillon et al 1988). Occasional false positive reactions (i.e. identification of non-pathogenic neisseria as *N.gonorrhoeae*) have been noted (Dillon et al 1988). This kit has been reported to be sensitive using a small inoculum and hence can identify successfully colonies direct from primary selective plates (Brown & Thomas 1985, Janda et al 1985).

### 3. Immunological identification

In recent years it has become popular to use specific antibodies raised to *N.gonorrhoeae* to identify colonies directly from primary isolation plates. A pure culture of the organism is not necessary and the result is obtained within an hour. Initially polyclonal antibodies raised in rabbits were used and were found to be useful (Young & Reid 1984) but cross-reactivity with other species of the genus, particularly *N.meningitidis*, was sometimes encountered. This is not surprising as these two species are closely related genetically and share many common antigens. The advent of monoclonal antibodies promised a greater specificity but there was the concern that the high specificity would affect the sensitivity of the reagents. In practice this would mean that while other neisseria might not cross-react with the monoclonal antibodies and give false positives, some strains of *N.gonorrhoeae* might not carry the epitope for the antibody and give a false negative reaction.

The monoclonal antibodies that have been used in such tests have been raised to the major outer membrane protein, PI. Panels of antibodies directed at epitopes on the two types of PI, IA and IB, have been used to give a broad range of reactivity. They have been linked either to staphylococcal Protein A (Phadebact Monoclonal GC OMNI Test, Pharmacia, Sweden and GonoGen, New Horizons Diagnostics, Columbia, USA) or to flourescein (Syva Micro-Trak, Palo Alto, USA). The Phadebact Test is the only coagglutination test available in Europe and has two reagents which allow the strains to be serogrouped into IA (WI) or IB (WII/III). All three tests have been found to be highly specific and sensitive (Dillon et al 1988, Anand et al 1988, Ison et al 1988b, Young & Moyes 1989). False positive reactions have been encountered with *N.lactamica* and *N.meningitidis* (Anand et al 1988) using the Phadebact Monoclonal kit as well as *B.catarrhalis* and *N.cinerea* (Dillon et al 1988). The sensitivity of these reagents has varied from 92–100% when tested by the same workers (Anand et al 1988, Dillon et al 1988). The presence of non-reactive strains will always be a possibility when a mixture of antibodies is used rather than a single antibody to a conserved epitope although no such epitope has yet been identified in *N.gonorrhoeae*. Evins et al (1988) developed a reference panel of 52 strains of *N.gonorrhoeae* for testing serological reagents that were antigenically diverse and had been isolated worldwide. This must be the ideal approach for detecting non-reactive strains but the emergence of new serotypes cannot be anticipated and will still give negative results. Unless a cluster of such strains should occur within one clinic it is not a major problem. In our experience when these reagents are used for the confirmation of *N.gonorrhoeae* the specificity is so high that the identity of any unexpected negatives can be confirmed by biochemical methods.

### 4. DNA probes

DNA probes were first used for the detection of *N.gonorrhoeae* in clinical samples using radiolabelled probes of the cryptic 2.6 MD plasmid (Totten et al 1983). The absence of this plasmid in up to 10% of strains in some areas, together with the lack of sensitivity of radiolabelled probes, has restricted their use to research groups (Perine et al 1985). More recently a biotinylated DNA probe for the identification of *N.gonorrhoeae* has been developed which detects chromosomal sequences in gonococcal strains (Knapp 1988b). DNA probes offer a greater specificity and differentiation between the species of Neisseria but at this time have not been evaluated for culture confirmation as rigorously as the tests described above.

### In summary

It is common in most laboratories to use only one or two types of test for the identification of *N.gonorrhoeae*. However, if there is confusion whether a strain belongs to a non-pathogenic species or is *N.gonorrhoeae*, Knapp (1988a) has recommended the use of eight tests together. These are production of acid from glucose and maltose, superoxol, hydroxyprolylaminopeptidase, glutamylaminopeptidase, nitrate reduction, deoxyribonuclease and colistin susceptibility. In practice at this stage most laboratories would probably send the strain to a reference centre.

## Susceptibility testing

Susceptibility testing of *N.gonorrhoeae* is performed to detect strains resistant to standard therapy and/or to establish patterns of susceptibility that may influence the choice of therapy. In most diagnostic laboratories susceptibility testing is aimed at the detection of organisms resistant to standard therapy. As discussed later in this chapter *N.gonorrhoeae* exhibits both plasmid and chromosomally mediated resistance and, therefore, different tests are required to ensure that both types of resistance are detected.

Plasmid mediated resistance to penicillin is generally detected by use of a chromogenic cephalosporin which in the presence of gonococcal penicillinase causes a colour change from yellow to red (O'Callaghan et al 1972). This test is simple and reproducible (Snell & Brown 1988) but requires a pure culture of the organism which delays detection for 24 hours. If the patient has received penicillin as first line therapy identification of a penicillinase producing strain requires the patient to be recalled for further therapy. This delay also allows time for spread of an antibiotic resistant organism.

Rapid methods for detection of penicillinase in clinical specimens have been described. Chen et al (1984) used the production of fluorescent endproducts from beta-lactamase activity on ampicillin and cephalexin to develop a rapid test which was more sensitive than the chromogenic cephalosporin (nitrocefin) method when used on cultured organisms. This has been further developed into a spot test and shows high specificity and sensitivity when used on urethral exudates from men with gonococcal urethritis (Chen & Holmes 1986). Two assays have been described recently (Sanchez-Pescador et al 1988) for the detection of the TEM-1 B-lactamase in clinical specimens which use oligonucleotide probes that hybridize to the target DNA captured on a solid phase and are detected using an amplified chemiluminescent method. This non-radioactive technique was found to be 100 times more sensitive than a commercially available colourimetric test for beta-lactamase activity. Another method described by Herve et al (1989) uses the substrate pyridine-2-azo-p-dimethylalanine cephalosporin (PADAC; Diagnostic Pasteur, Marnes-La-Coquette, France). Beta-lactamase positive strains are orange-yellow and negative strains are violet. The main limitation of these approaches is that they are not specific for gonococcal beta-lactamase and other genital tract organisms could also produce this enzyme. Hence these tests are probably unsuitable and have seldom been used in women. Detection of resistant organisms in this way would be ideal for large numbers of specimens, for instance in major STD clinics, but would be too technically demanding and expensive in small hospitals with only a limited number of cases. The time and expense of these tests is difficult to justify except in parts of the world where the prevalence of penicillinase producing *N.gonorrhoeae* is high. Unfortunately, it is in areas of the world such as West Africa where there is a need for this test that the facilities and finance are not available. In areas with a high prevalence of PPNG it may be more economic to use an alternative first line therapy. A rapid, economic and simple system is still urgently required to control the spread of this type of antibiotic resistant gonorrhoea.

Since the description of high level tetracycline resistance due to the presence of a plasmid of 25.2 Megadaltons (MD) carrying a *tetM* determinant (see below) it is now advisable to screen all clinical isolates particularly in countries where tetracycline is used to treat gonorrhoea to prevent dissemination of these strains. Unfortunately there is no analogous test for tetracycline resistance to the chromogenic cephalosporin test for penicillinase. There are two recommended methods for detection of TRNG, either a 10 µg tetracycline disc on a lawn of the test organism or subculture onto a GC agar plate containing 10 mg/1 tetracycline (Center for Disease Control 1987, Communicable Disease Report 1987). The presence of growth on the latter indicates a resistant strain. However, plasmid mediated high level tetracycline resistance can only be confirmed by isolation of the 25.2 MD plasmid or by the use of DNA probes specific for the *tetM* determinant in hybridisation experiments (Morse et al 1986).

The detection of chromosomal resistance to antibiotics such as penicillin, spectinomycin and cephalosporins is considerably more difficult. No rapid method exists and a pure culture of the infecting organism is required for susceptibility testing and at least a further 24 hours incubation until the result is known. In managing gonorrhoea it is not possible to delay therapy until this procedure has been completed. It is, therefore, necessary to choose a suitable first line regimen that will produce cure rates of about 95%. The primary function of susceptibility testing of *N.gonorrhoeae* is, in most diagnostic laboratories, to detect any organisms which are highly resistant to the chosen therapy and to enable the patient to be recalled and given an alternative.

In most clinical laboratories in the United Kingdom resistant organisms are detected using a disc diffusion test. For penicillin susceptibility this will be achieved, in most instances, using three discs of differing concentration, 1.0 unit (u), 0.25 u and 0.03 u. The zone sizes are then measured and an estimate of the minimum inhibitory concentration (MIC) determined from regressions of MICs (Phillips 1978). In our experience it has been difficult to find a direct correlation between the size of the zone of inhibition of growth in a disc susceptibility test and the MIC as determined by agar dilution for gonococci. However a large zone is usually obtained for very sensitive strains and no zone of inhibiton for totally resistant strains but this technique has little discriminative value for strains of reduced susceptibility.

The major problems with disc diffusion tests lie with the standardisation of the inoculum and type of media used which affects the growth rate and subsequently the zone size. However, it has also been shown that the antibiotic content of the disc can be a source of error. In the UKNEQAS study of susceptibility testing of *N.gonorrhoeae* laboratories using high content tetracycline discs (25, 30 or 100 µg) made proportionately more errors than those using low content discs (2, 5 or 10 µg). In contrast, laboratories using low content spectinomycin discs (10 or 16 µg) made more errors than those using higher content discs (25, 30 or 100 µg) (Snell & Brown 1988). Despite the problems associated with this technique it still remains for many the method of choice because agar dilution methods for MICs are considered too difficult and time consuming.

We have examined the feasibility of using agar dilution breakpoint susceptibility testing where a few select antibiotic concentrations are used as a compromise between conventional MIC determination and disc testing for use in diagnostic laboratories (Gill & Ison 1988). We used media containing three concentrations of penicillin, 0.06, 0.5 and 1mg/l, which enabled strains to be categorised as 'sensitive' (MIC   0.06mg/l), of 'intermediate resistance' (MIC 0.12–0.5mg/l) , or 'resistant' (MIC 1.0mg/l). Different concentrations of spectinomycin were also evaluated, 16, 32 and 64mg/l. We found that breakpoint susceptibility testing gave reliable results that could be used for immediate clinical benefit and also allowed long term epidemiological studies.

This technique, however, in common with disc diffusion and agar dilution susceptibility testing is dependant on the protocol used.

The monitoring of antimicrobial susceptibility to establish patterns of resistance over time to determine the efficacy of the standard regimens has invariably used MICs determined by an agar dilution technique. In 1976, the World Health Organization recommended a standard method that would enable results to be compared between different laboratories. The medium suggested was a 'chocolate' agar containing proteose No. 3 (Difco) agar supplemented with 1% (v/v) IsoVitaleX (BBL) and 1% (v/v) haemoglobin (Difco). It was recommended that the inoculum should be $10^3$ colony forming units (cfu) and that the results should be read after 20–24 hours incubation at 36°C in a moist carbon dioxide enriched atmosphere. The MIC was defined as the lowest dilution inhibiting growth (World Health Organisation 1976). Despite this recommendation a number of different modifications have been used including various media such as Mueller-Hinton, Diagnostic Sensitivity Test (DST) Agar and GC agar base and different inocula ranging from $10^3$ to $10^5$ cfu. Several groups have shown that the results obtained can be highly variable depending on the method used (Members of the Australian Gonococcal Surveillance Programme 1984, Dillon et al 1987, Woodford & Ison 1988). For example, the use of a GC agar medium for susceptibility testing has been shown to give significantly different results for erythromcycin and tetracycline in comparison with agars developed for sensitivity testing. Gonococci appeared less sensitive to erythromycin and more sensitive to tetracycline on GC medium when compared to DST Agar (Woodford & Ison 1988). The 'chocolate' medium recommended by the WHO compared well with DST agar in our own studies except for erythromycin on which the gonococci also appeared more resistant.

Recently the Center for Disease Control, Atlanta has changed its procedure to include GC agar supplemented with 1% IsoVitaleX instead of the WHO medium (Knapp 1988b). Dillon et al (1987) have also recommended the use of GC agar for susceptibility testing. This medium is simple to prepare in comparison to the 'chocolate' medium and the results are clear and easy to read and it is, therefore an understandable decision. It is also true that the effects of GC agar already noticed by various groups are relatively minor on the drugs such as penicillin, cephalosporins and spectinomycin, the main therapeutic choices. However, if the discrepancies found with erythromycin and tetracycline are ignored the effects on new antibiotics introduced in the future may not be considered.

Chromosomal resistance to many antibiotics is increasing worldwide and constant surveillance is necessary if the spread of these organisms is to be controlled. At this time in the absence of one accepted method comparison of results between centres is almost impossible. The Australian Gonococcal Surveillance Programme (1984) has shown that a single protocol can be adopted that allows strains to be tested in a number of laboratories, and the reproducibility has proved good enough to allow comparison of gonococcal sensitivity patterns in different states.

In the United States of America the problem of variation in technique has been overcome in the past by testing representative strains isolated from a number of centres in a single laboratory (Jaffe et al 1976, Rice et al 1986). However, in the future this approach will not be feasible if the different geographical locations and larger numbers of strains are to be tested.

## Typing schemes

A reproducible and discriminative typing scheme is needed to study the epidemiology of *N.gonorrhoeae* particularly of antibiotic resistant strains. There have been numerous attempts to do this of which typing by nutritional requirement, auxotyping, has been one of the most successful. The method described by Catlin (1973) has been used extensively but of the 35 auxotypes described the majority of strains in most studies fall into only four auxotypes, prototrophic, proline requiring, arginine requiring and arginine, hypoxanthine and uracil (AHU) requiring. Strains belonging to the AHU auxotype have been shown to be hypersensitive to penicillin (Knapp & Holmes 1975) and proline requiring strains to show increased resistance (Ison et al 1987). However, this technique is time consuming and technically demanding and shows insufficient discrimination for detailed studies of movement of strains within and between populations.

There have been many attempts over the last 50 years to develop a serological typing scheme most of which are based on the major outer membrane protein, PI. This protein is an ideal candidate because it is expressed in large amounts and shows no intra-strain variation. Early attempts used polyclonal antibodies raised in rabbits with techniques such as micro-immunofluorescence (Wang et al 1977), enzyme linked assays (Buchanan & Hildebrandt 1981) and coagglutination (Sandstrom & Danielsson 1980). The use of these schemes, however, was limited by the availability of the antisera or the complexity of the technique. It was not until monoclonal antibodies were raised to the types of PI, PI-A and PI-B (Tam et al 1982) that a serological classification scheme evolved which has been disseminated worldwide. Knapp et al (1984) described the use of a panel of 12 monoclonal antibodies, 6 of which were PI-A specific and 6 were PI-B specific, linked to staphylococcal Protein A and used in a coagglutination test. The pattern of reactivity with this panel denotes the serovar. Since the use of this serotyping scheme was described in the previous volume of this book (Danielsson 1986) two sets of similar antibodies (Bygdeman et al 1985) have been used for typing gonococci which were not totally interchangeable and with different nomenclatures. This confusion has made comparison of data from different groups around the world difficult. However, since 1986 a single panel of 12 monoclonal antibodies (Syva Company, Palo Alto, USA) as originally described (Knapp et al 1984) has been used by the majority of workers with the nomenclature of Knapp et al (1984). The antibodies are supplied through a small number of distributors located in the USA, Europe and Australia who are responsible for the storage of the antibodies, supplying research groups, training of new users and problem solving. The aim of this distribution system is to help ensure the standardisation and reproducibility of the technique. As a result it is becoming evident that serotyping used alone or in combination with auxotyping can be a powerful epidemiological tool. Serotyping has proved useful for the identification of co-infections at multiple sites and of treatment failure and reinfection (Knapp et al 1987a). This is particularly important in the evaluation of new antimicrobial agents for the treatment of gonorrhoea. Serotyping is also useful for the identification of strains from sexual partners and can be applied to sexual abuse cases. This application should be carefully controlled and used in combination with other typing systems such as auxotyping and antibiotic susceptibility profiles. It is easier to eliminate a contact when strains are different but any link between two similar isolates should be tempered by knowledge of the frequency of that type of isolate in the overall population.

We have been using serotyping to examine the association to susceptibility of a number of antibiotics and host characteristics. We have demonstrated that strains belonging to serovar IA-1/2 show increased susceptibility and strains of serovar IB-5/7 show increased resistance to a number of antibiotics including penicillin, cefuroxime, erythromycin and tetracycline (Woodford et al 1989). Other serovars are associated with intermediate levels of resistance. These results suggest that it may be possible to use serotyping prospectively to indicate the likelihood of a resistant strain before the susceptibility testing has been completed and hence giving a quicker result to the clinican. In addition we have shown that strains belonging to serovar IB-2 are more common and those of serovar IB-3 less common in both rectal and homosexual infections. This could suggest that the serovar could be a marker for differences in survival of gonococci at various anatomical sites.

The power of this technique has only recently become evident. When used in combination with auxotyping producing auxotype/serovar (A/S) classes the detailed movement of strains can be monitored. However, it does remain a subjective technique and needs to be carefully controlled. The position of most of the epitopes of these antibodies has now been determined within the DNA sequence of the PI gene (Carbonetti et al 1988) which may in the future allow the antibodies to be replaced by oligonucleotide probes in the same typing scheme. This could result in a more objective technique.

## TREATMENT

### Development of antibiotic resistance in *N.gonorrhoeae*

The sulphonamides were the first modern antibacterial agents to be active against *N.gonorrhoeae*. However, resistance to sulphonamides developed rapidly. Within 15 years of their introduction most gonococci showed increased resistance to sulphonamides with a high proportion of treatment failures (Dunlop 1949).

The importance of penicillin as therapy for gonorrhoea was recognised early. Indeed, an early batch of penicillin made in Britain and detained for a trial of the treatment of battlefield injuries in North Africa was used to treat gonorrhoea instead. In a broadcast in 1945 Fleming predicted that penicillin would play a major role in treating gonorrhoea. Before the widespread use of penicillin most strains of gonococci were susceptible to less than 0.03 mg penicillin/l (Romanovsky 1946). A single dose of 150 000 units gave cure rates in excess of 90%. In 1958 Reyn et al (1958) reported that gonococci isolated in 1957 showed a bimodal distribution of penicillin susceptibility not seen in strains isolated in 1944. Some strains were now resistant to 0.2 mg/1, a tenfold rise in MIC over fully sensitive strains. This increased resistance to penicillin was closely associated with increased resistance to unrelated antibiotics such as streptomycin and tetracycline (Reyn et al 1958, Reyn 1961).

The slow but steady decrease in gonococcal susceptibility to penicillin could be overcome by increasing the dose of the penicillin and by the use of probenecid. In the 1960s the introduction of acid stable semi-synthetic penicillins such as ampicillin allowed the use of single dose oral therapy. However, this also increased the likelihood of inadequate therapy especially where antibiotics were freely available to the general public (Willcox 1970). By the early 1970s a significant percentage of gonococci isolated in parts of the Far East and Africa were not susceptible to 1 mg/1 penicillin (Hart 1973, Ayra & Phillips 1970). Even the maximum dose of penicillin and probenecid was no longer reliably effective against such strains.

In Britain levels of gonococcal resistance were far lower but the same basic process was happening. Nicol et al (1968) reported that over one third of the gonococci isolated at St Thomas' Hospital in 1966 were resistant to 0.1 mg/1 of penicillin while 5% of strains were resistant to 0.5 mg/1. Leigh et al (1969) found similar levels of resistance among gonococci isolated at St Mary's Hospital.

By the mid 1970s penicillin resistance had become a major problem in the Far East and parts of Africa (Jaffe et al 1976) but a relatively small and stable problem elsewhere. Resistance to other useful agents such as tetracycline, co-trimoxazole, chloramphenicol and thiamphenicol followed a similar pattern. However, in 1976 the situation changed with the first isolation of penicillinase producing N.gonorrhoeae (PPNG) in Britain and the United States (Ashford et al 1976, Phillips 1976, Percival et al 1976).

Penicillin resistance in these strains was plasmid controlled. PPNG appear to have originated in the Far East and West Africa and are still most common in these areas. In the years following 1976 there were numerous reports of PPNG isolations. Where these could be studied in detail, PPNG appeared to be acquired in areas of high prevalence and then imported into Western Europe and the United States. However, in the 1980s there was a significant change in the epidemiology of PPNG in these areas with marked increases in prevalence and evidence of indigenous spread (McCutchan et al 1982, Center for Disease Control 1983, Ansink-Schipper et al 1984).

PPNG containing the 4.4MD plasmid are known to be more resistant to non-beta lactam antibiotics (Van Klingeren et al 1985) but all PPNG infections require treatment with beta-lactamase stable antibiotics. Spectinomycin and the newer cephalosporins such as cefuroxime and cefotaxime became the agents of choice. The control of PPNG infections depends as much on good epidemiological back-up as on the use of suitable antibiotics (Rothenberg & Voigt 1988).

Adler (1986) described the pattern of PPNG infections in various countries up to 1983. Since then there has been a decline in the prevalence of these infections in Britain. The distribution of PPNG in Europe and the United States is patchy with concentrations in large urban areas. However, overall in the United States infections with PPNG have continued to increase (Whittington & Knapp 1988).

Although spectinomycin resistance had been described in gonococci (Thornsberry et al 1977), it became a cause for concern with the first reports of resistance in PPNG following spectinomycin therapy (Ashford et al 1981, Easmon et al 1982). Sporadic outbreaks of gonorrhoea caused by spectinomycin resistant PPNG and non-PPNG have been reported since, but at present there is no evidence of a sustained worldwide increase in spectinomycin-resistant gonococcal infection.

Concern over PPNG has tended to divert attention away from the more insidious but less spectacular non-enzymic resistance to beta-lactam antibiotics. As discussed in greater detail below this resistance is chromosomally rather than plasmid-mediated. Strains with MICs of 1 mg/l or more are known as chromosomally mediated resistant *N.gonorrhoeae* or CMRNG to distinguish them from PPNG.

CMRNG strains continue to be a problem not only in parts of the Far East and Africa, but also in some centres in the United States and Europe. Faruki et al (1985) described an outbreak of gonorrhoea caused by CMRNG in the USA in 1985. Over 150 CMRNG have since been reported from 22 States between 1983 and 1984 (Rice et al 1986). CMRNG are now more common than PPNG among strains of gonococci isolated at St Mary's Hospital and since we published our findings in 1987 (Ison et al 1987) the prevalence of CMRNG has risen above 10%. Fortunately this level of resistance is still atypical for much of Europe and North America.

As discussed later in this chapter, CMRNG tend to be relatively resistant to non-beta lactam antibiotics such as tetracycline and erythromycin (Ison et al 1987). In addition there is increasing evidence that CMRNG also show decreased sensitivity to cephalosporins such as cefuroxime (Ison et al 1987) and even to the most active anti-gonococcal cephalosporin, ceftriaxone (Whittington & Knapp 1988).

Low level tetracycline resistance evolved alongside resistance to penicillin (Reyn et al 1958). A significant level of treatment failure could be correlated with a tetracycline MIC of 1 mg/l. As discussed below this type of resistance rarely produces MICs above 8 mg/l and is chromosomally mediated. Recently, however, strains of gonococci have been isolated with high level plasmid-mediated resistance to tetracycline. These new tetracycline resistant *N.gonorrhoeae* (TRNG) were first recognised in the United States (Center for Disease Control 1985, Knapp et al 1987b) but have now been found in Europe (Waugh et al 1988, Roberts et al 1988, Ison et al 1988a). Tetracycline is still used to treat gonorrhoea but the worrying feature about this new development is that it is plasmid-controlled and thus more likely to spread rapidly. Its occurrence could not have been predicted easily.

The 4-quinolones are the latest antimicrobial agents to be used for treating *N.gonorrhoeae*. While gonococcal resistance to earlier quinolones such as acrosoxacin has been described (Macaulay 1982), there is a single reported case of resistance to one of the newer agents, enoxacin (Wagen Voort et al 1986). Gonococci increasingly resistant to 4-quinolones are being seen in the Far East, but it is too early to say whether this is likely to prove a significant problem. Quinolone resistance is unlikely to be plasmid mediated and this should minimise the risk of rapid spread among gonococci.

### Genetic control of antibiotic resistance in *N. gonorrhoeae*

Antibiotic resistance in *N.gonorrhoeae* can be controlled by plasmid or chromosomal DNA. While this is not the place for an exhaustive review of such control mechanisms, it is becoming increasingly important for clinical microbiologists and clinicians to understand something of the basis of antibiotic resistance and its implications for the spread of clinically significant resistance in organisms like the gonococcus. This in turn allows the most effective use of antibiotics not only to treat individual cases of gonorrhoea, but also prevent the spread of resistant strains.

*Plasmid mediated resistance*

Five main plasmids have been described in *N.gonorrhoeae*. The smallest is a cryptic plasmid of 2.6MD with no known role in antibiotic resistance. The 3.2 MD and 4.4 MD plasmid both control the production of a TEM-1 type-beta lactamase. Gonococci carrying the 4.4 MD plasmid appear to have originated from the Far East, those with the 3.2 MD from West Africa. DNA hybridisation has shown that they are closely related, the smaller appearing to have a deletion of about 7 kilobases from the larger. The same is true of other recently described beta-lactamase plasmids (Yeung et al 1986, Van Embden et al 1985, Brett 1989).

None of these beta-lactamase encoding plasmids are self-transmissable. They require the presence of the fourth gonococcal plasmid which at 24.5 MD is much larger. This acts as a conjugal plasmid allowing transfer of the beta-lactamase plasmid between strains (Brunton et al 1986). The only good thing about PPNG is that they are simple rapid tests for detecting beta-lactamase production.

Although the 24.5 MD plasmid does not control antibiotic resistance, recently the streptococcal *tetM* tetracycline resistance determinant (Burdett et al 1982) has become integrated into the gonococcal 24.5 MD plasmid. The resultant 25.2 MD plasmid codes for tetracycline resistance and is found in the TRNG described above (Morse et al 1986). The *tetM* determinant has also been found in other genital tract organisms (Roberts et al 1986).

The importance of plasmid mediated resistance lies in the speed with which it may spread. It is not simply dependant on transfer of a resistant organism between patients but can equally result from the spread of the resistant plasmid between strains. Furthermore, such spread may involve genital tract commensals as well as gonococci.


*Chromosomal resistance*

Low level penicillin resistance of the type that developed slowly in the gonococcus between 1945 and 1976 results from mutations at multiple loci on the chromosome. A mutation at each locus results in a small increase in the MIC of penicillin. CMRNG will contain many such mutations (Sparling et al 1975).

Mutations at some loci mediate resistance to a single antibiotic. Examples are *penA* for penicillin and *tet* and *chl* for tetracycline and chloramphenicol (Sparling et al 1975, Sarubbi et al 1974). Mutations at other loci e.g. *penB* and *mtr* result in increased resistance to more than one antibiotic (Sparling et al 1975, Maier et al 1975).

*penA*, *penB* and *mtr* act additively to increase penicillin resistance 120 fold compared with levels found in fully sensitive strains (MIC $\leqslant 0.008$ mg/l). Two further genes have been described, *pem* and *tem*. Neither mutation is expressed alone but rather they modify the expression of existing mutations such as *penA, mtr* and *tet* to further increase resistance to penicillin and tetracycline.

These complex interactions partly explain why CMRNG are often relatively resistant to other unrelated antibiotics such as tetracycline, erythromycin and chloramphenicol. Resistance to streptomycin and spectinomycin also results from chromosomal mutation, but the loci involved are remote from those described above. Much of this work has been done on highly characterised laboratory strains. Work with fresh clinical isolates, especially CMRNG with high penicillin MICs, may reveal other important resistance loci.

In CMRNG penicillin resistance is expressed partly through a reduced affinity for penicillin in the cell membrane penicillin binding proteins (PBP) 1 and 2 (Dougherty et al 1980, Barbour 1981). Alterations to other outer membrane proteins and lipopolysaccharide may also contribute to non-enzymic penicillin resistance.

In addition to increasing resistance to penicillins the *penA*, *penB* and *mtr* loci also appear to increase resistance to cephalosporins. There is epidemio- logical evidence for this (Rice et al 1986, Ison et al 1987) as well as shared mechanism of expression in reduced affinity for PBPs (Johnson & Morse 1988). Using DNA from CMRNG to transform fully sensitive gonococci, we have been able to demonstrate reduced sensitivity to second and third generation cephalosporins closely associated with reduced sensitivity to penicillin itself.

Chromosomal spectinomycin and aminoglycoside resistance results from changes to the gonococcal 30S ribosome which prevent antibiotic binding. The mechanism of expression of chromosomally mediated tetracycline resistance is not known.

Chromosomal resistance to antibiotics tends to develop more slowly than plasmid mediated resistance. Transformation is the only known mechanism of inter-strain transfer of such resistance in gonococci. The build up of resistance to some agents which have been used extensively, such as spectinomycin, has not been seen. In contrast resistance to penicillins and tetracyclines has been slow and remorseless. Chromosomal cross resistance between penicillins and beta-lactamase stable cephalosporins may eventually negate the usefulness of the latter for treating gonorrhoea caused by PPNG. In any case chromosomal resistance can also exist in PPNG. Finally, there is no rapid test for detecting CMRNG equivalent to those available for beta-lactamase detection. A programme of sensitivity testing has to be introduced with all the attendant logistical and technical problems.

**Current therapy**

For many cases of ano-genital gonorrhoea, standard therapy with a penicillin (benzylpenicillin, ampicillin, or amoxycillin) plus probenecid continues to be highly effective. The continuing problem areas are gonococcal infection caused by antibiotic resistant strains such as CMRNG, PPNG (or indeed TRNG if it spreads to areas where tetracycline is used commonly); together with male rectal and pharyngeal gonorrhoea. Antibiotic resistant strains can cause complicated gonococcal infections, but the main problem here is diagnosis rather than therapy.

New therapeutic agents against gonorrhoea fall into two main groups. First, beta-lactamase-stable beta lactams. These include on the one hand third generation cephalosporins, monobactams, and thienamycins and on the other combinations of a beta-lactamase inhibitor such as clavulanic acid with an established beta lactam antibiotic like amoxycillin. The inhibitor protects the active beta lactam against the TEM-1 beta-lactamase produced by PPNG. The second group consists of the newer 4-quinolones such as norfloxacin, ciprofloxacin, enoxacin, pefloxacin. These agents are descendents of nalidixic acid, but unlike this urinary antiseptic have useful systemic activity. Quino- lones are thought to act on bacterial DNA gyrase. They are well absorbed when given orally, have excellent pharmacokinetics and tissue distribution and are thought not to stimulate plasmid mediated resistance. Each of these groups of agents will be considered in terms of treating CMRNG, PPNG, pharyngeal infection and complicated gonococcal disease. As with any survey of therapy, direct comparisons between studies are complicated by variations in study design and definitions of treatment failure, re-infection etc.

First the combinations of beta-lactamase inhibitor and an active beta lactam. The most widely used combination is that of the inhibitor clavulanic acid and amoxycillin. For general use the ratio of amoxycillin to clavulanate is 2:1. However, only a relatively low dose of clavulanate can be tolerated without causing nausea. Most single dose regimens for gonorrhoea have combined amoxycillin 3 g with 125 mg of probenecid. A few studies have used amoxycillin/clavulanate in combination with aqueous procaine penicillin and probenecid. Results have been variable and not always predictable. One would predict that amoxycillin/clavulanate or penicillin/clavulanate would be successful in treating gonorrhoea (including that caused by PPNG) in areas where CMRNG were not common, but of lesser efficacy where CMRNG were endemic. Here the inhibitory effect of clavulanate on beta lactams would be irrelevant. This was borne out by Lawrence & Shanson (1985) working with sensitive nonPPNG in London. However, Lim et al (1984, 1985), working in an area with a high prevalence of CMRNG strains, found a surprisingly high cure rate with this combination. As might be expected, single dose amoxycillin/clavulanate regimens are not effective in pharyngeal or male rectal gonorrhoea.

The main beta-lactamase stable cephalosporins used in the treatment of gonorrhoea have been cefuroxime, cefoxitin, cefotaxime and now ceftriaxone. Ceftriaxone is one of the cephalosporins with greatest intrinsic activity against gonococci. Good results have been obtained in ano-genital infection with single doses ranging from 32.25 mg to 250 mg, although the latter is most generally recommended (Rajan et al 1982, Zajdowicz et al 1983, Panikabutra et al 1985). Ceftriaxone has a long half life and unlike most other cephalosporins is effective against pharyngeal and male rectal infection (Judson et al 1985) and gonococcal ophthalmia (Haase et al 1986). Unfortunately ceftriaxone is not yet licensed in Britain.

The beta-lactamase stability of second and third generation cephalosporins make them ideal antibiotics for treating infections caused by PPNG. However, this property is of no value in treating gonorrhoea caused by CMRNG, where only the intrinsic activity of the cephalosporin is important. As mentioned earlier, there is considerable epidemiological and genetic evidence that resistance to penicillin in CMRNG is closely linked to cephalosporin resistance. In recent years there has been a decrease in susceptibility to agents such as cefuroxime and cefoxitin (Ison et al 1987, Rice et al 1986) and a significant increase in the MICs of some CMRNG to cefotaxime and ceftriaxone (Whittington & Knapp 1988). Low doses of ceftriaxone, 32–64 mg, which will cure individual cases of gonorrhoea and be attractive because of the lower costs, may accelerate this process. The introduction of an oral form of cefuroxime, cefuroxime axetil, could have the same effect.

Monobactams such as aztreonam have beta-lactamase stability similar to the new cephalosporins. A single dose of aztreonam too can be used to treat antibiotic resistant gonococcal infections (Easmon et al 1985, McLean & Harris 1985). It has not been used widely and its relationship to non-enzymic gonococcal resistance to penicillin is unknown.

The 4-quinolones are the latest group of antimicrobial agents to be used to treat gonorrhoea. Their mode of action on DNA gyrase is unrelated to that of any other agents used in this area. Quinolones have the advantage of oral administration with a long half life and good penetration. They have good in vitro activity against sensitive gonococci, PPNG and CMRNG. Ciprofloxacin appears to be the most active of this group when tested against *N.gonorrhoeae* in vitro (Easmon et al 1987).

Crider et al (1984) used two doses of 600 mg norfloxacin successfully. Belli et al (1985) used doses of ciprofloxacin ranging from 100 mg to 500 mg with equal success while Loo et al (1985) used 250 mg. Quinolones such as ciprofloxacin will deal with pharyngeal gonorrhoea.

Although antibiotics have been used to treat gonococcal infection, third generation cephalopsorins, such as cefotaxime and ceftriaxone, spectinomycin and 4-quinolones, are the agents of choice for managing gonorrhoea caused by PPNG or CMRNG. There are advantages and disadvantages with each. Quinolones can be given orally and they and ceftriaxone eradicate pharyngeal infection. However, neither spectinomycin nor quinolones will eradicate concurrent early syphilis while only the quinolones offer some hope of dealing with chlamydial infection (not as a single dose). With ceftriaxone there is the possibility of increasing resistance among CMRNG. Cost and ease of administration are the key factors. With ceftriaxone in particular, cost reduction by using low doses is tempting. It may well accelerate the increase in non-enzymic resistance.

### The future

The gonococcus has proved itself a highly versatile pathogen, responding to the various types of chemotheraphy used to treat gonorrhoea. This will continue and therefore we need to use current and future therapies so as to minimise the development of gonococcal resistance in the future. Several points need to be considered:

1. What is likely to be the future pattern of established mechanisms of resistance?
2. Can the biological characterisation of gonococcal strains within a population help to predict future patterns of resistance?

3. What new forms of antibiotic resistance may arise in the gonococcus?

PPNG and CMRNG constitute the majority of resistant gonococcal isolates. As with many types of plasmid mediated antibiotic resistance, PPNG will continue to have the potential for explosive spread in areas where the normal prevalance is low. However, the lessons learnt in Europe and America over the past 10 years should enable us to control PPNG. CMRNG are a greater problem, particularly in view of the cross resistance between penicillin and the new cephalosporins. Increasingly spectinomycin and 4-quinolones, together with any new antimicrobial agents where resistance is not closely linked on the chromosome to penicillin resistance, will be preferred. TRNG have the potential for spread as the 25.2 MD plasmid involved is self-transmissable. Of course, none of these resistant mechanisms is mutually exclusive. Many CMRNG contain penicillinase plasmids. Sooner or later we shall probably see CMRNG with both 3.2/4.4 and 25.2 MD plasmids.

As mentioned earlier in this chapter, serological classification on the basis of monoclonal antibodies raised against epitopes on protein IA and IB is now available. There is increasing evidence of association between serovar and chromosomally mediated antibiotic resistance in the gonococcus. Overall gonococci isolated at St Mary's Hospital show the characteristic bimodal distribution of susceptibility to penicillin. The penicillin susceptibility of the five most commonly isolated serovars has been shown to differ (Woodford et al 1989).

Strains belonging to the IA-1/2 group are clustered at the sensitive end of the spectrum. Those belonging to serovars IB-2 and IB-3 are mainly of intermediate resistance while the IB-5/7 isolates constitute the majority of CMRNG. Cephalosporin and erythromycin resistance is also associated with these serovars. Our experience with CMRNG suggests that strains of intermediate penicillin resistance (MIC 0.06–0.5 mg/l) form a source from which CMRNG can emerge by the acquisition of further mutations. In 1984 61% of gonococci isolated at St Mary's showed intermediate suscepti-bility to penicillin while 7% were resistant. By 1987 the figures were 46% and 16.5% respectively. Over the same time the percentage of sensitive strains (MIC >0.06 mg/l) remained the same at 32% in 1984 and 38% in 1987.

It may even be that only some gonococcal strains have the potential to develop chromosomally mediated resistance. Serology may provide a marker for it. At present this is speculation but it does warrant further investigation. There is also recent evidence (Hook et al 1989) that introduction of CMRNG into a community may be due to a subset of patients. These patients have repeated infections, more sexual partners, prostitute contact and are involved in drug abuse. Serology might be used to define the gonococci being isolated in a clinic or geographical area and if used together with good patient information may allow patterns of resistance to be monitored and to predict the future emergence of CMRNG.

Finally, what new forms of antibiotic resistance may emerge in the gonococcus? It is impossible to predict plasmid and transposon mediated events. The TEM-1 beta-lactamase can be overcome relatively easily with third generation cephalosporins and related compounds. However, modification of TEM-1 could render the resultant enzyme more effective against TEM-1 stable beta lactam antibiotics. Other beta-lactamases again with greater activity against 'stable' antibiotics could be transferred into the gonococcus. We have seen the recent acquisition of the *tetM* tetracycline determinant by gonococci. Plasmid mediated low level resistance to aminoglycosides and aminocyclitols could also be acquired, jeopardising the use of spectinomycin.

Antibacterial agents need to reach their substrate if they are to be effective. The existence of permeability barriers can be an effective means of resistance to a wide range of antibiotics. In the gonococcus such a development could result in resistance to any of the agents currently in use. Alternatively, reduced permeability could work together with other resistance mechanisms to produce highly resistant strains.

This might appear to be unduly pessimistic. However, it is important to be realistic. Antibiotic susceptibility surveillance programmes which examine strains from different parts of the world are the only way in which such developments can be detected early. This is an important area for future international collaboration.

REFERENCES

Adler M W 1986 Epidemiology and treatment of penicillinase-producing *Neisseria gonorrhoeae*. In: Oriel JD, Harris JRW (eds) Recent advances in sexually transmitted diseases 3. Churchill Livingstone, New York. pp23–38

Anand C M, Gubash S M, Shaw H 1988 Serologic confirmation of *Neisseria gonorrhoeae* by monoclonal antibody-based coagglutination procedures. Journal of Clinical Microbiology 26: 2283–2286

Ansink-Schipper M C, van Klingeren B, Huikeshoven M H, Woudstra R K, Dessens-Kroon M, Wijngaarden L J 1984 Epidemiology of PPNG infections in the Netherlands: analysis by auxanographic typing and plasmid identification. British Journal of Venereal Diseases 60: 141–146

Arya O P, Phillips I 1970 Antibiotic sensitivity of gonococci and treatment of gonorrhoea in Uganda. British Journal of Venereal Diseases 46: 149–152

Ashford W A, Golash R G, Hemming V G 1976 Penicillinase producing *Neisseria gonorrhoeae*. Lancet 2: 657–658

Ashford W A, Potts D W, Adams H J U et al 1981 Spectinomycin-resistant penicillinase-producing *Neisseria gonorrhoeae*. Lancet 2: 1035–1037

Australian Gonococcal Surveillance Programme 1984 Penicillin sensitivity of gonococci isolated in Australia 1981–6. Genitourinary Medicine 64: 147–151

Barbour A G 1981 Properties of penicillin-binding proteins in *Neisseria gonorrhoeae*. Antimicrobial Agents and Chemotherapy 19: 316–322

Belli L, Castro J M, Casco R 1985 Ciprofloxacin in the treatment of non-complicated urethritis. 14th International Congress of Chemotherapy. Abstract P-38-98

Brett M 1989 A novel gonococcal B-lactamase plasmid. Journal of Antimicrobial Chemotherapy 23: 653–654

Brown W J 1974 Modification of the rapid fermentation test for *Neisseria gonorrhoeae*. Applied Microbiology 27: 1027–1030

Brown J D, Thomas K R 1985 Rapid enzyme system for the identification of pathogenic
*Neisseria* spp. Journal of Clinical Microbiology 21: 857-858

Brunton J, Meier M, Ehrman N, Clare D, Almawy R 1986 Origin of small beta-lactamase
specifying plasmids in *Haemophilus* species and *Neisseria gonorrhoeae*. Journal of
Bacteriology 168: 374-379

Buchanan T M, Hildebrandt J F 1981 Antigen-specific serotyping of *Neisseria gonorrhoeae*:
characterization based upon principal outer membrane protein. Infection and Immunity 32:
985-994

Burdett V, Inamine J, Rajagopalan S 1982 Heterogeneity of tetracycline resistance
determinants in Streptococcus. Journal of Bacteriology 149: 995-1004

Bygdeman S M, Gillenius E C, Sandstrom E G 1985 A comparison of two different sets of
monoclonal antibodies for the serological classification of *Neisseria gonorrhoeae*. In:
Schoolnik GK et al (eds) The pathogenic Neisseriae. American Society for Microbiology,
Washington DC. pp31-36

Carbonetti N H, Simnad V I, Siefert H S, So M, Sparling P F 1988 Genetics of protein I of
*Neisseria gonorrhoeae*: construction of hybrid porins. Proceedings of the National Academy
of Sciences USA 85: 6841-6845

Catlin BW 1973 Nutritional profiles of *Neisseria gonorrhoeae, Neisseria meningitidis* and
*Neisseria lactamica* in chemically defined media and the use of growth requirements for
gonococcal typing. Journal of Infectious Diseases 128: 178-194

Center for Disease Control 1983 Penicillinase-producing *Neisseria gonorrhoeae* -Los Angeles.
Morbidity & Mortality Weekly Report 32: 181-182

Center for Disease Control 1985 Tetracycline-resistant *Neisseria gonorrhoeae* — Georgia,
Pennsylvania, New Hampshire. Morbidity and Mortality Weekly Report 34: 563-570

Center for Disease Control 1987 Antibiotic resistant strains of *Neisseria gonorrhoeae*.
Morbidity & Mortality Weekly Report 36 (suppl 5S): 1S-18S

Chen K C S, Knapp J S, Holmes K K 1984 Rapid, inexpensive method for specific detection
of microbial B-lactamases by detection of fluorescent end products. Journal of Clinical
Microbiology 19: 818-825

Chen K C S, Holmes K K 1986 Enhancement of fluorescence development of endproducts
by use of a fluorescence developer solution in a rapid and sensitive fluorescent spot test for
specific detection of microbial B-lactamases. Journal of Clinical Microbiology 23: 539-544

Communicable Disease Report 1987 Tetracycline-resistant *Neisseria gonorrhoeae* CDR
1987/46

Crider S R, Colby S D, Miller L K, Harrison W O, Kerbs S B J, Berg S W 1984 Treatment
of penicillin-resistant *Neisseria gonorrhoeae* with oral norfloxacin. New England Journal of
Medicine 311: 137-140

D'Amato R F, Eriquez L A, Tomforde K M, Singerman E 1978 Rapid identification of
*Neisseria gonorrhoeae* and *Neisseria meningitidis* by using enzymatic profiles. Journal of
Clinical Microbiology 7: 77-81

Danielsson D 1986 Biology of *Neisseria gonorrhoeae*. In: Oriel J D, Harris J R W (eds)
Recent advances in sexually transmitted diseases 3. Churchill Livingstone, New York. p
1-22

Danielsson D, Moi H, Forslin L 1983 Diagnosis of urogenital gonorrhoea by detecting
gonococcal antigen with a solid phase enzyme immunoassay (Gonozyme). Journal of
Clinical Pathology 36: 674-677

Dillon J R, Tostowaryk W, Pauze M 1987 Effects of media and methods of inoculum
preparation on results of antimicrobial susceptibility testing of *Neisseria gonorrhoeae* by agar
dilution. Antimicrobial Agents and Chemotherapy 31: 1744-1749

Dillon J R, Carballo M, Pauze M 1988 Evaluation of eight methods for identification of
pathogenic *Neisseria* species: Neisseria-Kwik, RIM-N, Gonobio-Test, Minitek, Gonochek
II, GonoGen, Phadebact Monoclonal GC OMNI Test and Syva MicroTrak Test. Journal
of Clinical Microbiology 26: 493-497

Dougherty T J, Koller A E, Tomasz A 1980 Penicillin-binding proteins of
penicillin-susceptible and intrinsically resistant *Neisseria gonorrhoeae*. Antimicrobial Agents
and Chemotherapy 18: 730-737

Dunlop E M C 1949 Gonorrhoea and the sulphonamides. British Journal of Venereal
Diseases 25: 81-83

Easmon C S F, Ison C A, Bellinger C M, Harris J R W 1982 Emergence of resistance after
spectinomycin treatment for gonorrhoea due to beta-lactamase-producing strain of *Neisseria*

*gonorrhoeae*. British Medical Journal 284: 1604–1605

Easmon C S F, Ison C A, Gedney J 1985 In vitro activity of aztreonam against penicillin and spectinomycin resistant *Neisseria gonorrhoeae* In: Williams JD, Woods P (eds) Aztreonam the antibiotic discovery for Gram-negative infections. Royal Society of Medicine, London. pp 75–78

Easmon C S F, Woodford N, Ison C A 1987 The activity of the 4 quinolone Ro 23 6240 and the cephalosporins Ro 15 8074 and Ro 19 5247 against penicillin sensitive and resistant gonococci. Journal of Antimicrobial Chemotherapy 19: 761–765

Evins G M, Pigott N E, Knapp J S, DeWitt W E 1988 Panel of reference strains for evaluating serologic reagents used to identify gonococci. Journal of Clinical Microbiology 26: 354–357

Faruki H, Kohmescher R N, McKinney W P, Sparling P F 1985 A community-based outbreak of infection with penicillin resistant *Neisseria gonorrhoeae* not producing penicillinase (chromosomally mediated resistance). New England Journal of Medicine 313: 607–611

Flynn J, Waitkins S A 1972 A serum-free medium for testing fermentation reaction in *Neisseria gonorrhoeae*. Journal of Clinical Pathology 25: 525–527

Gill M J, Ison C A 1988 Susceptibility testing of *Neisseria gonorrhoeae* to penicillin and spectinomycin in a diagnostic laboratory. Journal of Clinical Pathology 41: 978–982

Goodhart M E, Ogden J, Zaidii A A, Kraus S J 1982 Factors affecting the performance of smear and culture tests for the detection of *Neisseria gonorrhoeae*. Sexually Transmitted Diseases 9: 63–69

Granato P A, Roefaro M 1985 Comparative evaluation of enzyme immunoassay and culture for the laboratory diagnosis of gonorrhoea. American Journal of Clinical Pathology 83: 613–618

Haase D A, Nash R A, Nsanze H et al 1986 Single-dose ceftriaxone therapy of gonococcal ophthalmia neonatorum. Sexually Transmitted Diseases 13: 53–55

Handsfield H H, Lipman T O, Harnisch J P, Tronca E, Holmes K K 1974 Asymptomatic gonorrhoea in men. Diagnosis, natural course, relevance and significance. New England Journal of Medicine 290: 117–123

Hart G 1973 Penicillin resistance of the gonococcus in South Vietnam. Medical Journal of Australia 2:638

Herve V M A, Georges A J, Massanga M, Martin P M V 1989 Evaluation of a method for the rapid detection of penicillinase-producing *Neisseria gonorrhoeae* in urethral exudates. Journal of Clinical Microbiology 27: 227–228

Hook E W III, Brady W E, Reichart C A, Upchurch D M, Sherman LA, Wasserheit J N 1989 Determinants of antibiotic-resistant *Neisseria gonorrhoeae*. Journal of Infectious Diseases 159: 900–907

Ison C A, McLean K, Gedney J et al 1985 Evaluation of a direct immunofluorescence test for diagnosing gonorrhoea. Journal of Clinical Pathology 38: 1142–1145

Ison C A, Gedney J, Easmon C S F 1987 Chromosomal resistance of gonococci to antibiotics. Genitourinary Medicine 63: 239–243

Ison C A, Terry P, Bindayna K, Gill M J, Adams J, Woodford N 1988a Tetracycline-resistant gonococci in UK. Lancet 1: 651–652

Ison C A, Tanna A, Easmon C S F 1988b Evaluation of a fluorescent monoclonal antibody reagent for identification of cultured *Neisseria gonorrhoeae*. Journal of Medical Microbiology 26: 121–123

Jaffe H W, Biddle J W, Thornesberry C, Johnson R E, Reynolds G H, Weisner P J 1976 National gonorrhoea therapy monitoring study: in vitro susceptibility and its correlation with treatment results. New England Journal Medicine 294: 5–9

Janda W M, Ulanday M G, Bohnhoff M, LeBeau L J 1985 Evaluation of the RIM-N, Gonochek II and Phadebact systems for the identification of pathogenic *Neisseria* spp. and *Branhamella catarrhalis*. Journal of Clinical Microbiology 21: 734–737

Janda W M, Zigler K L, Branda J J 1987 API QuadFERM + with rapid DNase for identification of *Neisseria* spp. and *Branhamella catarrhalis*. Journal of Clinical Microbiology 25: 203–206

Johnson S R, Morse S A 1988 Antibiotic resistance in *Neisseria gonorrhoeae*: genetics and mechanisms of resistance. Sexually Transmitted Diseases 15: 217–224

Judson F N, Ehret J M, Handsfield H H 1985 Comparative study of ceftriaxone and spectinomycin for treatment of pharyngeal and anorectal gonorrhoea. Journal of the

American Medical Association 253: 1417–1419

Knapp J S 1988a Historical perspectives and identification of *Neisseria* and related species. Clinical Microbiological Reviews 1: 415–431

Knapp J S 1988b Laboratory methods for the detection and phenotypic characterisation of *Neisseria gonorrhoeae* strains resistant to antimicrobial agents. Sexually Transmitted Diseases 15: 225–233

Knapp J S, Holmes K K 1975 Disseminated gonococcal infections caused by *Neisseria gonorrhoeae*. Journal of Infectious Diseases 132: 204–208

Knapp J S, Tam M R, Nowinski R C, Holmes K K, Sandstrom E G 1984 Serological classification of *Neisseria gonorrhoeae* with use of monoclonal antibodies to gonococcal outer membrane protein I. Journal of Infectious Diseases 150: 44–48

Knapp J S, Zenilman J M, Biddle J W et al 1987a Frequency and distribution in the United States of strains of *Neisseria gonorrhoeae* with plasmid-mediated, high-level resistance to tetracycline. Journal of Infectious Diseases 155: 819–822

Knapp J S, Holmes K K, Bonin P, Hook E W III 1987b Epidemiology of gonorrhoea: distribution and temporal changes in auxotype/serovar classes of *Neisseria gonorrhoeae*. Sexually Transmitted Diseases 14: 26–32

Lairsey R C, Kelly M T 1985 Evaluation of a one-hour test for the identification of *Neisseria* species. Journal of Clinical Microbiology 22: 238–240

Lawrence A G, Shanson D C 1985 Single dose oral amoxycillin 3 g with either 125 mg or 250 mg clavulanic acid to treat uncomplicated anogenital gonorrhoea. Genitourinary Medicine 61: 168–171

Leigh D A, Le Franc J, Turnbull A R 1969 Sensitivity to penicillin of *Neisseria gonorrhoeae*: relationship to the results of treatment. British Journal of Venereal Diseases 45: 151–153

Lieberman R W, Wheelock J B 1987 The diagnosis of gonorrhoea in a low-prevalence female population: enzyme immunoassay versus culture. Obstetrics & Gynecology 69: 643–646

Lim K B, Rajan V S, Giam Y C, Lui E O, Sng E H, Yeo K L 1984 Two dose augmentin treatment of acute gonorrhoea in men. British Journal of Venereal Diseases 60: 161–163

Lim K B, Thirumoorthy T, Lee C T, Sng E H, Tan T 1985 Three regimens of procaine penicillin G, Augmentin and probenecid compared for treating acute gonorrhoea in men. Genitourinary Medicine 62: 82–85

Loo P S, Ridgway G L, Oriel J D 1985 Single dose ciprofloxacin for treating gonococcal infections in men. Genitourinary Medicine 61: 302–305

Macaulay M E 1982 Acrosoxacin resistance in *Neisseria gonorrhoeae*. Lancet i: 171–172

McCutchan J A, Adler M W, Berrie J H 1982 Penicillinase-producing *Neisseria gonorrhoeae* in Great Britain 1977–1981: alarming increase in incidence and recent development of endemic transmission. British Medical Journal 285: 337–340

McLean K A, Harris J R W 1985 Treatment of uncomplicated anogenital gonorrhoea with single dose aztreonam. In Williams JD, Woods P (eds) Aztreonam the antibiotic discovery for Gram-negative infections. Royal Society of Medicine, London. pp 69–74

Maier T W, Zubrzycki L, Coyle M B, Chila M, Warner P 1975 Genetic analysis of drug resistance in *Neisseria gonorrhoeae*: production of increased resistance by the combination of two antibiotic resistance loci. Journal of Bacteriology 124: 834–842

Manis R D, Harris B, Geiseler P J 1984 Evaluation of Gonozyme, an enzyme immunoassay for the rapid diagnosis of gonorrhoea. Journal of Clinical Microbiology 20: 742–746

Members of the Australian Gonococcal Surveillance Programme 1984 Penicillin sensitivity of gonococci in Australia: development of the Australian gonococcal surveillance programme. British Journal of Venereal Diseases 60: 226–230

Morse S A, Johnson S R, Biddle J W, Roberts M C 1986 High-level tetracycline resistance in *Neisseria gonorrhoeae* is result of acquisition of streptococcal *tetM* determinant. Antimicrobial Agents and Chemotherapy 30: 664–670

Nachamkin I, Sondheimer S J, Barbagallo S, Barth S 1984 Detection of *Neisseria gonorrhoeae* in cervical swabs using the Gonozyme enzyme immunoassay. Clinical evaluation in a university family planning clinic. American Journal of Clinical Pathology 82: 461–465

Nicol C S, Ridley M, Symonds M A 1968 The problem of penicillin resistant gonococci. British Journal of Venereal Diseases 44: 315–318

O'Callaghan C H, Morris A, Kirby S M, Shingler A H 1972 Novel method for detection of beta-lactamases by using a chromogenic cephalosporin substrate. Antimicrobial Agents and Chemotherapy 1: 283–288

Panikabutra K, Ariyarit C, Chitwarakorn A, Saensanoh C, Wongba C 1985 Randomised comparative study of ceftriaxone and spectinomycin in gonorrhoea. Genitourinary Medicine 61: 106–108

Percival A, Rowlands J, Corkhill J E et al 1976 Penicillinase-producing gonococci in Liverpool. Lancet 2: 1379–1382

Perine P L, Totten P A, Holmes K K et al 1985 Evaluation of a DNA-hybridisation method for detection of African and Asian strains of *Neisseria gonorrhoeae* in men with urethritis. Journal of Infectious Diseases 152: 59–63

Phillips I 1976 Beta-lactamase producing, penicillin resistant gonococcus. Lancet 2: 656–657

Phillips I 1978 *Neisseria gonorrhoeae* In: Reeves D S, Phillips I, Williams J D, Wise R (eds) Laboratory methods in antimicrobial chemotherapy. Churchill Livingstone, London. pp 103–105

Rajan V S, Sng E H, Thirumoorthy T, Goh C L 1982 Ceftriaxone in the treatment of ordinary and penicillinase-producing strains of *Neisseria gonorrhoeae*. British Journal of Venereal Diseases 58: 314–316

Reyn A 1961 Sensitivity of *Neisseria gonorrhoeae* to antibiotics. British Journal of Venereal Diseases 37: 145–157

Reyn A, Korner B, Benzton M W 1958 Effects of penicillin, streptomycin and tetracycline on *Neisseria gonorrhoeae* isolated in 1944 and in 1957. British Journal of Venereal Diseases 34: 227–239

Rice R J, Biddle J W, JeanLoius Y A, De Witt W E, Blount J H, Morse S A 1986 Chromosomally mediated resistance in *Neisseria gonorrhoeae* in the United States: results of surveillance and reporting. Journal of Infectious Diseases 153: 340–345

Roberts M C, Hillier S L, Hale J, Holmes K K, Kenny G E 1986 Tetracycline resistance and *tetM* in pathogenic urogenital bacteria. Antimicrobial Agents and Chemotherapy 30: 810–812

Roberts M C, Wagenvoort J H T, van Klingeren B, Knapp J S 1988 *TetM*- and beta-lactamase-containing *Neisseria gonorrhoeae* (tetracycline resistant and penicillinase-producing) in the Netherlands. Antimicrobial Agents and Chemotherapy 32: 158

Romanovsky M J 1946 The current status of calcium penicillin in beeswax and peanut oil. American Journal of Medicine 1: 395–411

Rothenberg R, Voigt R 1988 Epidemiologic aspects of control of penicillinase-producing *Neisseria gonorrhoeae*. Sexually Transmitted Diseases 15: 211–216

Sanchez-Pescador R, Stempien M S, Urdea M S 1988 Rapid chemiluminescent nucleic acid assays for detection of TEM-1 B-lactamase-mediated penicillin resistance in *Neisseria gonorrhoeae* and other bacteria. Journal of Clinical Microbiology 26: 1934–1938

Sandstrom E G, Danielsson D 1980 Serology of *Neisseria gonorrhoeae*. Classification by coagglutination. Acta Pathologica Microbiologic Scandanavia Section B 88: 27–38

Sarubbi F A Jr, Blackman E, Sparling P F 1974 Genetic mapping of linked antibiotic resistance loci in *Neisseria gonorrhoeae*. Journal of Bacteriology 120: 1284–1294

Schachter J, McCormack W M, Smith R F, Parks R M, Bailey R, Ohlin A C 1984 Enzyme immunoassay for diagnosis of gonorrhoea. Journal of Clinical Microbiology 19: 57–59

Snell J J S, Brown D F J 1988 Antimicrobial susceptibility testing of *Neisseria gonorrhoeae:* a trial organised as part of the United Kingdom national external quality assessment scheme for microbiology. Journal of Clinical Pathology 41: 97–102

Sparling P F, Sarubbi F A Jr, Blackman E 1975 Inheritance of low-level resistance to penicillin, tetracycline and chloramphenicol in *Neisseria gonorrhoeae*. Journal of Bacteriology 124: 740–749

Sprott M S, Kearns A M, Neale M W 1989 Non-radioactive DNA probe to identify *Neisseria gonorrhoeae*. Genitourinary Medicine 65: 60–61

Tam M R, Buchanan T M, Sandstrom E G et al 1982 Serological classification of *Neisseria gonorrhoeae* with monoclonal antibodies. Infection and Immunity 36: 1042–1053

Thomason J L, Gelbart S M, Sobieski V J, Anderson R J, Schulen M B, Hamilton P R 1989 Effectiveness of Gonozyme for detection of gonorrhoea in low-risk pregnant and gynecologic populations. Sexuallly Transmitted Diseases 16: 28–31

Thornsberry C, Jaffe H W, Brown S T, Edwards T, Biddle J W, Thompson S E 1977 Spectinomycin-resistant *Neisseria gonorrhoeae*. Journal of the American Medical Association 237: 2405–2406

Totten P A, Holmes K K, Handsfield H H, Knapp J S, Perine P L, Falkow S 1983 DNA hybridisation technique for the detection of *Neisseria gonorrhoeae* in men with urethritis.

Journal of Infectious Diseases 148: 462–471

van Embden J D A, Dessens-Kroon M , van Klingeren B 1985 A new beta-lactamase plasmid in *Neisseria gonorrhoeae*. Journal of Antimicrobial Chemotherapy 15: 247–258

van Klingeren B, Dessens-Kroon M, Verheuvel M 1985 In vitro activity of quinolones against penicillinase-producing and non-penicillinase-producing gonococci. Proceedings of the Fourth Mediterranean Congress on Chemotherapy. Chemotherapia 4 (supplement 2): 464–465

Wagen Voort J H T, van der Willigen A H, van Vliet H J A, Michel M F, van Klingeren B 1986 Resistence of *Neisseria gonorrhoeae* to enoxacin. Journal of Antimicrobial Chemotherapy 18: 429

Wang S P, Holmes K K, Knapp J S, Ott S, Kyzer D D 1977 Immunologic classification of *Neisseria gonorrhoeae* with microimmunofluorescence. Journal of Immunology 119: 795–803

Waugh M A, Lacey C J N, Hawkey P M, Heritage J, Turner A, Jephcott A E 1988 Spread of *Neisseria gonorrhoeae* resistant to tetracycline outside the United States of America. British Medical Journal 296:898

Whittington W L, Knapp J S 1988 Trends in resistance of *Neisseria gonorrhoeae* to antimicrobial agents in the United States. Sexually Transmitted Diseases 15: 202–210

Willcox R R 1970 A survey of problems in the antibiotic treatment of gonorrhoea with special reference to South-East Asia. British Journal of Venereal Diseases 46: 217–242

Woodford N, Ison C A 1988 The effect of media on antimicrobial susceptibility testing of *Neisseria gonorrhoeae*. Journal of Antimicrobial Chemotherapy 22: 463–471

Woodford N, Bindayna K M, Easmon C S F, Ison C A 1989 Associations between serotype and susceptibility to antibiotics of *Neisseria gonorrhoeae*. Genitourinary Medicine 65: 86–91

World Health Organization 1976 *Neisseria gonorrhoeae* and gonococcal infection, Report of a WHO Scientific Group. World Health Organization Technical Report Series no. 616: 65–91

Yeung K H, Dillon J R, Pauze M, Wallace E 1986 A novel 4.9 kilobase plasmid associated with an outbreak of penicillinase-producing *Neisseria gonorrhoeae*. Journal of Infectious Diseases 153: 1162–1165

Young H, Reid K G 1984 Immunological identification of *Neisseria gonorrhoeae* with monoclonal and polyclonal antibody coagglutination reagents. Journal of Clinical Pathology 37: 1276–1281

Young H, Moyes A 1989 Utility of monoclonal antibody coagglutination to identify *Neisseria gonorrhoeae*. Genitourinary Medicine 65: 8–13

Zajdowicz T R, Sanchez P L, Berg S W, Kerbs S B J, Newquist R L, Harrison W O 1983 Comparison of ceftriaxone with cefoxitin in the treatment of penicillin resistant gonococcal urethritis. British Journal of Venereal Diseases 59: 176–178

Zenilman J M, Cates W Jr, Morse S A 1986 *Neisseria gonorrhoeae:* an old enemy rearms. Infectious Medical Disease Letters of Obstetrics and Gynecology 8 (suppl): 2–9

# 9

# Prostitution

*Helen Ward   Sophie Day*

'Historically, society has blamed prostitutes for spreading all kinds of disease. Syphilis was blamed on prostitutes. The plague was blamed on prostitutes. During World War One the government locked up prostitutes to protect enlisted men from VD... We prostitutes knew that, sooner or later, AIDS would spread into the heterosexual community and that when it did not only would we be blamed but, if history was any guide, we would also be arrested, quarantined, and worse.' (French 1989)

## INTRODUCTION

Prostitutes are concerned about sexually transmitted diseases. They are concerned for their own health, that of their children, their lovers and, indeed, their clients.

Clinicians, epidemiologists and public health policy makers are also concerned about infections in prostitutes. They are concerned about the current and potential role of prostitution in the dynamics of epidemics of sexually transmitted diseases, including AIDS.

Concern has focused on prostitutes in relation to HIV infection in so far as they are seen as a potential bridge across which HIV may reach the 'general population'.

Prostitution is an almost universal phenomenon which spans different cultures. It is widely practised but also widely feared and suppressed. Prostitutes are generally stigmatised for their work, and considered an immoral group responsible for corrupting or infecting their clients.

'An 'innocent' woman could only get venereal disease from a 'sinful' man. But the man could only get venereal disease from a 'fallen woman''. (Delacoste & Alexander 1988)

The conflation of moral evil and infectious disease ensures that prostitution is regarded by many as the source of disease. But just as it takes two to tango, so it takes two to transmit an infection through sex. Before she can infect the 'sinful' man, the 'fallen' woman must have been infected by someone else. The only way to both understand and anticipate the likely role of prostitution in any STD epidemic is to regard prostitutes as an integral part of the general population rather than a separate group.

The current levels of HIV and other STDs amongst prostitutes vary widely: the prevalence of HIV-1 ranges from zero to over 80% depending on geographical area and behavioural features such as injecting drug use. The significance of prostitution in the dynamics of any STD epidemic is dependent upon the wider nature of that epidemic in a particular area, and the local features of prostitution and sexuality.

Misconceptions and lack of knowledge about prostitution can lead to inappropriate targeting of prevention or control campaigns. By understanding more about prostitution, key professionals concerned with the prevention of HIV and STDs, as well as those who treat cases of disease, will be better able to make informed decisions about individual and community initiatives.

In this chapter we shall review current knowledge about the epidemiology of sexually transmitted diseases in prostitutes, their clients and their other sexual partners. The particular role of prostitution in both the transmission and prevention of disease will be discussed.

## THE NATURE OF PROSTITUTION

Prostitution is a social phenomenon. The idea that sexual services can be bought relates to a wider concept of society where services, like goods, become exchangeable commodities. And, like trade in any other commodity, prostitution involves the provider (or seller) of the sexual service (the prostitute or sex worker), and the buyer (the client). Prostitution frequently also involves third parties who may directly manage the prostitute, or be brokers who arrange an exchange for which they extract a fee.

Thus prostitution is not simply about the seller of sex for whom STDs are a potential occupational hazard. Prostitution is also about the clients, the mediators and, in most societies, the state which regulates prostitution in some way. Legal systems may involve registration, as in Greece, or the criminalisation and regular charging of fines for prostitution, the current situation in Britain.

Prostitutes themselves may be women or men, adults or children, coerced or 'free' workers. The majority of prostitutes are adult women providing sex for men, but significant numbers of male prostitutes service male clients, with a few servicing women. Child prostitution is thought to be a growing phenomenon, particularly in rapidly industrialising countries, just as it was in 19th century Britain (Walkowitz 1980).

The question is often asked, 'what forces women/men/children into selling their bodies?' The 'force' referred to should be clarified. Some people are literally coerced into prostitution under threat of violence or, in the case of many migrant workers, deportation. Such prostitutes have no real choice and often exist under conditions of slavery where they have no access to the money they earn. They may also have little or no control over the process of their work. But, for many other prostitutes, prostitution is a job chosen in favour of alternatives. The tens of thousands of women in the Philippines and Thailand, for example, who go into prostitution may be 'forced' to choose such work because of a lack of other employment opportunities and a need to support their families. It may be preferable to appalling sweat shop conditions in a factory.

Young people in Britain who have few job opportunities and no housing provision if they leave the parental home may turn to prostitution as a way of supporting themselves. Others with a greater degree of choice may decide that prostitution offers them better financial reward or preferable working conditions than other jobs for which they are qualified.

These considerations are relevant to any discussion of public health as they may influence the degree of control which prostitutes have over their work, their ability to insist on safer sex practices or not, and the extent to which re-training and the offering of alternatives to prostitution are appropriate parts of any public health campaign. They also illustrate how prostitution, and any diseases which may be associated with its practice, is related to wider social issues of poverty and work.

Prostitutes are thought to be at increased risk of contracting and transmitting STDs as a result of their high number of partners. As the figures presented later in the chapter demonstrate, the number of clients is not necessarily the most important risk factor for infection. Indeed very few studies have shown an association between numbers of clients and rates of infection (Padian 1988). At first this may seem puzzling, but it can be explained in part by looking at relationships with other partners.

Firstly, not all the sexual services involve penetrative intercourse. Masturbation may be the main service provided by people working in massage parlours and saunas, for example (Verlade & Warlick 1973). Oral sex on a male client (fellatio), which appears to involve less risk of HIV transmission, is the predominant service sold in certain areas of street prostitution in New York (Shedlin 1987).

Secondly, the degree of protection from infection on each encounter may vary between prostitutes. In London 80% of 146 prostitutes reported condom use with all clients for vaginal sex (Ward et al 1989). The clients with whom condoms were not used were almost invariably 'regulars', i.e. men who paid the same woman for sex repeatedly (Day & Ward 1989). Women with fewer different partners, but more regulars with whom they do not use condoms, may therefore be at increased risk of infection. Some studies have shown that condom use is lower amongst drug injecting prostitutes than others working in a similar area (Carmen & Moody 1985).

A third variable in prostitution is the particular place of work, i.e. how the prostitute meets the client. The most visible prostitutes are those who solicit on the streets of large cities, who work openly in the windows of a red light district, or who work in bars and brothels. But prostitutes work in many other ways—discreetly through personal referrals from previous clients or other prostitutes, through referrals from madams or agencies which openly advertise their escort services, massage parlours, saunas, health clubs, advertising in phone boxes, newspapers or newsagents—this partial list portrays the diversity. Each way of working may be associated with different types of clients and differing norms of work, which may have an impact on the risk of infection.

## METHODS OF STUDY

Prostitutes are a heterogeneous group. Any attempt to describe the epidemiology of STD and HIV must consider this variation in both the design of the study and the interpretation of results.

No-one knows how many prostitutes there are. Prevalence figures for a sexually transmitted disease (STD), that is the proportion of the group with the infection at a given point in time, are thus immediately problematic. Even if all cases were detected, the denominator, that is the total number in the group, remains unknown.

There are no accurate records of the total numbers working because of the criminalisation and stigmatisation of prostitution in all countries. Routine estimates are based either on the number of convictions for prostitution-related offences, on attenders at STD clinics or, in certain countries, on numbers of registered prostitutes. All these will be underestimates since they exclude those who work discreetly and avoid arrest, do not attend clinics, or, in the case of registration, those working outside the system (Papaevangelou 1989). These factors combine to ensure that the total population is unknown.

Most studies involve samples of prostitutes, which may in turn be subject to various forms of bias. They cannot be said to represent the total population of prostitutes whilst the parameters of the latter remain unknown. Samples have in general depended upon people who will attend a clinic, who are accessible to researchers through their method of work, or who are arrested, imprisoned or registered.

Efforts can be made to overcome such biases through combining varied recruitment methods and, if consideration is given to likely bias at the time of analysis and interpretation, useful conclusions may be reached.

Many surveys of STD in prostitutes are of a cross sectional design—they look for the number of people infected at any one time. Where a disease is thought to be on the increase such figures need to be interpreted alongside the incidence figures, that is, the number of new cases over time.

A disease with relatively low prevalence may still be a major public health problem if there is a high incidence. This is illustrated by the example of Nairobi prostitutes in the early 1980s. In 1981 the prevalence of HIV-1 was 4%; by 1985 it had risen to 61% (Piot et al 1987b).

Similarly where a disease has a high prevalence, such as HIV-1 amongst gay men in San Francisco in 1989, the incidence may be very low. In this example marked behaviour change has led to a declining incidence (Winklestein et al 1987).

Incidence figures are therefore particularly important for directing and monitoring the impact of public health programmes.

For the reasons outlined above in terms of the hidden nature of prostitution, incidence figures are even more illusive than prevalence ones, since they require regular screening of a cohort with, ideally, a standardised frequency. Where prostitutes attend for voluntary screening, achieving regularity and uniformity of follow-up is difficult. These problems do not occur where screening is compulsory in registered prostitutes, as in Greece, where women attend fortnightly for medical checks, but a large number of prostitutes will remain outside this sector and be missed (Papaevangelou 1989).

For true comparability of figures from different studies, the methods of identifying pathogens and the diagnostic criteria should be similar. Clinical and laboratory techniques will depend on local resources. False differences in STD prevalence may be found if standardised guide-lines are not used—for example if serological diagnoses are carelessly compared with culture positive diagnoses in the case of herpes virus infection.

Factors such as these should influence the interpretation of studies. For example a high level of HIV may be found in a group of prostitutes primarily because they were selected from imprisoned women and included many injecting drug users. The figure would then reveal little about prostitutes in the same area who did not use drugs or were not imprisoned. This note of caution is sounded before reporting any of the figures of STD in prostitutes to warn against inappropriate generalisations.

## SEXUALLY TRANSMITTED INFECTIONS IN PROSTITUTES

During the late 19th and early 20th centuries, very high levels of gonorrhoea and syphilis were reported amongst female prostitutes working in urban areas and ports. In New York City in 1911, 1563 women prostitutes were tested for STD; 66.3% were found to have gonorrhoea, 26.4% had syphilis (Kneeland 1913). As recently as 1953, 62.8% of 188 women prostitutes in British prisons were infected with gonorrhoea, 16% with syphilis (Keighly 1957).

Such alarming levels of infection and consequent morbidity are not merely of historical interest. Equally high levels can still be detected amongst certain groups of prostitutes, both in the industrialised countries of western Europe and North America, and in the urban areas of many of the developing countries in Africa, Latin America and the Far East.

Of 50 male prostitutes working in gay brothels in Amsterdam in 1987, 26% had syphilis (Coutinho et al 1988). 40% of 44 female and 6 male adolescent prostitutes in Toronto in 1987 had gonorrhoea (Read et al 1988). In one survey in Thailand in 1988, 29% of female prostitutes had an episode of STD in the month prior to interview (Sittitrai & Brown 1989). In Kinshasa, Zaire, it was estimated that 41% of prostitutes would have at least one episode of gonorrhoea each year, with 8% having some STD leading to genital ulceration. In the same study, only 25% of the prostitutes had no STD (Laga et al 1989).

Reported or documented past history of STD in many studies indicates that over the course of a working life the morbidity from STD for many prostitutes remains high.The numbers reporting a past history of STD reaches 90% in 20 female brothel workers in the Netherlands (Ruijs et al 1988). In Sydney 58% of 387 women prostitutes gave a history of past gonococcal infection, 46% chlamydial infection and 2% syphilis (Philpot et al 1988). Of the 50 male prostitutes studied in Amsterdam, 58% gave a history of gonorrhoea (Coutinho et al 1988). In Spain, 28% of 80 women prostitutes gave a history of STD (Caballero et al 1987).

The wide variation in STD prevalence is demonstrated by the figures in Table 9.1 for syphilis, gonorrhoea and hepatitis amongst selected groups of prostitutes.

As with any study, the particular factor under consideration, prostitution, should ideally be analysed in comparison with a control group of, in this case, non-prostitutes. Although there is no perfect control group of equally sexually active non-prostitutes for comparison, some studies have looked at general population prevalences, or STD clinic attenders.

In the Dominican Republic 14.6% of 2874 female sex workers had syphilis, 13.1% had gonorrhoea (see Table 9.1). These compare with estimated population prevalences of about 3 per 1000 for both infections in 1987 (de Moya 1988). Several studies of hepatitis B have shown a higher rate of infection amongst prostitutes than in the general population. In Australia, 30.7% of 163 prostitute women had serological markers of hepatitis B, compared with 5.5% in blood donors and 13.5% in female heterosexual STD clinic attenders (Christopher et al 1984). In Spain, 84% of 80 prostitutes had evidence of current or past hepatitis B, with 10% hepatitis B surface antigen positive, 7.5% were also e-antigen positive (Caballero et al 1987). In general these varied results reflect the prevalence of hepatitis B in the local

**Table 9.1** Variation in STD prevalence

| Disease | Place | Year | Number tested | % infected | Details | Reference |
|---------|-------|------|---------------|------------|---------|-----------|
| Syphilis | Amsterdam | 1988 | 50 | 26 | Male | Coutinho et al (1988) |
| | Dominican Republic | 1988 | 2874 | 14.6 | Clinic | de Moya (1988) |
| | California | 1979 | 512 | 6.3 | Female | Jaffe et al (1979) |
| | London | 1988 | 146 | 0 | Clinic | Ward et al (1989) |
| Gonorrhoea | Toronto | 1988 | 50 | 40 | Adolescents | Read et al (1988) |
| | Kinshasa | 1988 | 801 | 23 | Clinic | Laga et al (1989) |
| | California | 1979 | 512 | 21.7 | Female | Jaffe et al (1979) |
| | Amsterdam | 1985 | 280 | 14 | IVDU | van den Hoek (1982) |
| | Dominican Republic | 1988 | 2874 | 13.1 | Clinic | de Moya (1988) |
| | Netherlands | 1987 | 20 | 10 | Brothel | Ruijs et al (1988) |
| | London | 1988 | 146 | 5.5 | Clinic | Ward et al (1989) |
| Hepatitis B | Spain | 1987 | 80 | 84 | Female | Caballero et al (1987) |
| | Amsterdam | 1988 | 50 | 43 | Male | Coutinho et al (1988) |
| | Australia | 1984 | 163 | 30.7 | Clinic | Philpot et al (1988) |
| | Germany | 1985 | 79 | 20 | Female | Blutke (1985) |
| | London | 1988 | 146 | 0.7 | Clinic | Ward et al (1989) |

population, being slightly higher amongst the prostitutes. However, in Amsterdam only 43% of male prostitutes had hepatitis B markers, compared with 60% of gay men tested (Coutinho et al 1988). In general, levels of hepatitis B are sufficiently high for researchers to advocate vaccination programmes directed towards prostitutes.

The relatively high levels of infection amongst prostitutes with these and many other pathogens represents considerable morbidity for the women, men and children involved. Particularly worrying for the hundreds of thousands of women prostitutes world-wide is the reality or potential of infertility following pelvic infection with *Neisseria gonorrhoeae* or *Chlamydia trachomatis*, or the possibility of transmitting infection to their unborn or newborn children. And continuing high levels of STD even amongst relatively small groups of prostitutes represent a significant potential for transmission to their private and commercial sexual partners.

## AIDS AND PROSTITUTION

With continuing high levels of other STDs amongst some groups of prostitutes, the potential for epidemic spread of AIDS was clear as soon as the mode of HIV transmission was understood. However, the lack of knowledge about the local practices of prostitution has led to many false assumptions that prostitutes would be a 'high risk group' in all areas.

As with other STDs, the levels of HIV amongst prostitutes vary and can only be interpreted in relation to the broader features of the epidemic in a particular area, and in the context of the role of prostitution in relation to the wider organisation of sexual activity (Day 1988).

High levels of HIV-1 infection have been found among prostitutes in countries where the virus is predominantly transmitted through heterosexual contact. Explosive epidemics have been associated with prostitution in Kenya for example. As noted earlier, a rapid increase in the prevalence of HIV-1 in a group of prostitute women working in Nairobi was documented in the early 1980s (Piot et al 1987b).

Low or zero prevalence has been reported in many other areas, particularly in west European prostitutes who do not inject drugs, but also in parts of Africa and the far East (Smith & Smith 1986, Day et al 1988, Krogsgaard et al 1986).

There are a number of factors which influence the prevalence of HIV in any particular area and group of prostitutes. In Europe and North America the single most important risk factor for HIV in female prostitutes is a history of injecting drug use with shared equipment. In the US and Italy a seroprevalence of over 50% has been reported amongst drug injecting female prostitutes (Centre for Disease Control 1987, Tirelli et al 1986).

Amongst non-drug injectors, other risk behaviours may be associated with HIV. Many studies have found that the number of sexual partners was not related to the prevalence of HIV. This may indicate a low prevalence of HIV amongst the clients, or a high degree of protection by condom use. Where numbers of partners has been shown to be a factor, it is often the numbers of non-paying partners rather than clients which is significant (Darrow et al 1988, Fischl et al 1987).

Other factors related to HIV prevalence amongst prostitutes studied in North America and Western Europe include a past history of STD, notably gonorrhoea and syphilis. More recently, a strong association has been shown between the use of crack-cocaine (non-injected) and HIV infection in parts of the USA (Fischl et al 1987, van den Hoek et al 1988, Sterk 1988).

In these western countries prostitutes are at risk of HIV from behaviours which are not directly connected with their work, that is, it may not be the fact of multiple sexual partners that leads to HIV risk, but the degree to which prostitution is associated with drug use and contact with non-paying partners who may themselves be at increased risk of HIV (Day et al 1988). These factors are not independent of prostitution. For example, associations between prostitution and organised crime, notably the marketing of illicit drugs, have been documented from the early 20th century to today (Allen 1984, Perkins & Bennett 1985).

In sub-Saharan Africa where HIV infection amongst prostitutes is primarily related to heterosexual transmission rather than drug use, factors related to seropositivity include a past history of STD, particularly genital ulcer disease and chlamydia, numbers of sexual partners, use of the oral contraceptive pill and socio-economic status (Piot et al 1987a, Greenblatt et al 1988, Kreiss et al 1986).

In this situation, the actual number of sexual partners is still not the main determinant of HIV risk. When a cohort of sero-negative prostitutes in Nairobi was followed for 4 years, 71% seroconverted but the number of sexual partners was not found to be associated with seroconversion (Plummer et al 1988b).

Clearly the risks associated with high numbers of sexual partners must depend on a number of factors. Firstly, the prevalence of HIV amongst the clients and other partners, which varies widely, is likely to be important in determining levels amongst prostitutes. Where population prevalence is low, this has generally been reflected in prostitutes. This is true in Ghana, for example, where 1 of 98 prostitutes studied was HIV-1 antibody positive (Neequaya et al 1986).

Secondly, the likelihood of transmission of HIV during each prostitute-client contact will be important where there is a high level of HIV. This infectivity has been found to be dependent upon certain co-factors such as genital ulceration, other STD infections, lack of circumcision in the male and possibly oral contraceptive use in the female (Greenblatt et al 1988).

Transmission will also depend upon the degree to which condoms or other risk reduction methods are used. Whereas many groups of prostitutes in western Europe, the USA and Australia report that condom use had been practised with clients for many years before the advent of AIDS, this has not been reported in Nairobi and Kinshasa (Ward et al 1989, Laga et al 1989, Plummer et al 1988a).

As with other sexually transmitted diseases therefore, the prevalence of HIV amongst prostitutes will depend on a number of factors relating to wider aspects of behaviour, and the prevalence of HIV and other STDs amongst their clients and other sexual partners.

The varied forms of prostitution, discussed earlier in the chapter, have an impact on epidemiology. It is not only broad geographical differences in epidemic pattern that determine HIV levels in North America and sub-Saharan Africa. Within one country there is likely to be wide variation.

A few studies have considered levels of disease in relation to different types of prostitution. In relation to the method of meeting clients, Fischl found that women who worked on the streets in an economically depressed inner-city area in South Florida had an HIV-1 seroprevalence of 41%, whereas women in the same state who worked for escort agencies showed no evidence of HIV infection (Fischl et al 1989). A similar pattern is found in Nairobi, where 66% of prostitutes described as of low socio-economic status were HIV-1 positive, compared with 8% of those with a higher socio-economic status (Kreiss et al 1986).

These differences may again reflect the client group, other associated behaviours such as drug use, or it may be different practices in the actual work of the prostitutes.

Blutke reported on hepatitis B infection in four different groups of prostitutes and found the highest prevalence among women who worked in ways which meant they did not systematically use protection, 44.4% of women working privately, and 27.7% of women working in saunas were positive for anti-HBs and/or anti-HBc. Those who always used protection had rates of 12.5% (brothel workers) and 16% (private always using condoms) (Blutke 1985).

In Kinshasa, Nzila found higher levels of STD amongst hotel-based prostitutes than amongst those working on the streets. The latter had higher levels of education and fewer partners. Gonorrhoea was found in 29% of hotel prostitutes, 14% of street workers. Syphilis was also higher (14% hotel, 9% street) but not statistically significant. HIV-1 antibodies were found in 35% of hotel and 22% of street prostitutes (Nzila 1989).

## CLIENTS

Little is known about the large numbers of men who pay for sex. Particular social situations have been associated with widespread prostitute contact—military bases (peace and wartime), migrant workers including business travellers for example. Increasingly, tourism is associated with the purchase of sex.

Like prostitutes, clients are a heterogeneous group. There are few estimates of the numbers of people who pay for sex, although it is known to vary between cultures. The number of clients is far greater than the number of prostitutes. Identifying them for any study of STD prevalence is fraught with even greater problems than identifying prostitutes, as they do not form any socially or geographically distinct group in general. There are two main ways of studying clients. One is at the place where the prostitution occurs, but this is likely to be unpopular with client and prostitute alike. The second is through STD clinic attenders. This will introduce bias as it may over-represent those who have acquired an infection and are therefore seeking help.

Few studies have reported on STD prevalence amongst clients. For HIV, the available figures are as varied as with the prostitutes and depend largely on local factors.

In a New York STD clinic, Wallace found 3 out of 340 clients of prostitutes to be HIV-1 positive. They had no other identified risk for infection (Wallace et al 1988). A further study in New York found no association between prostitute contact and HIV seropositivity amongst heterosexual men with no other identified risk behaviours. The HIV-1 seroprevalence was 3.4% overall, with no difference between those reporting prostitute contact and those who did not (Chaisson et al 1988).

In London 117 men attending the STD clinic at St Mary's Hospital between 1986 and 1989 were tested for HIV where female prostitute contact was acknowledged as a risk. 3 (2.6%) were HIV positive, 2 having other recognised risk factors (sex with male partners), and the third reporting contact with female prostitutes in Thailand (C Donegan, personal communication).

In Nairobi Cameron has found a seroconversion rate of 8.2% amongst 293 sero-negative men who had contact with a group of prostitutes in whom the level of HIV was over 80%. Seroconversion in the men was associated with regular prostitute contact, current genital ulceration and lack of circumcision. In a sub-group of uncircumcised men who acquired a genital ulcer, the seroconversion rate was 43% after a single prostitute contact (Cameron et al 1989).

In a workplace survey in Zaire, 7068 male factory workers were tested for HIV-1. Seropositivity was associated with a history of genital ulceration and prostitute contact, but not related to prostitute contact alone (Ryder et al 1989).

## THE ROLE OF PROSTITUTION IN STD EPIDEMICS

We may now address the question—is prostitution a significant factor in STD epidemics?

The answer must be both cautious and qualified. In some areas, prostitutes are at great risk of acquiring infections as are their clients. In other areas there is far less infection in the prostitutes and little evidence that the client group is at risk from the prostitute.

In theoretical terms, models of epidemics suggest that where there are a small number of people having very high numbers of sexual partners, they will play a disproportionate role in transmission. Since prostitution involves a small sub-section of the population (the prostitutes) having sex with a larger sub-population (the clients), each prostitute is likely to have a relatively high rate of sexual partner change. Whatever the prevalence of an infection within the population, those with the highest number of new partners are most likely to come into contact with an infected person. If they become infected, then they can potentially transmit this infection to a large number of subsequent partners. The degree to which those with a high rate of partner change mix with those with a relatively low rate of partner change will have an important impact on the pattern of spread (Anderson 1989).

Auvert has attempted to use such a model to look at the role of prostitution in HIV epidemics in Zaire (Auvert et al 1988). But such models are based on various assumptions which we have little concrete data to support. To create a model for any population, we need to know the number of prostitutes, the total number of clients and other partners of prostitutes, the rate of partner change in clients, prostitutes and prostitutes' other partners. The proportion of contacts where condoms are used would also be essential to estimate infectivity. With such data, an accurate network of sexual contacts within the population could be developed, but until that is known, we are guessing about the likely impact of HIV in prostitutes upon the rest of the population (Klovdahl 1985).

Current models have to make assumptions about these parameters, and must therefore be used with care. Predictions based on such models can only be crude.

Empirical evidence can give some indication of the role of prostitution in STD epidemics. Some epidemics of gonorrhoea, syphilis and HIV-1 support the model outlined above in which prostitution plays a central role in transmission, others do not.

For example, in Sheffield in 1976, 17.7% of 1663 cases of locally (heterosexual) acquired gonorrhoea in men were traced to 60 prostitutes (Morton 1977). Similarly in a review of the epidemiology of penicillinase-producing *Neisseria gonorrhoeae* in the Netherlands the proportion of cases related to prostitution ranged from 21% to 79% in different regions (Ansink-Schipper et al 1984).

In 1981/2 an epidemic of chancroid was described in Orange County, California. 86% of the 271 patients with culture positive *Haemophilus ducreyi* reported recent sexual contact with prostitutes. Only 5 of the 271 patients were known prostitutes, but it was thought that undiagnosed infection in prostitutes was playing an important role in the continuing epidemic. The use of a prophylactic mass treatment programme, treating 287 prostitutes in the local jail, plus over 700 men reporting recent contact with prostitutes was followed by a steady decline in the numbers of new cases (Blackmore et al 1985).

As described earlier, local epidemics of HIV associated with prostitution have been described primarily in urban areas of sub-Saharan African (Piot et al 1987b).

Transmission of STD therefore clearly occurs through prostitution, but the contribution it makes to overall epidemics will vary. The predictive model developed by Auvert for HIV infection in Zaire suggested that whilst prostitutes would get rapidly infected early on in an epidemic, and play a key role in transmission, the elimination of prostitution would only decrease the predicted rate of transmission by 25% (Auvert et al 1988).

In the west, prostitution currently appears to play little role in HIV transmission, but the association of other STD epidemics with prostitution, such as the chancroid example, show that the potential for spread remains.

The lack of an association between prostitute contact and HIV amongst New York heterosexual men (Wallace et al 1988, Chaisson et al 1988), is indicative of the different role that prostitution may play. Many New York prostitutes are known to be HIV-1 antibody positive, mainly drug-related, so why are so few men apparently being infected? It may be that the sex involved is largely low risk—oral sex, masturbation—or that condoms are widely used and effective. It is also likely to be related to the prevalence of other STDs which facilitate transmission. In Nairobi and Kinshasa genital ulceration is common amongst prostitutes and clients. This may be less common in New York, but predictions of inner-city epidemics of STD in North America mean that we cannot be complacent (Holmes 1989).

## INTERVENTIONS

Whether prostitution is a major or minor factor in the epidemic spread of STD, interventions are urgently required to prevent further transmission. As stated at the beginning of the chapter, prostitutes are concerned about their own health and are conscious of risks at work. Given the knowledge, resources and support to adopt safer behaviour, they have been shown willing and able to both change their own behaviour and to educate clients and others in the practice of safer sex.

Historically a number of approaches have been developed by public health policy makers which have concentrated on the control of prostitution rather than the control of infectious diseases. Abolition, regulation, repression—none of these approaches has been found to be effective as a means of controlling STDs (Darrow 1984).

Prostitution will not disappear as a result of an act of parliament or a police crackdown. It may move to less visible places, making it harder to find for the purposes of health interventions, but it will continue to be practised as long as services are bought and sold and sex is seen as a marketable product. The demand for prostitutes remains—without it prostitutes would not exist—and reflects the way that sexuality and work are organised in society. As with other HIV-prevention campaigns, interventions need to be based on recognising such realities and developing strategies for risk reduction.

The key elements for any intervention are: educating those involved in prostitution about risk reduction; developing accessible health services; and, where applicable, offering alternatives to prostitution.

Promoting safer practices means reaching the clients, other sexual partners of prostitutes, the prostitutes and the managers of prostitutes. Interventions directed at all three groups have been successful in different areas of the world. In San Francisco Cal-PEP (California Prostitutes' Education Project) has been carrying out street based education for several years. Women who themselves have experience in the sex industry go into areas of prostitution and distribute free condoms, bleach for the cleaning of syringes and information on safer sex. They have organised many successful meetings in local hotels where they discuss safer sex strategies with prostitutes (Alexander 1988). Similar projects have been developed in the UK (Kinnell 1989). This approach involves peer education which creates an important incentive for behaviour change (Day & Ward 1989). Specific initiatives directed towards migrant women prostitutes have been developed in Amsterdam where tapes with information in the women's native language are distributed with personal stereos to the women.

Education initiatives directed towards clients are more difficult due to the diverse nature of the target group, but in Amsterdam a group of clients has been set up to discuss safer sex and they have been involved in handing out condoms to clients in the red light district (Visser 1988). In Sydney, where prostitution is legal in certain areas, the Australian Prostitutes Collective has been able to target prostitutes, clients and managers through schemes such as one called the Safe House scheme. Here the prostitutes' collective will award a safe house symbol to parlours in which all clients are required to use condoms and working conditions are adequate for the prostitutes. They have also encouraged the distribution of introductory letters to clients of escort services which explain, from the management, that condoms are required for all sexual contact. This prior notification by the management means that the responsibility for negotiating safer sex does not lie solely with each individual prostitute (Perkins & Bennett 1985).

This scheme in Australia is not based on legal registration of prostitutes which is what operates in a number of other countries. Rather than a legal coercion to have regular STD screening, these safe house schemes are based on voluntary participation and are much preferred by prostitutes themselves.

The provision of good health services for prostitutes is an important element of any intervention. Detecting and treating STDs will reduce morbidity amongst the prostitutes and help decrease transmission to sexual partners and vertical transmission to their children. In the context of HIV prevention, it is clear that a reduction in the prevalence of other infections can help to decrease the rate of transmission of HIV. In addition to genital ulceration, chlamydial infection and trichomoniasis have been said to increase transmission in some studies. Good control programmes for these infections will help to reduce the HIV epidemic.

Prostitutes are frequently reluctant to attend STD clinics or other medical services. They often experience judgemental responses if they disclose their profession. They fear that by identifying themselves to health workers they may be subject to 'state' interference—either through police action or social service intervention to remove their children.

The provision of STD care in Britain has been based on a recognition that accessibility is essential to reach people at risk. The service is intended to be free, confidential and non-judgemental. This should apply equally to prostitutes and their clients when they attend for care. Improvements in the service could be made by better training for staff in STD clinics on prostitution in their area. Relevant advice on safer sex and risk reduction needs to be given by people with an understanding of prostitution—guidelines offered for other patients may well be inappropriate for sex workers. The inclusion of prostitutes themselves in such training and the development of health promotion materials can be very valuable.

By offering regular voluntary screening to prostitutes in clinics where they feel confident that their work is understood, we can hope to encourage the widest range of prostitutes to utilise the service. The alternative form of medical control, legal registration and mandatory screening, may discourage participation from those who believe that they have an infection and might therefore be prevented from working by withdrawal of a medical certificate. Such prostitutes are unlikely to stop working, they will find their place in the unregistered sector of prostitution and be effectively excluded from health care. Voluntary health care increases the control that the prostitutes have over their own health which will in turn increase their commitment to protecting themselves from infection.

One of the reasons why prostitutes are reluctant to identify themselves is fear of being lectured about the need to stop work. When medical staff discuss ways of preventing STDs and HIV, it is important to recognise that prostitution can be practised safely with minimal risk of STD. But where prostitutes wish to stop working, and alternative training and employment would be appropriate, facilities for counselling should be made available in order to discuss alternatives.

The legal conditions which apply to prostitution are an important influence on the control of STD and HIV. Criminalisation does not end prostitution, but makes those who practise it unwilling to identify themselves to health workers. Repeated fining of prostitutes ensures that they have no alternative but to continue their work in order to earn the money to pay the fines. Restrictions on the collective working of prostitutes means that they may be very isolated and thus vulnerable to violence and abuse from clients. This in turn makes many prostitute women dependent upon 'minders' who offer protection on the streets and extract money in return. Reliance upon such protection also brings many prostitutes into close contact with other criminalised activities which themselves may carry risks of HIV—namely drug use. De-criminalising prostitution may prove to be an important public health intervention which would improve the control that prostitutes have over their own work, and the access that they have to medical care.

CONCLUSION

Effective interventions can promote the practice of safer prostitution which will in turn reduce the contribution of prostitution to epidemics of infectious diseases. In areas where STDs including HIV are common amongst prostitutes and their clients, campaigns to promote condom use, the detection and treatment of genital ulceration and other STD, and the offering of alternatives to prostitution are all important initiatives for public health programmes.

The World Health Organization has advocated such programmes as an urgent priority (WHO 1989). It is hoped that genito-urinary medicine and public health physicians will take up these issues and ensure that in the future prostitutes are not blamed for spreading disease but assisted in practising their profession safely.

REFERENCES

Alexander P 1988 Prostitutes prevent AIDS: a manual for health educators. Cal-PEP, San Francisco.
Allen J 1984 The making of a prostitute proletariat in early 20th century New South Wales. In : Daniels K (ed) So much hard work. Sydney, Fontana/Collins/
Anderson RM 1989 Editorial review: mathematical and statistical studies of the epidemiology of HIV. AIDS 3 : 333–346
Ansink-Schipper MC, van Klineren B, Huikeshoven MH et al 1984 Epidemiology of PPNG infection in the Netherlands. British Journal of Venereal Disease 60; 141–146
Auvert R, Moore M, Bertrand W, Kashala T-D 1988 Prostitutes and HIV transmission in Zaire: computer-based projections IV International Conference on AIDS, Stockholm, (abstract 5141)
Blackmore CA, Limpakarnianarat K, Rigau-Perez et al 1985 An outbreak of chancroid in Orange County California: descriptive epidemiology and disease control measures. Journal of Infectious Disease 151:840–844
Blutke G 1985 Hepatitis B infection in prostitutes. Off Gesundheitswes 47 (7):326
Caballero LR, Caballero CR, Caballero IR 1987 Prevalence and risk factors of hepatitis B in Spanish prostitutes. Epidemiol Infection 99(3): 767–774
Cameron DW, Simonsen JN, D'Costa LJ et al 1989 Female to male transmission of human immunodeficiency virus type 1:risk factors for seroconversion in men. Lancet ii: 403–407
Carmen A, Moody H 1985 Working women: the subterranean world of street prostitution. Bessie and Harper Row, New York
Centre for Disease Control 1987 Antibody to human immunodeficiency virus in female prostitutes. MMWR 36; 157–161
Chaisson NA, Stoneburner R, Lifson A et al 1988 No association between HIV-1 seropositivity and prostitute contact in New York City. IV International Conference on AIDS, Stockholm, (abstract 4053)
Christopher PJ, Crewe EB, Mailer PT et al 1984 Hepatitis B infection among STD clinic patients in Sydney. Australian and New Zealand Journal of Medicine 14:491–494
Coutinho RA,van Andel RLM, Rijsdijk TJ 1988 Role of male prostitutes in spread of sexually transmitted diseases and human immunodeficiency virus Genitourinary Medicine 64:207–208
Darrow WW 1984 Prostitution and sexually transmitted diseases. In: Holmes KK et al (eds) Sexually transmitted diseases. McGraw Hill, New York
Darrow WW, Bigler W, Deppe D et al 1988 HIV antibody in 640 US prostitutes with no evidence of intravenous drug abuse. IV International Conference on AIDS, Stockholm, (abstract 4054)

Days S 1988 Prostitute women and AIDS: anthropology AIDS : 421–428

Day S, Ward H 1989 The Praed Street Project: a cohort of prostitute women. In : Plant M (ed) Prostitution, drugs and AIDS. Tavistock Routledge

Day S, Ward H, Harris JRW 1988 Prostitute women and public health. British Medical Journal 297: 1585

de Moya EA 1988 Towards an epidemiology of sexually transmitted diseases in Latin American sex workers and their clients: early responses to the AIDS threat. Paper presented to WHO Consultation on STD and Prostitution, Geneva

Delacoste, Alexander (eds) 1988 Sex work. Writings of women in the sex industry. Virago, London

Fischl MA, Dickenson GM, Flanagans et al 1987 Human immunodeficiency virus among female prostitutes in South Florida. III International Conference on AIDS, Washington, (abstract W2.2)

French D 1989 Working: my life as a prostitute, Gollanz, London p240

Greenblatt RM, Lukehart SA, Plummer FA et al 1988 Genital ulceration as a risk factor for human immunodeficiency virus infection. AIDS 2: 47–50

Holmes KK 1989 State of the art plenary presentation, V International Conference on AIDS, Montreal

Jaffe HW, Rice DT, Voigt R et al 1979 Selective mass treatment in a venereal disease control program. American Journal of Public Health 69: 1181–1182

Keighly E 1957 Venereal disease in women prisoners. British Journal of Venereal Disease 33: 105–111

Kinnell H 1989 Prostitutes, their clients and risks of HIV infection in Birmingham. Occasional paper, Central Birmingham Health Authority

Klovdahl AS 1985 Social networks and the spread of infectious diseases: the AIDS example. Social Science Medicine 21: 1203–1216

Kneeland GJ 1913 Commercialised prostitution in New York City. Century, New York

Kreiss JK, Koech D, Plummer FA et al 1986 AIDS virus infection in Nairobi prostitutes: spread of the epidemic to East Africa. New England Journal of Medicine 314: 414–418

Krogsgaard K, Gluud C, Pederson C et al 1986 Widespread use of condoms and low prevalence of sexually transmitted diseases in Danish non-drug addicted prostitutes. British Medical Journal 293: 1473–1474

Laga M, Nzila N, Manoka AT et al 1989 High prevalence and incidence of HIV and STD among 801 Kinshasa prostitutes. V International Conference on AIDS, Montreal (abstract THAO21)

Morton RS 1977 Gonorrhoea., Saunders, London

Neequaya AR, Neequaya J, Mingle JA et al 1986 "Preponderance of females with AIDS in Ghana" Lancet ii: 978

Nzila N 1989 Reported in roundtable discussion on heterosexual transmission Fifth International Conference on AIDS, Montreal (abstract WAO6)

Padian N 1988 Prostitute women and AIDS: epidemiology. AIDS : 413–419

Papaevangelou G 1989 Effectiveness of interventions to prostitutes in Greece. Paper presented to WHO/GPA Consultation on HIV and prostitution, Geneva, 3–6 June

Perkins R, Bennett G 1985 Being a prostitute. George Allen and Unwin, Sydney

Philpot CR et al 1988 Human immunodeficiency virus and female prostitutes, Sydney, 1985 Genitourinary Medicine 64: 193–197

Piot P, Kreiss JK, Ndinya-Achola JO et al 1987a Heterosexual transmission of HIV. AIDS 1: 199–206

Piot P, Plummer FA, Rey MA et al 1987b Retrospective sero-epidemiology of AIDS virus infection in Nairobi populations. Journal of Infectious Disease 155: 1108–1112

Plummer F, Braddick M, Cameron W et al 1988a Durability of changed sexual behaviour in Nairobi prostitutes: increasing use of condom. IV International Conference on AIDS, Stockholm (abstract 5141)

Plummer F, Cameron W, Simonsen N et at 1988b Co-factors in male-female transmission of HIV. IV International Conference on AIDS, Stockholm (abstract 4554)

Read SE, Cave C, Goldberg E 1988 STDs including HIV infection in teenage prostitutes. IV International Conference on AIDS, Stockholm (abstract 4045)

Ruijs GJ, Schut IK et al 1988 Prevalence, incidence and risk of acquiring urogenital gonococcal or chlamydial infection in prostitutes working in brothels. Genitourinary Medicine 64: 49–51

Ryder R, Hassig S, Ndilu M et al 1989 Extramarital/prostitute sex and genital ulcer disease are important risk factors in 7068 Kinshasa factory workers and their 4548 wives. V International Conference on AIDS, Montreal (abstract MAO35)

Shedlin MG 1987 If you wanna kiss go home to your wife: sexual meanings for the prostitute and implications for AIDS prevention activities. Presented at Annual meeting of American Anthropological Association, Chicago

Sittitrai W, Brown T 1989 Sex workers in Thailand. Paper presented in WHO/GPA Consultation on HIV and Prostitution, Geneva, 3–6 June

Smith GL, Smith KF 1986 Lack of HIV infection and condom use in licensed prostitutes. Lancet ii: 1392

Sterk C 1988 Cocaine and HIV seropositivity. Lancet i: 1052

Tirelli U, Vaccher E, Sorio R et al 1986 HTLV-III antibodies in drug addicted prostitutes used by US soldiers in Italy. JAMA 256: 711–712

van den Hoek JA et al 1988 Prevalence and risk factors of HIV infection among drug users and drug using prostitutes in Amsterdam. AIDS 2: 55–60

van den Hoek JA, Jansen Schoonhoven F, van Arnherm Q et al 1984 Sexually transmissible diseases in heroin addicted prostitutes in Amsterdam 1982 Ned Tijdschr Geneeskd 128 (6): 272–274

Verlade AJ Warlick M 1973 Massage parlours: the sensuality business. Society 11: 63–73

Visser JH 1988 Safe prostitution: legalised prostitution and the spread of STD in the Netherlands. Presented at WHO Consultation on STD and prostitution, Geneva, 24–27 October

Walkowitz JR 1980 Prostitution and Victorian Society. Cambridge University Press

Wallace J, Mann J, Beatrice S 1988 HIV exposure among clients of prostitutes. IV International Conference on AIDS, Stockholm (abstract 4055)

Ward H, Day S, Donegan C, Harris JRW 1989 Sexually transmitted infections in London prostitutes. Spring meeting of MSSVD, Bordeaux

WHO 1989 Consensus statement from the GPA/STD programme Consultation on HIV and Prostitution, 3–6 June 1989

Winklestein W, Samuel M, Padian NS et al 1987 The San Francisco Mens Study: III. Reduction in human immunodeficiency virus transmission among homosexual/bisexual men, 1982–6. Amercian Journal of Public Health 77: 685–689

# 10

# Sexually transmitted diseases in the Third World

*André Meheus   Anthon De Schryver*

## INTRODUCTION

Awareness is increasing that sexually transmitted diseases (STD) are very common in most of the developing world. Evidence for this can be found in the rapidly rising number of publications on STD in scientific journals, and in the many reports on these diseases in the lay press in many countries. The actual incidence of the STD, however, is not known in most countries.

Two major new developments in the STD field have led to this changed attitude to the STD problem.

The first was the advent and the spread of penicillinase-producing *N. gonorrhoeae* (PPNG) which added a new dimension to gonorrhoea treatment. The cheap and widely available penicillin had to be replaced by more expensive antibiotics and this has not been implemented in many areas resulting in increased gonorrhoea morbidity. The second is the appearance of the acquired immunodeficiency syndrome (AIDS), which in a large part of the developing world is mainly a sexually transmitted disease, and now poses the most difficult challenge of all.

It is now clearly established that the epidemiology of STD in developing countries differs greatly from the situation in industrialized nations in at least four aspects (Arya & Lawson 1977), Osoba 1981, Piot & Meheus 1983, Antal & Meheus 1988):

1. The frequency rates of STD overall are much higher in both rural and urban areas.

For example, STD are among the top five causes of consultation at health services in many African countries. Ranking would even be higher if age-specific consultation rates were available for the 15–44 year-old age group. STD have a very high incidence and prevalence in specific population groups like female prostitutes and their clients (D'Costa et al 1985), while male homosexuals are not a significant group. Prostitution is still an important factor in the transmission of STD in developing countries, where prostitutes are named by up to 90% of men as the source of infection. They are named more frequently where they operate in a more easily identifiable pattern, such as in Asia (Thirumoorthy et al 1986) than in Africa where the dividing line between the typical prostitute and the casual sexual contact may be difficult to draw since the two groups overlap (Rotowa et al 1986).

2. Among the STD, genital ulcer disease is relatively much more frequent. The so-called tropical STD, in particular chancroid, and to a lesser degree lymphogranuloma venereum and granuloma inguinale are major causes of genital ulcers.

The proportion of genital ulcers caused by syphilis is also higher than in industrialized countries, while genital herpes accounts for only a small proportion of ulcerative disease.

3. The incidence of STD complications and sequelae is much higher, due to lack of resources for adequate diagnosis and treatment. The list of complications and late sequelae associated with STD has grown considerably during the last decade due to a better understanding of the natural history of STD.

Major STD complications and sequelae are, adverse pregnancy outcome for mother and newborn, neonatal and infant infections, infertility in both sexes, ectopic pregnancy, urethral stricture in males, blindness in infants due to gonococcal ophthalmia neonatorum and in adults due to gonococcal kerato-conjunctivitis, and genital cancers, particularly cancer of the cervix uteri and penile cancer (Laga et al 1986, Cates et al 1985, Brown et al 1985, Kestelyn et al 1987, Schulz et al 1987).

4. The epidemiology of AIDS is very different from that in Western countries: level of sexual activity, not sexual orientation is, apparently, the risk factor and heterosexual transmission of human immunodeficiency virus (HIV) is the predominant mode (Quinn et al 1986, Piot et al 1988). There is evidence, however, that genital ulceration, and perhaps also other STD as well facilitate the sexual transmission of HIV infection (Kreiss et al 1988, World Health Organization Working Group 1989, Pepin et al 1989).

Although the health, social and economical consequences of STD are huge, until recently, many governments and international donor agencies tended to ignore the real magnitude of the problem. It needed a fatal sexually transmitted infection to alert decision makers worldwide and the community to the STD problem and to generate resources for prevention and control.

STD control programmes should be strengthened (or initiated where they do not exist). This will not only reduce the incidence of STD and their severe complications and sequelae, but will also decrease the spread of HIV. What clearly should be avoided is to drain resources for AIDS prevention from the STD control budget, and to keep AIDS prevention isolated from STD control programmes (Cates 1988, Piot & Laga 1989).

## SURVEILLANCE OF STD—NEED FOR HEALTH INFORMATION SYSTEMS

STD are hyperendemic in many developing countries, often including rural areas where fewer facilities for appropriate diagnosis and treatment are available. This often results in a serious underestimation of the problem.

Health-policy planners require convincing evidence of the magnitude and seriousness of the problem to justify the allocation of an appropriate share of scarce resources for their control (Willcox 1976), and therefore an STD monitoring and surveillance system should be set up.

## Types of system

The first objective of a surveillance system is to define the size of the problem and its distribution in time, place and person. Three types of data systems can interact for this purpose: (1) clinician notification; (2) laboratory notification and (3) sentinel and ad hoc surveillance. The second important objective is a management-oriented information system that focuses on the process of control strategies rather than on their impact on disease epidemiology.

The following sections discuss briefly the nature and purpose of information systems for STD.

### 'Clinician' notification

A variety of clinicians see patients suffering from sexually transmitted diseases (specialists in venereology, other specialists, general practitioners, medical assistants, nurses, etc.) and are therefore potential reporters of cases. The precision and detail of the notification is a function of the interest and the sophistication of the clinician. On all levels, however, regular notification will occur only if the system is simple and provides periodic feedback to the clinicians.

Simplified notification systems have been proposed and are used by health care providers in areas without access to complex diagnostic tests (World Health Organization 1985, Meheus et al 1990). Cases notified should be subdivided by sex, by broad age-categories (under 15, 15–19, 20–29, 30 years and over) and by STD syndrome (urethral discharge, vaginal discharge, genital ulcer, etc.). This type of data allows for some estimate of the occurence of STD in a population, and projection of the medication supplies required for the health services. Such a simplified system can be useful for both assessing STD trends and for providing information on effectiveness of STD case management, by collecting data on cases referred to a next level of care. The quality of a system in general does not depend on the technology used but is related to the thoroughness with which the required data are obtained, the accessibility of the data, and the usefulness of the information to programme managers.

### Laboratory notification

The laboratory may provide important adjuncts to the reporting system based on the clinicians. The number of positive isolates, positive serological tests and specimens processed is a useful indicator of overall activity and gives some cross-check on official notification.

*Sentinel and ad hoc surveillance*

No routine notification system identifies all cases of infection. A method for identifying the notification biases is required in order to extrapolate the results obtained to the entire population. Sentinel surveillance systems and/or ad hoc surveys can be used to identify these biases, supplementing the notifications received.

**Sentinel surveillance.**   Sentinel surveillance is the identification of representative health care facilities that perform pre-defined disease tests on their patients and report the results to the control programme. Selection of the sentinel facilities will depend upon the setting but could include:

Random chosen health facilities

Private practitioners

Outpatient departments

Special group clinics (e.g. students, military, STD clinics if existing).

**Ad hoc surveys.**   Periodic studies can identify aetiological diagnoses among patients with urethral discharge, vaginal discharge or genital ulcer and this information is very useful for standardization of case management.

Epidemiological surveys may be used to identify prevalence and distribution of STD in the population. Such surveys are expensive and are of rather limited use for STD. However, when such surveys are being conducted for other health problems, it is worthwhile to add STD data to the survey.

Epidemiological surveys in selected population groups yield useful data on STD prevalence. Groups at different risk for STD that can be considered are:

1. Low risk: blood donors
2. Normal risk: antenatal patients
3. High risk: prostitutes, STD patients.


## EPIDEMIOLOGY OF STD

### Gonorrhoea and syphilis

As incidence rates are dependent on the accuracy of reporting, most comprehensive data on incidence are from a few industrialized countries. The incidence figures for developing countries are in general very unreliable, but estimates for large cities in Africa suggest an annual incidence rate for gonorrhoea of 3000–10 000 cases per 100 000 inhabitants (Arya & Lawson 1977). While in industrialized countries, gonorrhoea morbidity is gradually decreasing but is being replaced by genitourinary chlamydial infections, gonorrhoea prevalence in developing countries remains at a high level.

Table 10.1 summarizes the prevalence of gonorrhoea in women attending prenatal clinics; gonorrhoea prevalence varied from 0.5 to 15% in those studies and is generally between 5 and 10%, indicating an important risk of postpartum salpingitis and of transmission of the infection to the eyes of the newborn (gonococcal ophthalmia neonatorum).

**Table 10.1**   Prevalence of gonorrhoea in women attending
antenatal clinics

| Country | Gonorrhoea (%) | Reference |
|---|---|---|
| Cameroon | 15.0 | Nasah et al (1980) |
| Central African Republic | 9.5 | Widy-Wirsky & D'Costa (1980) |
| Fiji | 2.3 | Gyaneshwar et al (1987) |
| Gabon | 5.5 | Yvert et al (1984) |
| Gambia | 6.7 | Mabey et al (1984) |
| Ghana | 4.4 | Bentsi et al (1985) |
| Jamaica | 11.0 | George (1974) |
| Kenya | 6.6 | Laga et al (1986) |
| Malaysia | 0.5 | Goh et al (1981) |
| Nigeria | 5.2 | Okpere et al (1987) |
| South Africa | 11.7 | Welgemoed et al (1986) |
| Swaziland | 3.9 | Meheus et al (1980) |
| Tanzania | 6.0 | Urassa (1985) |
| Thailand | 11.9 | Goh et al (1981) |
| Zambia | 11.3 | Hira (1986) |

Reasons for the continued high infection rates are socio-behavioural
patterns associated with urban migratory movements, increasing treatment
failure rates which often go undetected and the virtual absence of contact
tracing.

The interpretation of the data on the prevalence of positive serological tests
for syphilis given in Table 10.2 is more difficult, as this may be due to
venereal syphilis (infectious or non-infectious), to biological false-positive
reactions, or in some areas, to past infection with a non-venereal treponema-
tosis.

**Table 10.2**   Prevalence of positive serological tests for syphilis in women attending antenatal
clinics

| Country | Positive syphilis serology | | Reference |
|---|---|---|---|
| | VDRL/RPR | TPHA/FTA-Abs | |
| | (%) | (%) | |
| Central African Republic | 9.5 | — | Widy-Wirski & D'Costa (1980) |
| Chili | 3.5 | — | Grinspun & Goldenberg (1977) |
| Ethiopia | 17.6 | 16.9* | Perine (1983) |
| Fiji | — | 8.9 | Gyaneshwar et al (1987) |
| Gabon | — | 14.0 | Mefane & Toung-Mve (1987) |
| Gambia | 15.0 | 11.0 | Mabey (1986) |
| Malawi | 17.6 | 13.7* | Watson (1985) |
| Malaysia | 3.3 | 2.0 | Jegathesan et al (1975) |
| Mozambique | 8.2 | 6.3* | Mabey (1986) |
| Nigeria | 0.7 | 2.1 | Fakeya et al (1986) |
| Rwanda | 4.4 | — | De Clercq (1982) |
| Saudi Arabia | 1.0 | 0.9 | Hossein (1986) |
| Somalia | 3.0 | 3.0 | Jama et al (1987a) |
| South Africa | — | 20.8 | Welgemoed et al (1986) |
| Swaziland | 10.0 | 33.3 | Meheus et al (1980) |
| Tanzania | 19.2 | 16.4* | Cooper-Poole (1986) |
| Zambia | 14.4 | 12.5 | Ratnam et al (1982) |
| Zimbabwe | 0.5 | — | Latif (1981) |

* TPHA/FTA-Abs performed only if VDRL was positive.

However, from a study on syphilis in pregnancy in Libreville, Gabon, it was concluded that most of the positive serological tests were due to venereal syphilis and that the country was facing a recrudescence of this disease. Of 47 seropositive pregnancies followed up to delivery, 1 resulted in a syphilitic stillbirth and 11 newborns developed early congenital syphilis. This convincingly demonstrates the presence of early syphilis in pregnant women in Libreville and also the inadequacy of appropriate treatment of infected patients (Mefane & Toung-Mve 1987).

In Zambia STD are the third most frequent cause for attending health care facilities. In both urban and rural pregnant women, 12.5% were found to have a positive treponemal test for syphilis but less than one-tenth of these women were routinely detected and treated (Hira 1986). Zambia has since implemented a control programme for maternal syphilis which decreased significantly adverse pregnancy outcome due to syphilis.

## Chlamydia trachomatis infections

Until recently the spectrum of STD commonly identified in developing countries was limited to the classical venereal diseases, including the tropical STD typically found under conditions of poverty and poor hygiene, i.e. chancroid, lymphogranuloma venereum, granuloma inguinale (donovanosis).

Sexually transmitted pathogens of the second generation have started to be identified in the tropical region. With the introduction of chlamydial antigen detection tests, which are easier to perform and are less costly than the culture procedure, many studies have been undertaken to investigate the prevalence of genital chlamydial infections and they are summarized in Tables 10.3 and 10.4.

In general, in developing countries, the prevalence of *C.trachomatis* infections in women is similar to the rates in industrialized countries, while infection rates for men with urethritis seem to be lower (World Health Organization Working Group 1986). As these agents cause a more indolent infection patients are not motivated to seek treatment, which is an important

**Table 10.3**  Prevalence of *C. trachomatis* infection in women attending antenatal clinics

| Country | Culture | Serology | Reference |
|---------|---------|----------|-----------|
| | (%) | (%) | |
| Fiji | 45.1 | ND | Gyaneshwar et al (1987) |
| Gabon | 8.3 | ND | Leclerc et al (1988) |
| Gambia | 6.9 | ND | Mabey & Whittle (1982) |
| Ghana | 7.7 | 25.3 | Bentsi et al (1985) |
| Kenya | 29.0 | ND | Laga et al (1986) |
| Nigeria | ND | 8.4 | Darougar et al (1982a) |
| Somalia | 18.8 | ND | Jama et al (1987b) |
| South Africa (urban) | 12.5 | ND | Ballard et al (1986) |
| South Africa (rural) | 1.3 | ND | Ballard et al (1986) |
| Thailand | 12.8 | ND | Niamsanit et al (1988) |

**Table 10.4** Prevalence of *C. trachomatis* infection in different population groups

| Population | Country | Culture (%) | Serology (%) | Reference |
|---|---|---|---|---|
| Men with urethritis | South Africa | 19.2 | ND | Ballard et al (1986) |
| | Swaziland | 3.7 | ND | Ballard et al (1986) |
| | Singapore | 30.2 | ND | Sng et al (1986) |
| | Gambia | 15.4 | ND | Mabey & Whittle (1982) |
| | Iran | 8.8 | 15.7 | Darougar et al (1982b) |
| | Gabon | 15.7 | ND | Leclerc et al (1988) |
| | Singapore | 19.2 | ND | Sng et al (1986) |
| Men treated for gonorrhoea | Central African Republic | 5.0 | ND | Meheus et al (1984) |
| | Kenya | 8.9 | 78.6 | Nsanze et al (1982) |
| Women with vaginal discharge | Gabon | 13.6 | ND | Leclerc et al (1988) |
| Gynaecologic outpatients | China | 1.0 | ND | Hodgson et al (1988) |
| | Ghana | 4.9 | ND | Bentsi et al (1985) |
| | Gambia | 13.6 | ND | Mabey & Whittle (1982) |
| Women at STD Clinics | South Africa | 13.3 | ND | Ballard et al (1986) |
| Patients with PID | Singapore | 14.0 | ND | Sng et al (1986) |
| | Gabon | 10.8 | ND | Leclerc et al (1988) |
| Patients at family planning clinics | South Africa | 16.1 | ND | Ballard et al (1986) |
| | Singapore | 14.0 | ND | Chaudhuri et al (1986) |
| Infertile women | Gabon | 7.0 | ND | Leclerc et al (1988) |
| Prostitutes | Kenya | 4.9 | ND | Nsanze et al (1982) |
| | Somalia | 32.8 | ND | Jama et al (1987b) |
| | Singapore | 10.0 | ND | Sng et al (1986) |

factor in the rapid spread of chlamydial infection and the development of complications.

The growing recognition of the major role that STD play in reproductive health, pregnancy outcome and perinatal infections has added a new dimension to the STD problem. There is increasing evidence that in Africa *C. trachomatis* and *N. gonorrhoeae* are responsible for a large proportion of salpingitis, puerperal sepsis and infertility in both sexes (Frost et al 1987, Mabey et al 1985).

## Chancroid

The global incidence of chancroid greatly exceeds that of syphilis (Lancet 1982). The disease is highly endemic in many tropical countries, in particular in South-East Asia and in East and Southern Africa. At the Nairobi Special Treatment Clinic, more than 5000 patients a year are seen with chancroid (D'Costa 1988).

A resurgence of interest in chancroid has occurred since a selective medium for the isolation of *Haemophilus ducreyi* was developed. This allowed a better identification of patients with the disease and further study of the epidemiology, clinical management and microbiology of the pathogen.

For this purpose an international research team established itself in Nairobi.

Hammond's gonococcal agar further enriched by the addition of 5% fetal calf serum was shown to grow *H. ducreyi* from 61% of males with presumed chancroidal ulcers (Dylewski et al 1986, Lubwama et al 1986).

An enriched Müller-Hinton agar which had shown similar sensitivity in Johannesburg was less efficient when used in Nairobi. However, 11% of Nairobi strains grew only on the enriched Müller-Hinton and these strains continued to grow poorly, if at all, when subcultured on the gonococcal agar medium. These findings were explained by strain-specific variations of nutritional requirements. The search for the classical 'school of fish' grouping of Gram-negative rods in the stained smear of exudate remains a controversial procedure because of its lack of sensitivity and specificity (Lubwama et al 1986, D'Costa et al 1986).

Recently, an enzyme immunoassay for detecting serum IgG antibody to *H. ducreyi* was developed using an ultrasonicated whole-cell antigen. The value of this test for diagnostic purposes has still to be assessed, but it could be a valuable tool for epidemiological studies on *H. ducreyi* infection (Museyi et al 1988).

Prostitutes play a very important role in the spread of chancroid (Blackmore et al 1985). In Nairobi, Kenya, prostitutes and casual sex partners accounted for 57% and 36% of sources of chancroid infection respectively (Plummer et al 1983). This study also indicated that women who transmit *H. ducreyi* have clinical chancroid lesions, as all female source contacts of men with chancroid had genital ulcers. Chancroid lesions are also highly infectious with 63% of secondary contacts of male chancroid cases being infected with *H. ducreyi* or showing genital ulcers.

These results, however, should be interpreted with caution because the number of source and secondary contacts was very small (10 female source contacts and 29 female secondary contacts for 300 index cases).

Genital ulcers are prevalent in lower and middle class prostitutes, the figure being 10% in Nairobi, of which 4% were culture-proven chancroid. A further 4% of prostitutes are symptomless genital carriers of *H. ducreyi,* but their role in transmission is not clear.

As for the situation in other areas, it was shown that in Singapore, the incidence of chancroid is declining, paralled with socio-economic development (Goh 1987) while in El Salvador, it seems to increase, parallel to socio-political problems there (Orellana-Diaz & Hernandez-Perez 1988).

The ability to isolate *H. ducreyi* now permits laboratories to determine the antimicrobial susceptibility pattern of circulating strains. This is an important method of surveillance of the rapidly spreading resistance of *H. ducreyi* to a wide range of antimicrobials. Pattern of antimicrobial resistance and treatment effectiveness were reviewed (D'Costa et al 1986, Schmid 1986). Recent studies confirmed a decreasing efficacy of sulphamethoxazole-trimethoprim at a single dose and the high efficacy of a single-dose 500 mg regimen of ciprofloxacine, which could become the first-line treatment (Naamara et al 1987).

Genital ulceration due to any of the three classical aetiological patho-gens—*H. ducreyi, Treponema Pallidum* or *Herpes Simplex virus*—can be extremely variable in appearance and in the absence of diagnostic tests the clinical diagnosis is unreliable. In Africa, even in areas where syphilis is highly prevalent, most genital ulcers are due to chancroid. In the Gambia, a very similar frequency of aetiologies of genital ulcerations was found as had previously been reported from Swaziland, Nairobi and Johannesburg (Mabey et al 1987). It was also found that 10% of patients with genital ulcers had both chancroid and syphilis; in Nairobi both infections occurred concurrently in 5% of patients with genital ulcers (D'Costa et al 1986). Due to unreliability of clinical diagnosis and the frequent presence of the two agents in the same genital ulcer, it was recommended to combine an appropriate chancroid treatment with benzathine penicillin therapy.

## COMPLICATIONS OF STD

### Complications in adults

*Pelvic inflammatory disease (PID)*

The frequency of PID in the third world is not very well documented but the yearly incidence in some parts of Africa has been estimated at 360 cases per 100 000 (Muir & Belsey 1980). In Papua New Guinea, it is thought that 15% of gynaecological admissions and 40% of attendances at gynaecological outpatients departments are due to PID (Mola 1987).

In Africa, *C. trachomatis* and *N. gonorrhoeae* are the two most isolated pathogens in PID (Adelusi et al 1987, Burchell & Welgemoed 1988).

The relative importance of *C. trachomatis* as an aetiologic agent was recently confirmed in a study in Gabon where 49% of women with laparoscopically confirmed acute salpingitis had evidence of chlamydial aetiology (Frost et al 1987).

*Maternal infection*

In developing countries postpartum endometritis is an important source of maternal morbidity and death.

In Kenya, it was recently shown in a prospective study that the incidence of postpartum upper genital tract infections was 20.3%, the development of which was significantly correlated with gonococcal infection, chlamydial infection, presence of ophthalmia neonatorum, labour lasting for more than 12 hours and area of residence.

Approximately 35% of these upper genital tract infection observed was due to *N. gonorrhoeae, C. trachomatis* or both agents (Plummer et al 1987).

*Ectopic pregnancy*

The risk of ectopic pregnancy increases approximately 7–10 fold after 1 or more episodes of PID (Weström & Märdh 1984). Incidence of ectopic pregnancy is higher in third world countries than in industrialized countries (Piot & Meheus 1983). In Jamaica, from 1981 to 1983 ectopic pregnancy was the third leading cause of maternal mortality (Walker et al 1986).

*Infertility*

**Infertility in women.**   STD and subsequent PID can lead to infertility in women due to postinfection tubal obstruction.

Incidence of infertility after first, second and third episodes of PID in women has been calculated to be 13, 35 and 75% respectively (Weström & Märdh 1984). There is increasing evidence that chlamydial infections play an important role because chlamydial PID is in general less symptomatic than gonococcal but tubal damages caused by chlamydial PID are equal or even larger than those caused by gonococcal PID (Cates 1984).

In Africa, the prevalence of infertility is remarkably widespread. It occurs in a broad zone of Central Africa including the Central African Republic, South-Western Sudan, North Zaire, Congo, Gabon and Cameroon, called the infertility belt (Frank 1983).

Also the pattern of infertility is different in Africa from the rest of the world. A WHO multicentre study has shown that the rate of bilateral tubal occlusions is three times higher in Africa than in Asia or industrialized countries; more than 85% could be attributed to PID. The aetiologic organisms are *N. gonorrhoeae* and, more and more *C. trachomatis* (Meheus et al 1986, Cates et al 1985, Mabey et al 1985, Collet et al 1988).

**Infertility in men.**   Urethritis in the male can lead to epididymitis, which is commonly bilateral and total azoospermia by complete obstruction may occur (Bernitsky & Roy 1986). This condition is extremely common in Africa.

In Uganda, 28% of a community sample of men had evidence of chronic epididymitis of which 6% was bilateral, while in Lagos, Nigeria, 40% of the husbands of women attending an infertility clinic were infertile themselves, and most of them gave a history of 2 or more attacks of urethritis which was either untreated or undertreated (Osoba 1984).

*Complications in children*

**Congenital syphilis.**   With the high rates of seropositivity to a serological test for syphilis in pregnant women, it should come as no surprise that congenital syphilis, which causes fetal and perinatal death of 40% of the infants affected, is rampant in developing countries (Centers for Disease Control 1988). Rates are 700/100 000 live births in Bangkok, Thailand, 850/100 000 in Lusaka and 3200/100 000 in Addis Ababa (Piot & Meheus 1983, Hira et al 1982, Perine 1983). In Zambia, 8.6% of the infants less than 3 months admitted to hospital had congenital syphilis, as had 7.5% of neonates admitted to intensive care units (Mabey 1986).

**Spontaneous abortion and stillbirth.**   The most common outcome of syphilis during pregnancy is probably spontaneous abortions during the second and early third trimester. In Zambia, 19% of miscarriages are attributed to syphilis, while in Ethiopia, pregnant women who were found to be seroreactive to syphilis were five times more likely to have an abortion or stillbirth than women who were seronegative (Ratnam et al 1982, Schulz et al 1986).

A case-control study from Zambia demonstrated a 28-fold increased risk for stillbirths among women with a high-titre RPR card test seroreactivity (Watts et al 1984).

**Perinatal, neonatal and infant deaths.**    In Zambia, congenital syphilitic infection is implicated in 20 to 30% of the total perinatal mortality which is 50 per 1000 births (Hira 1986).

This probably underestimates the problem because postneonatal infant deaths are not included and because many stillborn infants do not have clinical evidence of congenital syphilis.

In Ethiopia, syphilis was the fourth most common cause of perinatal death, accounting for 10% of the approximately 70 perinatal deaths per 1000 births and nearly 5% of all postneonatal deaths (Naeye et al 1977).

**Neonatal conjunctivitis.**    This complication which can lead to blindness has virtually disappeared from industrialized countries, mainly due to the introduction of Credé's silver nitrate eye prophylaxis.

*Chlamydia trachomatis* has replaced *N. gonorrhoeae* as the most important single aetiology even in developing countries, causing up to 32% of all cases (Laga et al 1986). The transmission rate from an infected mother to the newborn is 30-45% for *N. gonorrhoeae* and 30% for *C. trachomatis* (Galega et al 1984, Laga et al 1986).

In some developing countries, Credé's prophylaxis has been abandoned: the consequence has been a considerable increase in the incidence of gonococcal ophthalmia neonatorum up to 5% of births in some settings. Reintroduction of the prophylaxis drastically reduced the incidence by 83% when using silver nitrate and by 93% when using tetracycline ointment (Laga et al 1988) so it is clearly necessary to reintroduce the prophylaxis where it has been revoked and to enforce the practice where it exists.

**Prematurity, low birth weight, neonatal and infant infections.** Prematurity is still an important cause of neonatal death, mostly as a consequence of infection. The aetiologic link with *N. gonorrhoeae* and *C. trachomatis* is suspected but has not been clearly established (Gravett et al 1986, Sweet et al 1987, Berman et al 1987, Harrison et al 1983).

Apart from *T. pallidum*, other STD pathogens can also cause neonatal and infant infection. In a study in Kenya, 12% of the infants born to *C. trachomatis* culture-positive mothers developed pneumonia, while none in a control group of non-exposed did so (Datta et al 1988).

## ANTIBIOTIC SENSITIVITY OF N. GONORRHOEAE

Resistance to antimicrobial agents by the gonococcus has been evolving since the availability of sulphonamides (Dunlop 1949); and the same pattern has been seen for penicillin. While initially 150 000 units of penicillin cured gonorrhoea, this dose increased to 4 800 000 units of procaine penicillin G plus 1g of probenicid in the seventies (Meheus 1987).

A similar and genetically linked increase in tetracycline resistance has been observed. In many areas of Africa and Southeast Asia, tetracycline resistance has reached levels associated with unacceptable high treatment failure rates (Meheus et al 1984, Brown et al 1982).

Beginning in 1975, the first beta-lactamase producing strains of *N. gonorrhoeae* (PPNG) emerged in the Far East and in West Africa (Meheus 1987); the West African strain spread to West and Central Africa and to Europe while the Asian strain spread to all areas of the world, including West, Central and East Africa (Perine et al 1977). PPNG strains are now distributed worldwide and can be found in any country if laboratory capabilities allow for their identification. The prevalence of PPNG is highest in South East Asia and Subsaharan Africa, now ranging from 20 to 80%.

## Southeast Asia

Up to 35 to 60% of cases of gonorrhoea in South east Asia are now caused by PPNG (Lim et al 1986). In Singapore, at one clinic, the proportion of gonococcal isolates which produced beta-lactamase increased from 0.1 in 1976 to 35.3 in 1985 (Chan & Thirumoorthy 1987). In the Philippines, as early as 1977, 30–50% of gonococcal isolates among bar girls or prostitutes around military camps were PPNG (Perine et al 1979). In Thailand, prevalence of beta-lactamase producing strains increased from 7% in 1978 to 42% in 1981 (Brown et al 1982). In India between 12 and 16% of gonococcal isolates are PPNG (Kulkarni et al 1987).

## Africa

The subject has been reviewed recently (Osoba 1986) and the presence of PPNG strains was confirmed in at least 30 of 45 African countries. Once PPNG strains were introduced in an African country they increased quickly and nearly exponentially and reached levels of 10–30% prevalence in 2 or 3 years. In Ibadan, Nigeria, PPNG strains were first detected in 1979 and by 1984, 81% of gonococci were PPNG (Osoba 1986).

Similarly in Nairobi, Kenya, PPNG strains increased from 4% in 1981 to 50% in 1984 (Laga et al 1986).

Whereas outbreaks of PPNG could be contained in most European countries, these strains established themselves quickly and very firmly in African countries, where they are now highly endemic. An explanation for this is the poor effectiveness of gonorrhoea control programmes in sub-Saharan Africa. In particular the abandonment of treatment of gonorrhoea with penicillin in favour of the more effective antimicrobials such as spectinomycin or the newer cephalosporins has not been implemented.

Another factor has probably been that the 'Africa' PPNG strains acquired the large 24.5 MDa conjugative plasmid in addition to the small 3.2 MDa plasmid promoting greater stability.

## CONCLUSION

Although the health and economic consequences of STD remain enormous, particularly in developing countries, many governments and international donor agencies still tended to ignore the real magnitude of the STD problem, until recently. Unfortunately, a fatal sexually transmitted infection, AIDS, was needed to alert worldwide decision makers and the community alike to the STD problem and to generate resources for the control of these infections. This is particularly true in developing countries because the AIDS epidemic has been increasing more rapidly there than anywhere else and evidence is accumulating that other sexually transmitted diseases, in particular genital ulcers, enhance HIV transmission. For optimal efficiency, AIDS prevention should be closely linked or integrated with comprehensive STD control. Separating AIDS and the other STD in national control programmes creates a false dichotomy which detracts from the commonality of intervention strategies.

REFERENCES

Adelusi B, Adetoro O, Adewole F, Osoba A O 1987 Epidemiology of acute pelvic inflammatory disease in a female population attending an STD clinic in Ibadan. African Journal of Sexually Transmitted Diseases 3: 9–11
Antal G M, Meheus A 1988 Sexually transmitted diseases in developing countries. Current Opinion in Infectious Diseases 1: 26–32
Arya O P, Lawson J B 1977 Sexually transmitted diseases in the tropics. Epidemiological, diagnostic, therapeutic and control aspects. Tropical Doctor 7: 51–56
Ballard R C, Fehler H G, Piot P 1986 Chlamydial infection in the eye and genital tract in developing societies. In: Oriel J D, Ridgway G, Schachter J, Taylor-Robinson D, Ward M (eds) Chlamydial infections. Cambridge University Press. pp 479–486
Bentsi C, Klufio C A, Perine P L et al 1985 Genital infections with *Chlamydia trachomatis* and *Neisseria gonorrhoeae* in Ghanaian women. Genitourinary Medicine 61: 48–50
Berman S M, Harrison H R, Boyce W T, Haffner W J, Lewis M, Arthur J B 1987 Low birth weight, prematurity and postpartum endometritis. Journal of the American Medical Association 257: 1189–1194
Bernitsky L G, Roy J B 1986 Male infertility and genitourinary infections. Infertility 9: 129–144
Blackmore C A, Limpakarnjanarat K, Rigau-Perez J G, Albritton W L, Greenwood J R 1985 An outbreak of chancroid in Orange County, California: descriptive epidemiology and disease-control measures. Journal of Infectious Diseases 151: 840–844
Brown S, Warnnissorn T, Biddle J, Panikabutra K, Traisupa A 1982 Antimicrobial resistance of *Neisseria gonorrhoeae* in Bangkok: is single-drug treatment passé. Lancet ii: 1366–1368
Brown S T, Zacarias F, Aral S O 1985 STD control in less developed countries: the time is now. International Journal of Epidemiology 14: 505–509
Burchell H J, Welgemoed N C 1988 Die mikrobiologiese etiologie van akute bekken — infektiewe siekte in Pelonomi-hospitaal, Bloemfontein. South African Medical Journal 73: 81–82
Cates W Jr 1984 Sexually transmitted organisms and infertility: the proof of the pudding. Sexually Transmitted Diseases 11: 113–116

Cates W 1988 The 'other' STD's: do they really matter ? Journal of the American Medical
   Association 259: 3606–3608
Cates W Jr, Farley T M, Rowe P J 1985 Worldwide patterns of infertility: is Africa different?
   Lancet ii: 596–598
Centers for Disease Control 1988 Guidelines for the prevention and control of congenital
   syphilis. Morbidity and Mortality Weekly Report 37: S1: 1–13
Chan R K, Thirumoorthy T 1987 A decade of PPNG in Singapore. Annals of the Academy
   of Medicine 16: 639–643
Chaudhuri P, Sng E H, Yuen W S 1986 Chlamydia trachomatis infection in unmarried
   women seeking abortion. Genitourinary Medicine 62: 17–18
Collet M, Reniers J, Frost E et al 1988 Infertility in Central Africa: infection is the cause.
   International Journal of Gynecology & Obstetrics 26: 423–428
Cooper-Poole B 1986 Prevalence of syphilis in Mbeya, Tanzania—the validity of the VDRL
   as a screening test. East African Medical Journal 63: 646–650
Darougar S, Forsey T, Osoba A O, Dines RJ, Adelusi B, Coker G O 1982a Chlamydial
   genital infection in Ibadan, Nigeria. British Journal of Venereal Diseases 58: 366–369
Darougar S, Jones B R, Cornell L, Treharne J D, Dwyer RS, Aramesh B 1982b Chlamydial
   urethral infection in Teheran. British Journal of Venereal Diseases 58: 374–376.
Datta P, Laga M, Plummer F A et al 1988 Infection and disease after perinatal exposure to
   Chlamydia trachomatis in Nairobi, Kenya. Journal of Infectious Diseases 158: 524–528
D'Costa L J 1988 Personal communication
D'Costa L, Plummer F A, Bowmer I et al 1985 Prostitutes are a major reservoir of sexually
   transmitted diseases in Nairobi, Kenya. Sexually Transmitted Diseases 12: 64–67
D'Costa L J, Bowmer I, Nsanze H et al 1986 Advances in the diagnosis and management of
   chancroid. Sexually Transmitted Diseases 13 (Suppl.) 189–191
De Clercq A 1982 Problèmes en obstétrique et gynécologie In: Meheus A, Butera A,
   Eylenbosch W, Gatera G, Kivits M, Musafili I (eds) Santé et maladies en Rwanda AGCD,
   Bruxelles. pp 627–656
Dunlop E M 1949 Gonorrhoea and the sulphonamides. British Journal of Venereal Diseases
   25: 81–83
Dylewski J, Nsanze H, Maitha G, Ronald A 1986 Laboratory diagnosis of Haemophilus
   ducreyi: sensitivity of culture media. Diagnostic Microbiology in Infectious Diseases 4:
   241–245
Fakeya R, Onile B, Odugbemi T 1986 Antitreponemal antibodies among antenatal patients at
   the University of Ilorin Teaching Hospital. African Journal of Sexually Transmitted
   Diseases 1:9–10
Frank O 1983 Infertility in sub-Saharan Africa: estimates and implications. Population and
   Development Review 9: 137–144
Frost E, Collet M, Reniers J, Leclerc A, Ivanoff B, Meheus A 1987 Importance of
   chlamydial antibodies in acute salpingitis in Central Africa. Genitourinary Medicine 63:
   176–178
Galega F P, Heymann D L, Nasah B T 1984 Gonococcal ophthalmia neonatorum: the case
   for prophylaxis in tropical Africa. Bulletin of the World Health Organization 62: 95–98
George W F 1974 An approach to VD control based on a study in Kingston, Jamaica. British
   Journal of Venereal Diseases 50: 222–227
Goh C L 1987 Chancroid — a review. Annals of the Academy of Medicine 16: 680–682
Goh T, Ngeow Y F, Teoh S K 1981 Screening for gonorrhea in a prenatal clinic in
   Southeast Asia. Sexually Transmitted Diseases 8: 67–69
Gravett M G, Nelson H P, De Rouen T, Critchlow C, Eschenbach D A Holmes KK 1986
   Independent associations of bacterial vaginosis and Chlamydia trachomatis infection with
   adverse pregnancy outcome. Journal of the American Medical Association 256: 1899–1903
Grinspun M S, Goldenberg R V 1977 Epidemiologia y control de la sifilis en el area sur,
   Santiago, Chile. Boletin de la Oficina Sanitaria Panamericana 83: 48–55
Gyaneshwar R, Nsanze H, Singh K P, Pillay S, Seruvatu I 1987 The prevalence of sexually
   transmitted disease agents in pregnant women in Suva. Australian and New Zealand
   Journal of Obstetrics and Gynaecology 27: 213–215
Harrison H R, Alexander E R, Weinstein L, Lewis M, Nash M, Sim D A 1983 Cervical
   Chlamydia trachomatis and mycoplasmal infections in pregnancy. Journal of the American
   Medical Association 250: 1721–1727
Hira S K 1986 Sexually transmitted diseases — a menace to mothers and children. World

Health Forum 7: 243–247

Hira S K, Bhat C J, Ratnam A V, Chintu C, Mulenga R C 1982 Congenital syphilis in Lusaka — II. Incidence at birth and potential risk among hospital deliveries. East African Medical Journal 59: 306–310

Hira S K, Bhat G J, Ratnam A V, Chintu C 1987 Maternal and congenital syphilis in Zambia — some epidemiological aspects. African Journal of Sexually Transmitted Diseases 3: 3–6

Hodgson J E, Shi Y F, Goa Y-L, Wu K-J, Jiang B Y, Chen Y L 1988 Chlamydial infection in a Chinese gynecologic outpatient clinic. Obstetrics & Gynecology 72: 96–100

Hossein A 1986 Serological tests for syphilis in Saudi Arabia. Genitourinary Medicine 62: 293–297

Jama H, Hederstedt B, Osman S, Omar K, Isse A, Bygdeman S 1987a Syphilis in women of reproductive age in Mogadishu, Somalia: serological survey. Genitourinary Medicine 63: 326–328

Jama H, Ismail S O, Isse K, Omar K, Lidbrink P, Bygdeman S 1987b Genital *Chlamydia trachomatis* infection in pregnant women and female prostitutes in Mogadishu, Somalia. African Journal of Sexually Transmitted Diseases 2: 17–25

Jegathesan M, Fan Y H, Ong K J 1975 Seroreactivity to syphilis in Malaysian blood donors and expectant mothers. Southeast Asian Journal of Tropical Medicine and Public Health 6: 413–418

Kestelyn P, Bogaerts J, Meheus A 1987 Gonorrheal keratoconjunctivitis in African adults. Sexually Transmitted Diseases 14: 191–194

Kreiss J, Caraël M, Meheus A 1988 Role of sexually transmitted diseases in transmitting human immunodeficiency virus (Editorial). Genitourinary Medicine 64: 1–2

Kulkarni M G, Mehta P R, Rairikar S V, Murti P K, Banker DD 1987 Incidence of penicillinase producing *Neisseria gonorrhoeae* (PPNG) and their antibiotic sensitivity pattern in Bombay. Indian Journal of Sexually Transmitted Diseases 8: 7–9

Laga M, Plummer F A, Nzanse H et al 1986 Epidemiology of ophthalmia neonatorum in Kenya. Lancet 2: 1145–1148

Laga M, Plummer F A, Piot et al 1988 Prophylaxis of gonococcal and chlamydial ophthalmia neonatorum. New England Journal of Medicine 318: 653–657

Lancet Editorial 1982 Chancroid 2: 747–748

Latif A S 1981 Sexually transmitted diseases in clinic patients in Salisbury, Zimbabwe. British Journal of Veneral Diseases 57: 181–183

Leclerc A, Frost A, Collet M, Goeman J, Bedjabaga L 1988 Urogenital *Chlamydia trachomatis* in Gabon: an unrecognised epidemic. Genitourinary Medicine 64: 308–311

Lim K B, Thirumoorthy T, Lee C T, Sng E, Tan T 1986 Clinical experience in the use of clavulanic acid/penicillin regimens in the treatment of uncomplicated gonorrhoea. Annals of the Academy of Medicine 15: 258–261

Lubwama S W, Plummer F A, Ndinya-Achola J, Nsanze H, Naamara W 1986 Isolation and identification of *Haemophilus ducreyi* in a clinical laboratory. Journal of Medical Microbiology 22: 175–178

Mabey DCW 1986 Syphilis in SubSaharan Africa. African Journal of Sexually Transmitted Diseases 2:61–64

Mabey D C W, Whittle H C 1982 Genital and neonatal chlamydial infection in a trachoma endemic area. Lancet 2: 300–301

Mabey D C W, Lloyd-Evans N E, Conteh S, Forsey T 1984 Sexually transmitted diseases among randomly selected attenders at antenatal clinic in the Gambia. British Journal of Venereal Diseases 60: 331–336

Mabey D C W, Ogbaselassie G, Robertson J N, Heckels J E, Ward M E 1985 Chlamydial and gonococcal serology in women with tubal occlusion compared with pregnant controls. Bulletin of the World Health Organization 63: 1107–1113

Mabey D C W, Wall R A, Bello C S 1987 Aetiology of genital ulceration in the Gambia. Genitourinary Medicine 63: 312–315

Mefane C, Toung-Mve M 1987 Syphilis chez la femme enceinte à Libreville (Gabon). Bulletin de la Société de Pathologie Exotique 80: 162–170

Meheus A 1987 Gonorrhoea in Osoba A O (ed) Balliére's Clinical Tropical Medicine and Communicable Diseases 2: 17–31

Meheus A, Friedman F, Van Dyck E, Guyver T 1980 Genital infections in prenatal and family planning attendants in Swaziland. East African Medical Journal 57: 212–217

Meheus A, Widy-Wirski R, D'Costa J, Van Dyck E, Delgadillo R, Piot P 1984 Treatment of gonorrhoea in males in the Central African Republic with spectinomycin and procaine penicillin. Bulletin of the World Health Organization 62: 89–94

Meheus A, Reniers J, Collet M 1986 Determinants of infertility in Africa. African Journal of Sexually Transmitted Diseases 2: 31–35

Meheus A, Schulz K F, Cates W Jr 1990 Development of prevention and control programs for sexually tramsmitted diseases in developing countries. In: Holmes KK et al (eds) Sexually transmitted diseases, 2nd Edn. New York, McGraw-Hill pp 1041–1046

Mola G 1987 Pelvic inflammatory disease. Papua New Guinea Medical Journal 30: 1–2

Muir D G, Belsey M A 1980 Pelvic inflammatory disease and its consequences in the developing world. American Journal of Obstetrics and Gynecology 138: 913–928

Museyi K, Van Dyck E, Vervoort T, Taylor D, Hoge C, Piot P 1988 Use of an enzyme immunoassay to detect serum IgG antibodies to *Haemophilus ducreyi*. Journal of Infectious Diseases 157: 1039–1043

Naamara W, Plummer F A, Greenblatt R M, D'Costa L J, Ndinya-Achola J O, Ronald A R 1987 Treatment of chancroid with ciprofloxacin: a prospective, randomized clinical trial. American Journal of Medicine 82 (suppl 4A): 317–320

Naeye M, Tafari N, Marboe C, Judge D M 1977 Causes of perinatal mortality in an African city. Bulletin of the World Health Organization 55: 63–65

Nasah B T, Nguematcha R, Eyong M, Godwin S 1980 Gonorrhea, trichomonas and candida among gravid and nongravid women in Cameroon. International Journal of Gynecology & Obstetrics 14: 48–52

Niamsanit S, Nunthapisud P, Limpongsanurak S 1988 Prevalence of *Chlamydia trachomatis* among women attending an antenatal clinic in Bangkok. Southeast Asian Journal of Tropical Medicine and Public Health 19: 609–613

Nsanze H, Waigwa S R, Mirza N, Plummer F, Roelants P, Piot P 1982 Chlamydial infections in selected populations in Kenya. In: Mardh P A, Holmes K K, Oriel J D, Piot P, Schachter J (eds) Chlamydial infections. Elsevier, Amsterdam pp 421–424

Okpere E E, Obaseiki-Ebor E E, Oyaide S M 1987 Type of intrauterine contraceptive device (IUCD) used and the incidence of asymptomatic *Neisseria gonorrhoeae*. African Journal of Sexually Transmitted Diseases 3: 7–8

Orellana-Diaz O, Hernandez-Perez E 1988 Chancroid in El Salvador. Increasing incidence, clinical features and therapeutics. International Journal of Dermatology 27: 243–245

Osoba A O 1981 Sexually transmitted diseases in tropical Africa. British Journal of Venereal Diseases 57: 89–94

Osoba A O 1984 A review of sexually transmitted diseases and male infertility in Subsaharan Africa. African Journal of Sexually Transmitted Diseases 1: 67–70

Osoba A O 1986 Overview of Penicillinase producing *Neisseria gonorrheae* in Africa. African Journal of Sexually Transmitted Diseases 2: 51–64

Pepin J, Plummer F A, Brunham R C, Piot P, Cameron D W, Ronald A R 1989 Editorial review. The interaction of HIV infection and other sexually transmitted diseases: an opportunity for intervention. AIDS 3: 3–9

Perine P L 1983 Congenital syphilis in Ethiopia. Medical Journal of Zambia 17: 12–14

Perine P L, Thornsberry C, Schalla W et al 1977 Evidence of two distinct types of penicillinase-producing *Neisseria gonorrhoeae*. Lancet 2: 993–995

Perine P L, Morton R S, Piot P, Siegel M S, Antal G M 1979 Epidemiology and treatment of penicillinase-producing *Neisseria gonorrhoeae*. Sexually Transmitted Diseases 6 (suppl): 152–158

Piot P, Laga M 1989 Genital ulcers, other sexually transmitted diseases and the sexual transmission of HIV. British Medical Journal 298: 623–624

Piot P, Meheus A 1983 Epidémiologie des maladies sexuellement transmissibles dans les pays en developement. Annales de la Société Belge de Médecine Tropicale 63: 87–110

Piot P, Plummer F A, Mhalu F S, Lambouray J L, Chin J, Mann J 1988 AIDS: an international perspective. Science 239: 573–579

Plummer F A, D'Costa L J, Nsanze H, Dylewski J, Karasira P, Ronald A R 1983 Epidemiology of chancroid and *Haemophilus ducreyi* in Nairobi, Kenya. Lancet ii: 1293–1295

Plummer F A, Laga M, Brunham R C et al 1987 Postpartum upper genital tract infections in Nairobi, Kenya: epidemiology, etiology and risk factors. Journal of Infectious Diseases 156: 92–98

Quinn T C, Mann J M, Curran J W, Piot P 1986 AIDS in Africa: an epidemiologic paradigm Science 234: 955–963

Ratnam A V, Din S N, Hira S K et al 1982 Syphilis in pregnant women in Zambia. British Journal of Veneral Diseases 58: 355–358

Rotawa N A, Ajayi I O, Osoba A O 1986 Casual contacts of the infective type — an infective pool of gonorrhoea in a developing country. African Journal of Sexually Transmitted Diseases 2: 16–18

Schmid G P 1986 The treatment of chancroid. Journal of the American Medical Association 255: 1757–1762

Schmid G P, Sanders L L, Blount J H et al 1987 Chancroid in the United States. Journal of the American Medical Association 258: 3265–3268

Schulz K F, Cates W, O'Mara P 1986 A synopsis of the problems in Africa of syphilis and gonorrhoea during pregnancy. African Journal of Sexually Transmitted Diseases 2: 56–60

Schulz K F, Cates W Jr, O'Mara P 1987 Pregnancy loss, infant death and suffering: the legacy of syphilis and gonorrhoea in Africa. Genitourinary Medicine 63: 320–325

Sng E, Thirumoorthy T, Yuen W S 1986 Isolation of *C. trachomatis* in Singapore. Annals of the Academy of Medicine 15: 3–5

Sweet R L, Landers D V, Walker C, Schachter J 1987 *Chlamydia trachomatis* infection and pregnancy outcome. American Journal of Obstetrics and Gynecology 156: 824–833

Thirumoorthy T, Lee C T, Lim K B 1986 Epidemiology of infectious syphilis in Singapore. Genitourinary Medicine 62: 75–77

Urassa E J N 1985 Some aspects of sexually transmitted diseases in obstetrics and gynaecology. Proceedings of the symposium on sexually transmitted diseases, Dar Es Salaam. pp 23–28

Walker G J, Ashley D E, McCaw A M, Bernard G W 1986 Maternal mortality in Jamaica. Lancet i: 486–488

Watson P A 1985 The use of screening tests for sexually transmitted diseases in a third world community. European Journal of Sexually Transmitted Diseases 2: 63–65

Watts T E, Larsen S A, Brown S T 1984 A case-control study of stillbirths at a teaching hospital in Zambia 1979–1980. Serological investigations for selected infectious agents. Bulletin of the World Health Organization 62: 803–808

Welgemoed N C, Mahaffey A, Van den Ende J 1986 Prevalence of *Neisseria gonorrhoeae* infection in patients attending an antenatal clinic. South African Medical Journal 69: 32–34

Weström L, Märdh P A 1984 Salpingitis. In: Holmes K K, Mardh P A, Sparling P F, Wiesner P J (eds) Sexually transmitted diseases. McGraw Hill New York. pp 615–632

Widy-Wirski R, D'Costa L J 1980 Prévalence des maladies transmises par voie sexuelle dans la population des femmes enceintes en milieu urbain en Centrafrique: In Rapport final, 13ème Conférence technique OCEAC, Yaoundé. pp 655–660

Willcox R R 1976 VD education in developing countries. British Journal of Venereal Diseases 52: 88–93

World Health Organization 1985 Simplified approaches for STD control at the primary health care level. WHO/VDT/85.437 Geneva

World Health Organization Working Group 1986 Extra-ocular chlamydial infection. Bulletin of the World Health Organization 64: 481–492

World Health Organization 1989 Consensus statement from consultation on sexually transmitted diseases as a risk factor for HIV transmission. WHO/GPA/INF/89.1, Geneva

Yvert F, Riou F Y, Frost E, Yvanoff B 1984 Les infections gonococciques au Gabon, Haut Oguoúe Pathologie Biologie 32: 80–84

# 11

# Genital chlamydial infections: clinical aspects, diagnosis, treatment and prevention

*David Taylor-Robinson*

This chapter is not intended as a complete account of chlamydiae and the infections caused by them. The aim is to present the salient features of investigations undertaken and observations made mainly since the previous review in this series by Schachter (1986a). The bulk of the bibliography, which comprises referenced publications, reflects this. Attention is also drawn to the proceedings of meetings (Oriel et al 1986, Oriel & Waugh 1988) including the first meeting of the European Society for Chlamydia Research (Proceedings 1988) and publications by Baron (1988) and Mårdh et al (1989). Emphasis will be, of course, on *Chlamydia trachomatis* but mention of *C. psittaci* and *C. pneumoniae* will be made where appropriate.

## CHLAMYDIAL TAXONOMY

The order Chlamydiales comprises one family, Chlamydiaceae, and one genus, *Chlamydia*, containing three species. *Chlamydia trachomatis* contains 15 serovars, serovars A, B and C causing endemic trachoma; the latter serovars will not be considered further because there is scant evidence for their sexual transmission. Serovars D to K do not seem to be associated with trachoma (Mabey et al 1987) but cause paratrachoma and a variety of genital-tract diseases, and serovars L1–L3 cause lymphogranuloma venereum (LGV). The species *C. psittaci* and *C. pneumoniae*, the latter being the recent designation (Grayston et al 1988) for strains hitherto termed TWAR, are responsible primarily for respiratory disease. *C. pneumoniae* has 10% or less relatedness with the two other species (Cox et al 1988) and can be distinguished also by its restriction endonuclease pattern (Campbell et al 1987) and by the use of specific monoclonal antibodies (Kuo et al 1986). A gene encoding a protein recognised during human TWAR infection has been isolated (Campbell et al 1989), but it contains some sequences shared among *Chlamydia* spp.

## FEATURES OF CHLAMYDIAE

The main features of chlamydiae (Taylor-Robinson & Thomas 1980, Ward 1983, 1986, 1988) compared with those of bacteria and viruses are shown in

**Table 11.1** Some features of chlamydiae present or absent in bacteria and viruses

| Feature considered | Presence ( + ) or absence ( – ) of feature in | | |
|---|---|---|---|
| | Chlamydiae | Bacteria | Viruses |
| Size (<500nm) | + | – | + |
| Cell wall | + | + | – |
| DNA and RNA | + | + | – |
| Ribosomes | + | + | – |
| Metabolism | + | + | – |
| Energy production | – | + | – |
| Inhibited by antibiotic | + | + | – |
| Obligate intracellular | + | – | + |

Table 11.1. Although chlamydiae possess peptidoglycan cell wall material like bacteria, the size of the infectious chlamydial particles (elementary bodies: EBs) is much smaller (about 300nm) and, like viruses, they have an obligate intracellular existence. The intracellular reproductive cycle (Taylor-Robinson & Thomas 1980) comprises several phases (Ward 1988): attachment and uptake of the EB, conversion to a metabolically active reticulate body (RB), increase in the number of the RBs by binary fission (cytoplasmic 'inclusion' formed), reorganisation of RBs to new EBs (larger inclusion) and, finally, release of the EBs from the cell. Apart from being metabolically inactive, the EBs differ from the RBs in several other respects (Ward 1983) and comprise the major constituents of late inclusions, the recognition of which by various staining or immunocytological techniques forms the basis of chlamydial detection in cell culture. The inclusions produced by *C. trachomatis* contain glycogen and, therefore, stain with iodine, whereas those of the other chlamydial species do not. Furthermore, EBs can be detected by specific fluorescent antibodies, detection of those in the extracellular phase enabling chlamydial infections to be diagnosed rapidly (vide infra). The EBs of *C. pneumoniae* are pear-shaped and have large periplasmic spaces (Chi et al 1987), unlike those of the other species which are typically round with narrow or barely discernible periplasmic spaces.

*C. trachomatis* EBs (serotype D) have been shown to enter and exit from cells in vitro without causing obvious damage (Todd & Caldwell 1985). This observation may have a bearing on the ability of chlamydiae to produce asymptomatic or latent infections. Support for the existence of a latent chlamydial state and the reactivation of chlamydiae by concurrent gonorrhoea has been provided by Batteiger et al (1989).

## GENITAL TRACT INFECTION

Chlamydial infections continue to occur more frequently than gonococcal infections (Swinker et al 1988, Hughes et al 1989) even in some parts of Africa (Bentsi et al 1985) and are common. For example, they were found in 16% of adolescent girls in residential care in the UK (Mulcahy & Lacey 1987)

and in 59% of women with non-gonococcal cervicitis in Poland (Zdrodowska-Stefanow & Manikowska-Lesinska 1988).


## Non-gonococcal urethritis (NGU)

In the past few years the number of studies concerned with NGU in men has diminished probably because it is now well established that *C. trachomatis* may be isolated from up to 50% of cases. However, there is no assurance that *C. trachomatis* is the aetiological agent in all the cases in which it is identified. That it is so is an assumption that is rarely, if ever, questioned. It could be that *C. trachomatis*, either alone or in conjunction with other micro-organisms, is the cause of disease only in those patients in whom it produces sufficient damage to elicit an antibody response; the notion that it is the cause of the disease only in those patients who develop antibody might, however, be difficult to establish. Although it has never been possible to isolate chlamydiae from all patients with NGU, nor for early workers to show that all chlamydia-positive men had urethritis, there was satisfaction that, in general, the organisms could be isolated from those with disease but not from those without; in other words, that there was fulfillment of the first of Koch's postulates. The widely held belief that NGU is quite a good marker of chlamydial infection and that, in the main, infection does not occur in men without disease has spawned the idea that screening for *C. trachomatis* in men is unnecessary. The truth of the matter, however, may be quite different. In a study by Stamm et al (1984), nearly 25% of men with a urethral chlamydial infection were reported to be asymptomatic and such chlamydia-positive asymptomatic men remained so for at least 21–45 days (Stamm & Cole 1986). In another study (Karam et al 1986), 11% of young heterosexual asymptomatic men were found to have a urethral chlamydial infection. Furthermore, 8–9% of teenage boys in San Francisco were found to have asymptomatic urethral chlamydial infections (Shafer et al 1987). Indeed, if sought assiduously by sensitive methods, it is possible that inapparent infections would be found to occur much more frequently than generally believed. If so, could the inapparent infections be caused by serovars different from urethritis-producing ones? Because serotyping is laborious it is rarely done, but the introduction of serovar-specific monoclonal antibodies (Wang et al 1985) might enable this issue to be resolved. Another question which has not been answered is whether chlamydial strains that produce inapparent infections are truly non-pathogenic or whether they are able to produce disease at other sites. For example, are such strains just as likely to infect the female genital tract and cause ascending infection as strains which produce NGU? A direct answer is not available, but experiments in animal models should provide a clear idea of whether one strain, even within a serovar, is more pathogenic than another. The suspicion is that this is the case. However, the immunological status of the individual (vide infra) may be of even more importance than the organism itself in determining the outcome of infection.

In women, there is still debate as to whether chlamydial urethral infection and urethritis are causally related (Bradley et al 1985), but chlamydiae would seem to have no part to play in chronic urological complaints in women (Bump & Copeland 1985).

## Prostatitis

Claims in the past of recovery of chlamydiae from expressed prostatic fluids have been open to strong criticism, this being that the results have not allowed a distinction to be made between chlamydiae in the prostate, if there, and those in the urethra. More recently, Poletti et al (1985) claimed to have isolated chlamydiae from the prostatic tissue of patients with 'non-acute abacterial prostatitis' following digitally guided needle aspiration of tissue. However, the surprisingly large proportion of patients reported to be chlamydia-positive, indeed as much as might be expected for acute NGU, and the completely negative results obtained by Doble et al (1989b), cast serious doubts on these observations. The latter investigators studied 50 patients with a diagnosis of chronic abacterial prostatitis, as defined by the Stamey procedure, and examined them by transrectal prostatic ultrasound. By such means, abnormal areas of echogenicity were defined and biopsy specimens were then taken from them, the needle being introduced transperineally and being guided under ultrasound control. Subsequent histological examination of the tissues confirmed their chronic inflammatory nature, but microbiological examination failed to reveal chlamydiae in any of them. These observations are supported by further negative results obtained in a study by Berger et al (1989). Thus, despite claims for the active involvement of chlamydiae in chronic prostatitis (Weidner et al 1988), there is no evidence that chlamydiae are implicated directly in the disease, although it is not possible to eliminate an active role for them at an earlier stage.

## Epididymo-orchitis

The condition has been linked primarily to chlamydial infection in men under the age of 35 years. This contention is based on a study more than a decade ago in the USA in which epididymal aspirates were examined (Berger et al 1978) and has not been under threat from subsequent comprehensive studies which, nevertheless, were inevitably less informative because of their 'non-aspiration' approach (Hawkins et al 1986, Grant et al 1987, Mulcahy et al 1987, De Jong et al 1988). Somewhat similar conclusions were drawn by Melekos & Asbach (1988) who examined epididymal tissues from patients, not all of whom had acute disease. In developing countries, *N. gonorrhoeae* is still a major cause of acute epididymitis, although chlamydiae are important too (Fehler et al 1989). The first study in the UK and, indeed, the only other one anywhere in which epididymal aspirates have been examined microbiologically was undertaken recently by Doble et al (1989a). Chlamydiae were detected in at least one-third of these specimens and the existence of chlamydial disease, almost all of which occurred in young men, was supported by serological investigations (vide infra). It is possible that chlamydiae might infect the testis, but the veracity of this having occurred in a man with sterile pyospermia (Hartmann et al 1986) is open to question, and past chlamydial infection (Close et al 1987, Torode et al 1987) or asymptomatic chlamydial infection as a cause of male infertility is most unlikely (Hellstrom et al 1987).

## Bartholin's gland abscess

Saul & Grossman (1988) reported that a Chlamydiazyme test on a swab taken from such an abscess was positive. However, a single result unconfirmed by other procedures is insufficient to deduce that chlamydiae were the cause.

## Cervicitis

The cervix would seem to be the primary target for chlamydial infection but its removal by hysterectomy does not necessarily mean that chlamydiae will not be found in the vagina (Barton et al 1985), although their ability to cause vaginitis in the adult is unlikely. Infection of the cervix by *C. trachomatis* is often asymptomatic (Glenney et al 1988, Leclerc et al 1988, Swinker et al 1988, Soren & Willis 1989). Rahm et al (1988) noted that one-sixth of asymptomatic infected adolescents developed symptoms within 3 months. Indeed, chlamydiae are well-known to cause mucopurulent/follicular cervicitis, a condition that has been examined in detail (Paavonen et al 1986, Dunlop et al 1989). Nevertheless, some outstanding epidemiological questions remain unanswered; for example, the question of how common chlamydial cervical infection is in the UK is difficult to answer because it is not clear what proportion of infections are asymptomatic. It is assumed that many are, but this notion may be warped because studies have involved predominantly STD clinic populations where most chlamydial infections are detected in sexual contacts of men with gonorrhoea or NGU, that is in women who have attended the clinic because of their contact history and not because of symptoms. In the community at large, the situation may be different. It is noteworthy that the majority of infected women in a general practice setting had symptoms (Longhurst et al 1987). Factors influencing the initial acquisition of chlamydiae are numerous and must include age, frequency of exposure, use of contraceptives (Rosenberg et al 1987, Ruijs et al 1988), the role of which is still debated (Edelman 1988), and spermicides (Benes & McCormack 1985, Kappus & Quinn 1986, Knight et al 1987, Ehret & Judson 1988a). In addition, the hormonal state and the presence of ectopy and host defences influence acquisition. The mix is so complex and doubtless variable that in an individual case it would probably be unrewarding and perhaps impossible to determine the relative contribution of each, although certain risk/factors have been outlined (Harrison et al 1985, Handsfield et al

1986, Magder et al 1988, Ruijs et al 1988). Although postmenopausal
chlamydial cervicitis has been purported to occur (Nagashima 1987), patients
under 25 years old, those who use oral contraceptives (Louv et al 1989) and
those who have signs of cervicitis are more likely to have a chlamydial
infection (Lefèvre et al 1988), although these factors are not always predictive
(Kent et al 1988). One would also like to think that host defences, in terms
of both cell-mediated immunity and pre-existing antibody, have an important
role in determining acquisition because it may be possible to enhance any
protective influence they have. Of course, knowing who is most likely to be
infected based on a multiplicity of historical and clinical characteristics
(Lindner et al 1988) is helpful in deciding who should be screened. Selection
may be required because routine testing may only be cost-effective if the
prevalence of chlamydial infection is relatively high (Phillips et al 1987a).

Reid (1985) has put forward arguments to suggest that *C. trachomatis* is not
a cause of cervical intraepithelial neoplasia (CIN) and Meijer et al (1989)
found a correlation between *C. trachomatis* infection and inflammatory, but
not neoplastic, changes of cervical cells. Syrjänen et al (1986) believe that
chlamydiae are found more frequently in women with CIN (Guaschino et al
1988) because of their promiscuous sexual behaviour. However, mild cellular
atypia, reversible by tetracycline therapy, may be due to chlamydial infection
(Mecsei et al 1989).

**Pelvic inflammatory disease (PID)**

On clinical grounds, Judson & Tavelli (1986) were not able to distinguish
chlamydial from gonococcal PID, although Cromer & Heald (1987) found
that break-through vaginal bleeding, current use of an oral contraceptive and
an elevated erythrocyte sedimentation rate were more often related to the
former than the latter. Both appear to be less severe than PID not associated
with chlamydiae or gonococci (Kirshon et al 1988). Canalicular spread of
chlamydiae to the upper genital tract (Jones et al 1986b) leads to endometritis
(Temmerman et al 1988), often plasma-cell associated (Paavonen et al
1985a,b, Tomioka et al 1987) and sometimes intensely lymphoid in reaction
(Thomas 1986). Further spread causes salpingitis, perihepatitis (Katzman et al
1988), sometimes confused with acute cholecystitis in young women (Shanahan et al 1988), in addition to periappendicitis and other abdominal
complaints (Duffy et al 1985), although the organisms are not always found
in the cervix when these conditions are recognised (Møller et al 1986).
Factors contributing to the spread of the organisms are the time in the
menstrual cycle during which acquisition occurs (Sweet et al 1986), serovar
and infecting dose, duration of infection, presence of associated infections,
absence of antibody, hormonal status (Maslow et al 1988) and also the
integrity of the genital tract. The most important of these in an individual case
may be impossible to identify, although the trauma of surgery, for example
termination of pregnancy (Heisterberg et al 1985), or insertion or removal of

an intrauterine contraceptive device, are obvious predisposing factors. So too is chorionicvillus sampling, but routine screening before sampling is not cost-effective unless the procedure is being undertaken in a high-risk population (Moncada et al 1987).

Chlamydial infection is the major cause of salpingitis in Scandinavia (Mårdh 1986) but seems to be somewhat less dominant in the United States (Sweet 1986, Wasserheit et al 1986). In one study of acute salpingitis in the UK (Kinghorn et al 1986), chlamydiae were not detected in the fallopian tubes, but subsequently they have been detected in the endometrium (Fish et al 1988) and the endometrium and tubes (Munday et al 1987) of such patients. However, it is unknown exactly how common chlamydial salpingitis is in the UK because laparoscopy required for clinical diagnosis and for obtaining specimens to distinguish accurately between upper and lower genital-tract infection is not undertaken routinely. Whether it will be possible to undertake laparoscopy more often and/or develop non-invasive procedures of sufficient sensitivity and specificity to be helpful remains to be seen.

The eventual outcome of PID may be infertility, for which there is direct isolation evidence (Brunham et al 1988) and indirect serological evidence to link it with chlamydial infection (Brunham et al 1985, Svensson et al 1985, Tjiam et al 1985, Robertson et al 1987); sometimes, this may be asymptomatic (Sellors et al 1988). Other consequences are ectopic pregnancy, which also may arise as a result of a subclinical chlamydial tubal infection (Brunham et al 1986) and for which a serological association with chlamydiae has been seen (Robertson et al 1988, Walters et al 1988), and chronic pelvic pain. What factors determine precisely the development of such sequelae in chlamydial PID are unclear, although there is evidence from the Scandinavian studies that the number and severity of the infections influence subsequent fertility rates (Weström & Mårdh 1983). Infertility could be due to endometritis, some of the women having an active endometrial infection at the time of presentation (Cleary & Jones 1985), or blocked or damaged tubes resulting from cellular infiltrates, or perhaps abnormalities of ovum transportation, as suggested by the results of recent work on a mouse model (Tuffrey et al 1986).

## In vitro fertilization (IVF)

In addition to artificial insemination by a donor, IVF is a well-established approach to tackling the problem of infertility. Gamete intra-fallopian transfer (GIFT) is also a means of overcoming infertility in cases where the tubes are apparently normal. Chlamydiae may be found in donor semen (Nagel et al 1986, Tjiam et al 1987) and to believe that a current chlamydial infection or a past infection that has damaged the tubes or endometrium might interfere with the implantation and development of a fertilized ovum is not outrageous. However, there is only anecdotal evidence for this (Moss & Steptoe 1984) and the real contribution of chlamydiae is unknown. A report that the presence of chlamydial antibodies was associated with a decreased pregnancy rate following IVF (Rowland et al 1985) has not been supported by others (Torode et al 1987) undertaking IVF and GIFT. Nevertheless, screening of the donors of semen (Greenblatt et al 1986, Moss et al 1986) and ova would seem wise if facilities are available.

## INFECTION IN PREGNANCY

The factors which influence infection rates in non-pregnant women, such as age and marital and socio-economic status, also affect infection rates in pregnant women. It would seem prudent for obstetricians to know the extent to which chlamydial infection occurs in the population they serve, since reported infection rates vary widely; 37% in a population of pregnant adolescents in downtown Baltimore (Hardy et al 1984), 14% in unmarried women seeking abortions in Singapore (Chaudhuri et al 1986), 9% in women seeking abortions in Pittsburgh (Amortegui et al 1986), 0% in Harrow, UK (Ross et al 1981), the latter figure having barely changed in the past decade, being 0.5% in 1988 (PM Furr, D Taylor-Robinson, unpublished data). Whether the differences matter depends on the effect that chlamydiae have on the outcome of pregnancy and on the newborn. Infection in utero is possible (Bell 1988) and suspicion that such infection might have an adverse effect on the outcome of pregnancy has been based on the following indirect evidence: 1. *C. psittaci* causes foetal wastage in domestic and farmyard animals; (2) ovine strains of *C. psittaci* cause human abortion occasionally (Buxton 1986); (3) babies with conjunctivitis are sometimes of low birth weight; (4) tetracycline given in pregnancy was significantly more effective in increasing birth weight than was a placebo (Elder et al 1971) and (5) *C. trachomatis* was isolated from 4 of 22 spontaneously aborted fetuses (Schachter 1967). However, the latter meagre isolation data do not seem to have been consolidated in the last 20 years and support for chlamydiae affecting the fetus has been serological. Although Gibbs & Schachter (1987) could not detect a serological difference between women with intra-amniotic infection and those without, and elevated chlamydial antibody titres in recurrent aborters (Quinn et al 1987) were insufficient to suggest an aetiological association, Harrison (1986) and colleagues (Berman et al 1987) noted an association between low birth weight or prematurity and the presence of chlamydial IgM antibody in chlamydia-positive women. Likewise, Sweet et al (1987) observed an association between premature rupture of the membranes and preterm delivery and the occurrence of such antibody, and Alger et al (1988) isolated *C. trachomatis* significantly more often from women with premature rupture than from those without. Of course, *C. trachomatis* is not the only micro-organism to be considered and *Mycoplasma hominis* and ureaplasmas (Hillier et al 1986, Foulon et al 1986, Lamont et al 1987) and the various bacteria involved in bacterial vaginosis (Martius et al 1988) have been associated with preterm birth. It would seem that, at most, *C. trachomatis* is likely to contribute to a poor pregnancy outcome in only a small subset of women who are at risk and to an even smaller proportion of the total perinatal morbidity and mortality.

## POSTNATAL INFECTION

In contrast to rare or dubious chlamydial infection in utero, the fetus comes in contact with chlamydiae in the mother's infected cervix during labour and delivery and a transmission rate of more than 50% has been suggested (Harrison 1986). This leads to neonatal conjunctivitis (Schachter et al 1986a, Preece et al 1989) which is no more effectively prevented by erythromycin ointment than by silver nitrate (Bell et al 1987); indeed, neither treatments nor oxytetracycline ointment prevented the conjunctivitis in one study (Hammerschlag et al 1989), suggesting the need for better control of the maternal infection. Pneumonia (Schachter et al 1986a), which may be worse in the low birthweight neonate (Attenburrow & Barker 1985) or in antibody deficiency (Klingebiel et al 1989) is another outcome with the possibility of chronic lung disease ensuing (Harrison 1986, Numazaki et al 1986). Chronic eye disease also may occur (Stenberg & Mårdh 1986). The frequency of neonatal disease in any geographical location will dictate whether prophylactic measures should operate (Laga et al 1986); the frequency will depend on the infection rate in pregnancy which, as noted previously, varies widely from one location to another. Antenatal screening and treatment of the mother with erythromycin is cost effective when the infection rate is high (Schachter et al 1986b) and screening may be of value even when it is low, if directed at the main at-risk group (Sanyal & Oates 1987). In developing countries gonococcal ophthalmia still dominates (Fransen et al 1986b). Whether chlamydial or otherwise, however, the occurrence of ophthalmia neonatorum or chlamydial respiratory disease should be considered as a strong indicator of sexually transmitted disease in the parents (Fransen et al 1985, Medici et al 1988).

## CONJUNCTIVITIS

The difference between those cases of conjunctivitis which are truly infective and those which are reactive is now more clearly understood. In adults, inclusion conjunctivitis was estimated to occur in about 0.3% of those with a chlamydial genital-tract infection (Tullo et al 1981). The suggestion that occult eye infection might occur in every other man with NGU (Monteiro et al 1987) has been strongly questioned (Taylor-Robinson 1987a). When conjunctivitis is the presenting condition, chlamydial infections should be sought not only in other sites, despite the fact that they might not be provoking symptoms, but in the partners too (Mantell & Goh 1987). A combined chlamydial and herpetic conjunctivitis has been reported (Mantell et al 1988) and postgonococcal chlamydial conjunctivitis too (Scott &

Fortenberry 1986). The conjunctivitis occurring together with arthritis as part of Reiter's syndrome is considered to be reactive, but whether chlamydial antigen can be found in the conjunctiva by any of the antigen detection techniques has not been established.

## ARTHRITIS

Arthritis occurring together with or soon after NGU has been termed sexually acquired reactive arthritis (SARA) and, until recently, evidence that at least one-third of cases of SARA are initiated by chlamydial infection had been circumstantial (Keat et al 1983). However, this concept has been given credence by the finding of chlamydial elementary bodies in the joints of such patients using direct immunofluorescence (Keat et al 1987), an observation corroborated independently recently (J. Treharne, unpublished data). The detection of chlamydial antigen within joints by an immunoperoxidase technique (Schumacher et al 1988) and of particles by electron microscopy (Ishikawa et al 1986, Schumacher et al 1988) is apparently supportive, although the specificity of the former technique is open to question, as is the interpretation of the microscopic findings. A rheumatoid arthritis-like condition has also been associated with intra-articular occurrence of the antigen (Ford et al 1988). The failure to detect viable chlamydiae in the joints of patients with SARA may be due to their rapid disappearance, as suggested by observations on a mouse model of chlamydial arthritis (Hough & Rank 1989). Observations on the mouse model also suggest that cell-mediated immunity may be an important factor in the development of the disease (Rank et al 1988). Rapid disappearance of viable organisms from the joint, if this is the case, is not encouraging for the success of early antibiotic therapy, but the detection of chlamydial antigen in the joints does have implications for other arthritides and for understanding disease mechanisms. In regard to the former, similar elementary bodies have been found in the joints of women with 'seronegative' arthritis (Taylor-Robinson et al 1988). The notion that chlamydial cell walls taken up by polymorphonuclear leucocytes may accumulate in the joints and stimulate oxygen radicals which participate in joint destruction (Zvillich & Sarov 1989) is purely speculative.

## PHARYNGEAL AND RECTAL INFECTIONS

Jones et al (1985) isolated chlamydiae from the pharynx of 3.7% of heterosexual men and 3.2% of women; recovery was not associated with symptoms, but in women it was associated with fellatio. Therefore, the reported recovery of C. trachomatis from one-quarter of patients with tonsillitis (Ogawa et al 1988) certainly invites further investigation to establish the veracity of the claim. The isolation of chlamydiae from the rectum of 5.2% of women also could not be associated with symptoms by Jones et al (1985). Rompalo et al (1986) cultured rectal specimens from 1429 homosexual men; 8% had a gonococcal infection, 5% a chlamydial infection and 1% had both. Again, the majority of rectal infections with these organisms were asymptomatic.

A summary of the extent to which *C. trachomatis* is involved in the various genital-tract and associated diseases is presented in Table 11.2.

## CHLAMYDIA PNEUMONIAE INFECTIONS

The nature of the organism and the respiratory disease it causes have been reviewed by Grayston et al (1989) and it seems inappropriate to consider these aspects in a discussion of genital-tract disease. However, three points are worth making. First, *C. trachomatis* occurs rarely in the respiratory tract of

**Table 11.2** Assessment of the extent to which *C. trachomatis* is involved in various oculogenital and associated diseases. *Key:* + + + + overwhelming; + + + good; + + moderate; + weak

| Disease | Evidence that *C. trachomatis* is a cause | Proportion of disease due to *C. trachomatis* |
|---|---|---|
| *In men* | | |
| NGU | + + + + | Up to 50% |
| Postgonococcal urethritis | + + + + | Up to 50% |
| Prostatitis | – | |
| Epididymitis | + + + + | Up to 50% |
| Infertility | – | |
| *In women* | | |
| Urethritis | + + | ? |
| Bartholinitis | + | ? |
| Cervicitis | + + + + | About 50% |
| Cervical dysplasia | + | ? |
| Endometritis | + + + | ? |
| Salpingitis | + + + + | 40–60% |
| Periappendicitis | + + | ? |
| Perihepatitis | + + + | ? |
| Infertility | + + + | ≥8% due to chlamydial salpingitis |
| Ectopic pregnancy | + + + | ? |
| Abortion | – | |
| *In men or women* | | |
| Conjunctivitis | + + + + | ? |
| Arthritis (Reiter's syndrome) | + + + | About 40% |
| Endocarditis | + + | ? |
| Pharyngitis | – | |
| Proctitis | + + | ? |
| Crohn's disease | – | |
| Lymphogranuloma venereum | + + + + | 100% (by definition) |
| *In infants* | | |
| Conjunctivitis | + + + + | Up to 50% |
| Pneumonia | + + + + | 30%? |
| Chronic lung disease | + + | ? |
| Gastroenteritis | – | |

patients with the acquired immunodeficiency syndrome (Moncada et al 1986), although a case of pneumonia has been attributed to it (Kroon et al 1989). Obviously, greater attention should be given to *C. pneumoniae* in this regard. Second, *C. trachomatis* is a trigger for some cases of SARA but clearly not for all; the possibility of *C. pneumoniae* being a cause, urethritis being 'reactive' rather than the focus of origin, should be considered; and third, the likelihood that some of the serological patterns attributed to *C. trachomatis* are due, in part, to *C. pneumoniae* as a result of antigenic cross-reactivity (Schachter 1986b) should be kept in mind.

## DIAGNOSIS

In recent years, most genitourinary physicians in the British Isles have had complete or partial access to a chlamydial diagnostic service (Royal College of Physicians Committee on Genitourinary Medicine 1987). The service may offer one or more of a variety of methods of detecting chlamydiae but, as Smith et al (1987) remark, no method is ideal. They have been reviewed in detail by Stamm (1988) and Barnes (1989).

### Collection, source and nature of specimens

The use of a cytobrush to collect material from the cervix has attracted attention recently. Increasing the number of chlamydia-infected cells for examination (Judson & Lambert 1988) is intuitively a sound idea. An initial evaluation (Ciotti et al 1988) was inconclusive (Taylor-Robinson 1989), and although subsequently some have not found the cytobrush valuable (Weiland et al 1988) or cost-effective if tested by Chlamydiazyme (Kellogg et al 1989), others (Judson & Lambert 1988, Moncada et al 1989) have concluded that use of the cytobrush is superior to swabbing. The results of a comparison may be influenced by the type of swab since many swabs are not optimal for chlamydial isolation (Mahony & Chernesky 1985).

Bradley et al (1985) found no evidence to suggest that taking urethral swabs routinely from women would help in diagnosing a chlamydial infection, although Jones et al (1986a) and Manuel et al (1987) increased the chlamydial isolation rate by pooling cervical and urethral specimens, and Dunlop et al (1985) by taking three cervical specimens. Singal et al (1986) found that a second urethral swab from men improved the rate of *C. trachomatis* recovery, and Goh et al (1985) increased the isolation rate from the male urethra by using a meatal swab and an endourethral curette. The collection of a 'first-catch' urine specimen, a non-invasive procedure, and its examination, not new in concept, is a more attractive proposition that has received attention recently. Examination of the whole urine and/or the centrifuged deposit by an enzyme immunoassay has been undertaken (Caul et al 1988). This approach is probably not as sensitive as testing a urethral swab by culture (Matthews &

Wise 1989) but requires further evaluation. Any suggestion that it would be valuable in women seems illogical.


## Direct detection methods

It is generally agreed that seeking chlamydial inclusions in ocular or genital-tract cells after staining of smears by various methods is insensitive, notably with genital-tract specimens. Thus, examination of Papanicolaou-stained cervical smears is notoriously insensitive for detecting chlamydial infection (Forster et al 1985, Shafer et al 1985, Arroyo et al 1989) and should have been abandoned by cytologists; unfortunately this does not seem to have happened (Sekhri et al 1988, Ghirardini et al 1989). On the other hand, increased numbers of histiocytes and the presence of transformed lymphocytes in cervical specimens provide a clue to the existence of a chlamydial infection (Kiviat et al 1985a), one that can be confirmed by a direct immunofluorescence test (Kiviat et al 1985b). Indeed, detection of elementary bodies directly in cervical or other smears by use of fluorscein- conjugated monoclonal antibodies produced commercially, for example MicroTrak, Imagen, Pathfinder (Tilton et al 1988) and Monofluor (Phillips et al 1988), has gained wide acceptance. Antibodies against the major outer membrane proteins of *C. trachomatis* produce brighter and less non-specific staining than those against the lipopolysaccharide (Cles et al 1988) but a test (Clonatac) combining both types of antibody has been described (Pouletty et al 1988). MicroTrak can be at least as sensitive as culture (Thomas et al 1984, Foulkes et al 1985, Hawkins et al 1985, Mabey & Booth-Mason 1986 [ophthalmia neonatorum], Rapoza et al 1986) or almost so (Alexander et al 1985, Quinn et al 1985, Leclerc et al 1988, Pastorek et al 1988). On the other hand, some have considered the method less sensitive than culture (Grillner et al 1986, Lipkin et al 1986, Näher & Petzoldt 1986, Kent et al 1988), particularly for the detection of small numbers of organisms (Stary et al 1985, Larsen et al 1986, Hipp et al 1987) or in a low-prevalence population (Forbes et al 1986), although Pothier & Kazmierczak (1986) and Phillips et al (1987b) found the method valuable in their low-prevalence populations. Beyond dispute, perhaps, is the observation that MicroTrak staining is even more sensitive than culture for the detection of chlamydiae in endometrial or tubal specimens (Kiviat et al 1986). Furthermore, it has proved useful for examining rectal specimens (Rompalo et al 1987) and has the potential for detecting chlamydiae in semen samples (Sherman & Jordan 1985). Its success depends on the experience of the observer (Livengood et al 1988), which includes the ability to detect non-specific staining (Harper et al 1985, Krech et al 1985), and different laboratories may produce remarkably different results (Reed & Huck 1987). The ability of the anti-chlamydial antibody to stain *Gardnerella vaginalis* (GL Ridgway and G Mumtaz, personal communication) and parainfluenza 2 virus particles (Fox et al 1989) should be noted.

Outside expert hands, direct immunofluorescence may be no more sensitive or specific for examining urethral and cervical specimens than the enzyme immunoassays (B.J. Thomas and D. Taylor-Robinson, unpublished data) which are not subject to observer error. Apart from the ease of using direct immunofluorescence to test single specimens, and its value in looking at specimens that have lost viable chlamydiae through prolonged transport (Williams et al 1985), it may be used more widely and with cost benefit. In this regard, early detection programmes using direct immunofluorescence or an enzyme immunoassay were shown to be cost-effective in female populations where the prevalences of chlamydial infection exceeded 6% and 7%, respectively (Estany et al 1989). Direct immunofluorescence also may be used as a test of cure, but with caution. Thus, 7 to 10 days after doxycycline was commenced (100mg twice daily for 7 days) in culture-positive women, a negative fluorescence test was also culture negative, but 1 of every 6 women had a fluorescence-positive/culture negative test (Nachamkin et al 1987).

## Indirect detection methods

This term refers to methods that do not involve the direct examination of smears. Culture of specimens in sensitive cell lines has never been undertaken by all laboratories (British Co-operative Clinical Group 1987) and is practised less widely now since the advent of antigen detection systems. Up to five blind passages in culture increased sensitivity (Jones et al 1986a) but Schachter & Martin (1987) contend that one blind passage is sufficient and this certainly enhanced sensitivity in the hands of Smith et al (1987). The use of a DNA probe to detect inclusions in culture did not enhance sensitivity (Näher et al 1988) and in recent years, apart from the treatment of cell cultures with mitomycin C (Woodland et al 1987) and the use of polyethylene glycol (Mohammed & Hilary 1985), there have been no further developments to standard methods (Smeltzer et al 1985) that have resulted in increased sensitivity of culture. Micromethods may be more convenient and rapid but no more sensitive (Yong & Paul 1986). Any diminished sensitivity they may have may be improved by sonicating and vortexing clinical specimens (Jones et al 1989).

## Immunoassays

An immune dot blot technique with sensitivity and specificity akin to those of culture has been described (Storey et al 1987, Mearns et al 1988) but does not seem to be widely used. In contrast, various enzyme-linked immunosorbent assays (ELISAs) have flooded the microbiological scene. Their sensitivity and specificity have gradually improved, the results produced by the Pharmacia assay (Mumtaz et al 1988a) bearing witness to this. Nevertheless, arguments about these aspects have abounded and are inevitable when the results depend on the inherent capacity of the test under examination and how it has been read (Chisholm et al 1988, Thomas & Taylor-Robinson 1988), the sensitivity of the comparative procedure as well as the capabilities of the investigators. While some may consider ELISAs, Chlamydiazyme for example (Mumtaz et al 1985, Howard et al 1986, Levy & Warford 1986, Mohanty et al 1986, Moi & Danielsson 1986, Morgan-Capner et al 1986, Hammerschlag et al 1987 [ophthalmia neonatorum], Weismeier et al 1988), to be satisfactory, generally they are not as sensitive or as specific as the culture technique (Näher & Petzoldt 1986, Hipp et al 1987, Jensen et al 1988) or, in capable hands, direct immunofluorescence (Taylor-Robinson et al 1987, Taylor-Robinson & Tuffrey 1987, Stamm 1988). Lack of specificity would seem to be due to cross-reactivity with other organisms (Riordan et al 1986, Rothburn et al 1986, Saikku et al 1986, Taylor-Robinson et al, 1987, Goudswaard et al 1989). Recently, use of a blocking antibody has helped to detect false-positive results in the Chlamydiazyme assay and so improve specificity. The IDEIA assay (Pugh et al 1985), although considered unsuitable for examination of non-genital sites (Sulaiman et al 1987), in particular the rectum (Riordan et al 1986), was regarded as more specific (Thomas et al 1989) and more sensitive (Caul & Paul 1985, Bygdeman et al 1988) than Chlamydiazyme for testing genital specimens. Although less sensitive than culture (Tjiam et al 1986, Thomas et al 1989), it has been possible to increase the sensitivity of IDEIA without jeopardising specificity by taking multiple swabs from the cervix, pooling them and so increasing the concentration of antigen tested (Thomas et al 1989). For epidemiological purposes in assessing the incidence of infection within a particular population group, it would seem reasonable to assume that the high degree of sensitivity and specificity needed in making a diagnosis in an individual patient is not required, simply because patient management does not depend on it. However, a new test of whatever kind that, in comparison with culture, has a sensitivity, specificity, predictive positive value (PPV) and predictive negative value (PNV) of 90% or more in a high risk population (25% chlamydial infection) has a high PNV but a PPV of only about 50% in a low risk population (4.5% chlamydial infection). Thus, when Chlamydiazyme was used to test asymptomatic women with a chlamy-dial prevalence of 6.7%, the PPV was 57% (Lefebvre et al 1988). It is clear that grossly erroneous assessments will be provided by tests of lesser sensitivity and specificity and that even for epidemiological purposes high sensitivity and specificity should be the goal. Irrespective of whatever criticism is levelled at a particular method, some laboratories will continue to use it and clinicians should keep a constant vigil for results that in their judgement are either falsely positive or falsely negative simply because clinically they 'make no sense'. Furthermore, both clinician and laboratory worker should be aware that in cases of sexual abuse and other cases of litigation, non-cultural diagnostic methods are unlikely to stand-up in a court of law.

The ease of serotyping chlamydial isolates has been enhanced by the advent of monoclonal antibodies (Wang et al 1985) which may be used either in immunofluorescence tests and/or immunoassays (dot ELISA; radioimmunoassay) (Barnes et al 1985, Newhall et al 1986, Wagenvoort et al 1988).

## Chlamydial DNA probes

Several investigators have used such probes. Palva et al (1987) used chromosomal DNA from the L2 serovar of *C. trachomatis*. This was digested with the restriction enzyme Bam H1 and cloned into *E. coli* using the plasmid vector pBr322. In sandwich hybridisation, the probe detected DNA from other chlamydial serovars but not DNA from unrelated organisms and in tests on genital-tract specimens there was good sensitivity and acceptable specificity (85%). On the other hand, Hyypia et al (1985), although showing a reasonable correlation between culture and probe when the culture was strongly positive, were less successful when testing specimens which were weakly positive in culture. Indeed, they obtained both false negative and false positive results. Dean et al (1989) used a probe that employs a 7.0-kilobase cryptic plasmid from *C. trachomatis* and found that it had a sensitivity of 87% and a specificity of 91% compared with culture in screening a trachoma-endemic population. Horn et al (1986, 1988) used in situ DNA hybridisation to detect *C. trachomatis* in cervical scrapings and rectal biopsies, the results being more or less comparable with those obtained by culture. Pao et al (1987) came to the same conclusion when they used DNA hybridisation to test cervical specimens. Dutilh et al (1988) used the same approach with sulphonated total DNA as a probe and visualised labelled DNA with a commercial enzyme-linked monoclonal antibody. Only five genital specimens were tested by this procedure but the results were in agreement with those observed in culture. The overall impression that DNA probes are specific but, as yet, not quite sufficiently sensitive in comparison with other techniques, an impression confirmed by Meddens et al (1988) and LeBar et al (1989), may be changed by use of the polymerase chain reaction (PCR). This offers a new approach to increasing sensitivity in allowing massive amplification of a DNA sequence. The technique comprises repeated cycles of high temperature template denaturation, oligonucleotide primer annealing and polymerase-mediated extension. After 25 cycles a hundred-thousand-fold increase in the DNA sequence under investigation may be achieved. Several groups of workers are now using this method to study and detect chlamydial DNA. For example, Dutilh et al (1989) chose oligonucleotide primers in a sequence of a conserved domain of the major outer membrane protein of *C. trachomatis* to generate the amplification of a 129-base pair fragment. The sequence was amplified in the 15 serovars of *C. trachomatis*, although serovar J gave a weak signal. No cross reactions were detected with the DNAs of 11 different micro-organisms encountered in the genital tract so that the reaction seemed to be specific. Similar results have been obtained in my laboratory (H. Palmer et al, unpublished observations). Obviously the PCR is potentially a powerful tool for the specific detection of *C. trachomatis* in clinical samples but the extent to which it comes up to expectation remains to be seen.


**Chlamydial serology**

The role of serology in diagnosis continues to be a contentious issue. A variety of serological techniques has been applied to studying chlamydial infections: complement fixation is not sufficiently sensitive for detecting chlamydial antibodies, except in lymphogranuloma venereum infections and in psittacosis (Puolakkainen et al 1987). Immunofluorescence (IMF) and enzyme immunoassays (Numazaki et al 1985, Puolakkainen et al 1985), including a $\mu$-capture ELISA for chlamydia-specific IgM (Wreghitt et al 1988), are much more useful and immunoblotting is in vogue as a means of determining which antigens stimulate antibody production (Cevenini et al 1986a, 1986b, Hanuka et al 1988). A few general points are appropriate. In men with NGU, antibody may not develop in a fifth of them and although serum antibody titres are higher in those with disease than in those without, the titres are usually quite low and it is rare to detect an antibody response; certainly, a diagnosis of NGU cannot be made on the basis of serology, although, debatably it has been suggested as a complementary test (Hagay et al 1989). In women, the frequent occurrence of serum antibodies in those who do not have chlamydiae in the cervix illustrates the problems encountered. In cervical infections, although the titres are higher than those in men with NGU, it is rare to see a rising antibody titre and it would be foolhardy to make a diagnosis of a cervical infection based on serology or, indeed, on the presence of antibody in local secretions (Gump & Gibson 1985). The detection of a rising antibody titre in PID is uncommon but the titres tend to be higher in cases of PID than in uncomplicated cervical infections, and perhaps suggestive of an aetiological association if very high, a titre of $\geqslant 512$ being used by Kristensen et al (1985). Lower titres are used (Moss & Hawkswell 1987), but there should be reluctance to make a firm diagnosis of chlamydial salpingitis in an individual case on the basis of a single serum antibody titre. Indeed, one has to ask the question 'Under what circumstances can detection of antibody in a single serum be in any way helpful?' It may have value in cases of epididymitis; in the study mentioned previously (Doble et al 1989a), patients who were culture positive always had IgG IMF antibody titres equal to or greater than 64, whereas those who were culture negative had lower antibody titres. These data are more convincing than those presented by Kaneti et al (1988) and the contention by Kojima et al (1988) that antibody in semen is diagnostic needs further support. In the case of patients with SARA, chlamydial serum antibody titres tend to be higher than those in patients with uncomplicated NGU or other arthritides (Keat et al 1983). Of even greater interest, however, is the fact that recently it has been found that antibody titres in the synovial fluids of SARA patients are sometimes higher than those in the corresponding sera, indicating local production (J. Treharne, B.J. Thomas et al, unpublished observations). In babies, the occurrence of specific IgM antibody in association with pneumonia is pathognomonic of chlamydia-induced disease (Mahony et al 1986). Thus, so far as serology is concerned, the situation may be summarised by saying that although a fourfold or greater antibody response should always be sought, this is rarely detected. An elevated antibody titre in a single serum may be helpful in the conditions mentioned, but caution should be exercised because high titres do not always correlate with detection of chlamydiae (Meyer & Amortegui 1987). Indeed, seropositivity is not highly predictive of active infection (Nettleman & Jones 1988). High titres may be associated more with chronic (Frost et al 1987) or recurrent disease (Miettinen et al 1986). The absence of antibody in women determined by a sensitive serological test probably excludes an active chlamydial infection (Csángó et al 1988). Although it has been alleged that it is possible to distinguish between a current and a past infection by measuring IgA antibody in a single serum sample (Sarov et al 1986) it is dangerous to believe that this is so, particularly when such antibody has been seen to persist for several years in some patients who have had PID (Puolakkainen et al 1986). Unfortunately, the practice of using IgA as a marker continues (Cohen et al 1988).

In conclusion, chlamydial infections rarely produce specific clinical features and, therefore, laboratory help is required for their diagnosis. Culture has been the bed-rock in this regard, but non-cultural methods have improved, although the value of the much vaunted polymerase chain reaction remains to be seen. Serological procedures have a well defined but limited role.


## TREATMENT

A review of published reports on in vitro antimicrobial susceptibility studies and clinical treatment trials has been presented by Sanders et al (1986) and some of the problems encountered in treating chlamydial infections are outlined by Handsfield (1986). Chlamydiae are particularly sensitive to drugs that interfere with protein synthesis, for example tetracyclines and macrolides, but are sensitive also to a variety of other drugs, some of which have been tested both in vitro and in vivo in the last few years. The ELISA has been used as a more rapid and easier way of measuring in vitro activity than other methods (Cevinini et al 1987, Bianchi et al 1988) but standardisation of procedures is required (Ehret & Judson 1988b). Lack of standardisation to some extent accounts for the range of values shown in Table 11.3 in which antibiotics are listed in order of diminishing in vitro activity. The information is based on numerous publications including those by Ridgway (1986) and Ehret & Judson (1988b). Although some investigators may not agree with the exact order in which the antibiotics are placed, the overall pattern is likely to be correct. However, whatever the merit of a particular drug, the best treatment is achieved when patients and partners are part of an effective

**Table 11.3** Susceptibility of *Chlamydia trachomatis* to various antibiotics. The range of concentrations reflects observations made by different investigators more than differences between chlamydial strains.

| Antibiotic | Minimum inhibitory conc. (µg/ml) | Minimum bacterial conc. (µg/ml) |
|---|---|---|
| Rifampicin | 0.005– 0.25 | 0.015 –0.25 |
| Rosaramicin | 0.015– 0.25 | 0.05 –0.25 |
| Minocycline | 0.015– 0.5 | |
| Tetracycline | 0.02 – 0.5 | 0.02 –2.0 |
| Doxycycline | 0.025– 0.5 | |
| Oxytetracycline | 0.03 – 0.25 | 0.5 |
| Erythromycin | 0.03 – 0.5 | 0.1 –4.0 |
| Josamycin | 0.03 | |
| Roxithromycin | 0.03 | 0.06 |
| Miocamycin | 0.06 – 0.125 | |
| Chlortetracycline | 0.125– 2.5 | 0.125 –2.5 |
| Azithromycin | 0.125 | |
| Clindamycin | 0.25 – 2.0 | |
| Spiramycin | 0.5 | |
| Ofloxacin | 0.5 – 1.0 | 0.5 –1.0 |
| Ciprofloxacin | 1.0 – 2.0 | 1.0 –2.0 |
| Benzylpenicillin | 0.25 – 50 | 1.0– –>100 |
| Ampicillin | 0.25 – 50 | >100 |
| Sulphamethoxazole | 0.5 – 50 | |
| Chloramphenicol | 1.0 – 10 | >8 –10 |
| Augmentin | 2.0 | |
| Lomefloxacin | 2.0 – 4 | |
| Amoxycillin | 2.0 – >4 | |
| Rosoxacin | 4 – 8 | 4 –8 |
| Sulphisoxazole | 2.0 –200 | 2.0–500 |
| Amifloxacin | 8 | |
| Enoxacin | 8 | |
| Pefloxacin | 8 | |
| Trospectomycin | 8 | 16 |
| Sulphamethiazole | 8 – 16 | |
| Cloxacillin | 10 | |
| Norfloxacin | 16 | |
| Cephaloridine | 20 – >40 | 20–>40 |
| Trimethoprim | 20 –>100 | >1000 |
| Spectinomycin | 32 – 256 | ?–250 |
| Flumequine | 64 | |
| Novobiocin | >50 | |
| Nalidixic acid | >64 | |
| Kanamycin | >100 | |
| Lincomycin | 512 | |
| Colistin | >500 | |
| Gentamicin | >1000 | |
| Vancomycin | >1000 | |
| Metronidazole | >5000 | |
| Streptomycin | >10 000 | |

contact-tracing system (Katz et al 1988). If universal treatment of patients attending an STD clinic is not provided, the most cost-effective strategy appears to be empirical therapy for patients at high risk for chlamydial infections and therapy based on diagnostic test results for women at low risk (Nettleman et al 1986).

## Rifampicins

These are at least as active as the tetracyclines in vitro but are usually reserved for mycobacterial infections. Emergence of chlamydial resistance to rifabutin is negligible, or much slower than to rifampicin (Yearsley et al 1988).

## Tetracyclines

These remain the drugs most widely administered for chlamydial infections. Occasional anecdotal reports of tetracyclines failing (Midulla et al 1987) or of recovery of chlamydiae following such therapy are probably spurious (Taylor-Robinson 1987b) and Viswalingam et al (1987) and Mentis et al (1989) provide examples of the fact that no tetracycline-resistant strains have been encountered so far. However, certain tetracylines are secreted in low concentrations in the female upper genital tract and lymecycline 300mg twice daily and doxycycline 200mg (not 100mg) have been recommended (Forslin et al 1982). Tetracycline hydrochloride was effective in preventing chlamydial salpingitis in a mouse model if given before the chlamydiae, but less effective after the chlamydiae (Swenson et al 1986).

## Macrolides

Erythromycin is sometimes used as an alternative to tetracyclines and is the drug of choice for the treatment of chlamydial infections in infants, young children and in pregnant and lactating women (Chow & Jewesson 1985). The standard 2g does often produces gastrointestinal adverse effects that require discontinuation of therapy and a 1g dose is inadequate (Linnemann et al 1987). Thus, other macrolides vie for a therapeutic niche. The minimal inhibitory concentration (MIC) of roxithromycin (RU 28965) is similar to that of erythromycin and the MIC and minimal bactericidal concentration (MBC) of roxithromycin are identical according to some investigators (Stamm & Suchland 1986, Bowie et al 1987), but not others (Bianchi et al 1988). Roxithromycin 300mg daily for 7 days seems to be as efficacious as erythromycin in treating chlamydial infections in men and women (Worm et al 1989). A new macrolide, A-56268, is more active than roxithromycin, having MIC and MBC values similar to those of tetracycline (Bowie et al 1987). Another macrolide, CP-62,993, recently developed, has a prolonged half life and activity in vitro similar to erythromycin (Walsh et al 1987). Azithromycin has an MIC only a little greater than that of erythromycin (Slaney et al 1987), but a longer half life and greater tissue affinity. Spiramycin has some activity in vitro (Orfila et al 1988) but is not a drug of choice.

## Quinolones

These synthetic derivatives of nalidixic acid vary in their in vitro anti-chlamydial activity (Rettig et al 1986). Ofloxacin (Heppleston et al 1985,

Stamm & Suchland 1986, Maeda et al 1988) and, in particular, difloxacin (Liebowitz et al 1986, Segreti et al 1989) and new drugs, T-3262 (Maeda et al 1988), PD127,391 (Wise et al 1988) and temafloxacin (A-62254) (Segreti et al 1989), have quite low MIC values, the MICs of the three latter being similar to that of the tetracyclines. Other quinolones (NY-198 and AM-833) are not as active as ofloxacin (Nagayama et al 1988). In vivo, there have been conflicting reports of the therapeutic effectiveness of ofloxacin. Thus, the cure rate for genital chlamydial infection after a 5 day course of ofloxacin (200mg twice daily) was only 20% (Bischoff 1986) and a reliable cure was not provided by 300mg twice daily for 7 days (Boslego et al 1988). On the other hand, Perea et al (1989) were encouraged by its activity in a small number of chlamydia-positive NGU patients and Fransen et al (1986a), Nayagam et al (1988) and Ibsen et al (1989) considered it effective in the treatment of NGU in men. So too did Richmond et al (1988) for mixed gonococcal and chlamydial infections. Fleroxcin relieved the symptoms of NGU and cleared the chlamydiae, but caused a number of adverse reactions (Pust et al 1988). Norfloxacin was not sufficiently effective for treating chlamydial NGU (Bowie et al 1986), nor was ciprofloxacin (Arya et al 1986, van der Willigen et al 1988), its MIC being a little greater than that of ofloxacin, although ciprofloxacin seemed to be more effective in women (Ahmed-Jushuf et al 1987).

## Sulphonamides

Sulphonamides are ineffective in treating C. trachomatis infections, as is trimethoprim (Nielsen et al 1984) but there is synergy between sulpha-methoxazole and trimethoprim, demonstrated most strikingly when the concentration of trimethoprim exceeds that of the sulphonamide by at least a factor of eight (How et al 1985, Mumtaz et al 1988b). Thus, trimethoprim combined with a sulphonamide can be used for treating chlamydial infections in patients who suffer drug allergies and in those in whom a diagnosis of syphilis is in doubt since the combination does not mask a concomitant treponemal infection. It should be noted, however, that the ratio of trimethroprim to sulphamethoxazole is fixed at 1:5 in co-trimoxazole, a ratio that is not optimal for effective chlamydial therapy.

## Clindamycin

This antibiotic (6-chlorolincomycin) is strikingly more active in vitro than lincomycin, an MIC range of 0.25–2.0 µg/ml having been reported (Harrison et al 1984, Walsh et al 1987). It has behaved poorly as a means of treating chlamydial NGU (Bowie et al 1986), although Gjønnaess et al (1982) reported that there was a good clinical response of patients with PID, half of whom were infected by chlamydiae in the cervix.

**Penicillins**

The MIC values for various β-lactam antibiotics vary greatly (Hobson et al 1982, Martin et al 1986). Penicillin with metronidazole was far less effective than doxycycline with metronidazole for treating PID (Heinonen et al 1986). However, amoxycillin has been used apparently with some success to treat chlamydia-positive, mucopurulent cervicitis, and also urethritis in men (0.75mg thrice daily for 7 days) (Csángó et al 1985). Augmentin (amoxycillin plus clavulanic acid) together with doxycycline were effective in treating PID, some of which was chlamydial, but gastrointestinal side-effects were troublesome (Wølner-Hanssen et al 1988). Pivampicillin in a daily dose of 3.0g for 10 days was effective in treating uncomplicated genital chlamydial infections (Møller et al 1985), as, apparently, was 700mg twice daily for 7 days (Cramersø et al 1988). Bacampicillin 800mg twice daily for 7 days was used effectively by Lee et al (1989) to treat chlamydia-positive NGU. However, irrespective of these favourable results, the possibility of suppressing chlamydiae rather than eliminating them by such treatments should be kept in mind. Nevertheless, treating chlamydia-positive pregnant women with amoxycillin, or other β-lactam antibiotics with low MIC values, before delivery is an effective way of preventing chlamydial infection of the neonate (J Schachter, personal communication).

**Cephalosporins**

In general, these have quite high MIC values and not surprisingly, therefore, appear valueless for the treatment of chlamydial infections, for example chlamydial NGU (Stamm & Cole 1986).

Other antibiotics with similar or greater MIC values, for example, spectinomycin, or even its more active analogue trospectomycin (Zurenko et al 1988), cannot be contemplated for treating or preventing chlamydial infections.

PREVENTION

Prevention of sexually transmitted chlamydial infections would seem to be the ideal in view of the morbidity they cause and the enormous economic consequences of infection, estimated at 1.4 billion dollars per year in the United States (Washington et al 1987). Condom usage seems to lower the rate of transmission of chlamydiae between sexual partners (Worm & Petersen 1987), as does the use of the spermicide, monoxynol-9 (Louv et al 1988). In addition, other non-immune mechanisms may play an important part in preventing chlamydial infections. For example, the inhibitory effect on chlamydiae of spermine, copper, zinc (Greenberg et al 1985) and lysozyme in seminal plasma may prevent chlamydiae from becoming established in the prostate, and spread of chlamydiae from the lower to the upper genital tract in women may be influenced by hormones, the stage of the menstrual cycle and by trauma as occurs in hysterosalpingography. However, in a sense, apart from condom and spermicide usage, these points are academic; at a practical level, prevention is likely to be improved only by the institution of more widespread screening programmes, for example in family planning clinics (Trachtenberg et al 1988) for which Schachter (1989) makes a plea. These may never be fully effective, however, and inevitably vaccination becomes an issue. With this in mind, an important question is whether infection leads to immunity.

## Resistance to reinfection

### Observations on man

Some evidence for protection against reinfection has come from the observation that the chlamydial isolation rate for men with NGU is lower if they have a history of NGU than if they do not (Jones & Batteiger 1986). However, such presumed protection seems to be short-lived since it has been observed that chlamydiae are isolated more often in a second isolation attempt if the interval between cultures is more than 6 months than if it is less (Jones & Batteiger 1986). A similar indication of short-lived immunity has been seen in women (Katz et al 1987). Observations relating to immunity of the female upper genital tract have been made by Brunham et al (1986a,b). Fifty-two women with cervical chlamydial infection had a therapeutic abortion; of 10 who then developed salpingitis, none had prior IgM antibody and the geometric mean (GM) titre of serum IgG antibody was 14.9. In contrast, of the 42 women who remained well, the IgG GM titre was 41.6 and antibody to 100, 32 and 29 Kd antigens was demonstrated only in them, suggesting the involvement of these antigens in protection. It is worth noting at this juncture that the assessment of antibody by IMF (the usual procedure) may provide an inaccurate measure of its neutralising ability (Peterson et al 1989) and so lead to spurious conclusions about the role of antibody in immunity. In general, most genital infections with C. trachomatis may be attributed to a small number of serovars (Wagenvoort et al 1988). However, the role of serovar multiplicity in the failure to protect is unclear, although protection may not be afforded even by the same serovar (Barnes et al 1986).

### Observations on animals

There is agreement, as reviewed previously (Taylor-Robinson 1986, Tuffrey 1988, Taylor-Robinson & Ward 1989) that after rechallenge chlamydiae are cleared more quickly from the genital tract of various previously infected immunocompetent animals than they are from previously uninfected animals. The observations of Zhong et al (1989), although not concerned with the genital tract, suggest that gamma-interferon could have some role. However, such clearance is different from protection against reinfection. Although there is evidence that guinea pigs are resistant to reinfection of the genital tract with the guinea pig inclusion conjunctivitis (GPIC) agent, and that serum antibody from immune animals confers some degree of protection on recipients (Rank & Batteiger 1989), attempts to prevent *C. trachomatis* genital-tract infection in female mice have been unsuccessful (Tuffrey 1988, Taylor-Robinson & Ward 1989). Indeed, in recent experiments, although there was rapid elimination of organisms following reinoculation of mice with the same serotype, the frequency with which salpingitis occurred was not reduced and the disease was worse in some instances (Tuffrey et al 1990). Such evidence for hypersensitivity has been recorded by others. Thus, for example, primary inoculation of the oviducts of pig-tailed macaques with chlamydiae produced a self-limited salpingitis with minimal residual damage (Patton et al 1983), whereas repeat tubal inoculation caused hydrosalpinx formation with adnexal adhesions (Wølner-Hanssen et al 1986, Patton et al 1987). The exact nature of the antigens responsible for hypersensitivity is not clear but it is noteworthy that a detergent (Triton X-100) soluble extract of surface antigens of the GPIC agent produced ocular delayed hypersensitivity reactions in the guinea pig model (Watkins & Caldwell 1986).

## Vaccination

The comments above and the general failure of attempts to vaccinate in man and animals (Taylor-Robinson & Thomas 1980, Taylor-Robinson & Ward 1989), with at best only partial protection and at worst the induction of even more severe disease, has not been an encouragement to vaccine development. Clearly, the strategy should be the separation of protective chlamydial antigens from components of whole organisms that produce damaging, immunopathological reactions. There has been considerable progress in the molecular field in identifying protective surface antigens and defining the structure of the epitopes on these antigens which should stimulate protective immunity.

### Relevant surface antigens

The antigens relevant to vaccine development include the major outer membrane protein (MOMP), the cysteine-rich developmentally-regulated proteins (CRPs) and the eukaryotic cell-binding proteins. The serovar and subspecies epitopes of MOMP account for much of the specificity of antibody to whole chlamydiae produced in natural human infection. Furthermore, both of these epitopes are immunoaccessible and antibody to them neutralises chlamydial infectivity for cell cultures or for the primate eye (Zhang et al 1987a). A set of three CRPs of 60/62 and 15 Kd, present only in EBs, has been identified for *C. trachomatis* (Batteiger et al 1985, Newhall 1987, Zhang et al 1987b). Nucleotide and inferred amino acid sequences for the 60 Kd protein have been published recently (Clarke et al 1988, Allen & Stephens 1989). Although the CRPs form a developmentally regulated part of the outer membrane complex (Ward 1988) and the 60/62 Kd CRPs are highly immunogenic in man (Newhall et al 1982), there is no evidence to indicate that they are immunoaccessible, diminishing their importance as potential vaccine candidates. The eukaryotic cell-binding proteins (Hackstadt 1986, Wenman & Meuser 1986) are about 18 and 32 Kd. The 18 Kd protein has been sequenced and shares common domains with the 32 Kd protein (Kaul et al 1987). Although antiserum to these proteins neutralised chlamydial infection to some extent (Wenman & Meuser 1986), it is not certain that they are surface exposed. Thus, none of the surface proteins identified so far is as clear a vaccine candidate as MOMP.

## Epitope mapping

Monoclonal antibodies to MOMP with serovar or subspecies specificity neutralise *C. trachomatis* infectivity (Zhang et al 1987a) and attempts have been made to identify the binding sites for these antibodies. Comparison of inferred amino acid sequences for the MOMP genes of several *C. trachomatis* serovars shows that the protein consists of four variable regions (VS 1 to 4) plus constant domains (Stephens et al 1987, Yuan et al 1989). The species and sub-species epitopes relate to a 16 amino acid region of VS 4 (Stephens et al 1986) and serovar-specific epitopes to homologous 14 amino acid peptides within VS 2 (Stephens et al 1988). More precise localisation of MOMP serovar, subspecies, species and genus specific epitopes has been achieved recently by using solid phase peptide synthesis on polythene pins (Conlan et al 1988, 1989). The use of epitope mapping techniques, in conjunction with surface proteolysis of intact organisms and monoclonal antibody probes, has suggested that only the variable regions of MOMP, notably VS 1, 2 and 4, protrude externally and are immunoaccessible (Su et al 1988), a concept supported by the neutralisation data (Zhang et al 1987a).

The sub-species epitope on MOMP is of particular interest for vaccine development because of its potentially broad neutralising activity. The critical binding site for the immunoaccessible B sub-species epitope on serovar L1 has been shown to be *ile-phe-asp-thr* (IFDT). A shift in binding specificity of just one amino acid to the N-terminus was sufficient to abolish binding to viable chlamydiae. However, immunisation with a flexible peptide derived from this region resulted in a binding requirement for only IFD, giving broadened species specificity at the sub-species binding site. This suggests that it may well be possible to improve the utility of antibody to chlamydial epitopes using synthetic peptide vaccines (Conlan et al 1989). Recently, the frequency with which human subjects with genital infection or trachoma respond to overlapping hexameric or decameric peptides covering the whole MOMP and 60 Kd CRP sequence has been determined (Kajbaf M, Conlan W,

Clarke I, Ward M E, personal communication). The results indicate that humans generally respond well to epitopes also recognised by mice. Most importantly, they indicate that haplotype restriction of B cell responses, at least in the Caucasian or African populations studied, should not pose too great a threat to chlamydial vaccine development.

Ideally a chlamydial vaccine should generate an anamnestic response on exposure to infection as well as neutralising mucosal antibody. In practice, mucosal immunity may be difficult to sustain in the absence of replicating antigen, although oral immunisation with live chlamydiae has been shown to generate ocular immunity in experimental animals (Whittum-Hudson et al 1986). Certainly, in the absence of high concentrations of mucosal antibodies it will be difficult to prevent initial infection of host cells. Chlamydiae within cells are sheltered from antibodies and it remains to be seen whether chlamydial antigens at the host cell surface are targets for antibody dependent- or cell mediated-immune cytotoxic attack. Irrespective of this, high levels of anti-chlamydial circulating antibody should be achieved easily by vaccination and following initial infection might gain access to the epithelia by inflammatory transudation. Such antibody, while not preventing initial infection, might be capable of neutralising released chlamydiae, so modifiying the severity of disease and rendering the individual less infectious to others. The molecular approach to chlamydial vaccine development would seem to have a bright future.

## REFERENCES

Ahmed-Jushuf I H, Arya O P, Hobson D et al 1988 Ciprofloxacin treatment of chlamydial infections of urogenital tracts of women. Genitourinary Medicine 64: 14–17

Alexander I, Paul I D, Caul E O 1985 Evaluation of a genus reactive monoclonal antibody in rapid identification of Chlamydia trachomatis by direct immunofluorescence. Genitourinary Medicine 61: 252–254

Alger L S, Lovchik J C, Hebel J R, Blackman L R, Crenshaw M C 1988 The association of Chlamydia trachomatis, Neisseria gonorrhoeae, and group B streptococci with preterm rupture of the membranes and pregnancy outcome. American Journal of Obstetrics and Gynecology 159: 397–404

Allen J E, Stephens R S 1989 Identification by sequence analysis of two-site posttranslational processing of the cysteine-rich outer membrane protein 2 of Chlamydia trachomatis serovar L2. Journal of Bacteriology 171: 285–291

Amortegui A J, Meyer M P, Gnatuk C L 1986 Prevalence of Chlamydia trachomatis and other micro-organisms in women seeking abortions in Pittsburgh, Pennsylvania, United States of America. Genitourinary Medicine 62: 88–92

Anestad G, Lunde O, Moen M, Dalaker K 1987 Infertility and chlamydial infection. Fertility and Sterility 48: 787–790

Arroyo G, Linnemann C, Wesseler T 1989 Role of the Papanicolaou smear in diagnosis of chlamydial infections. Sexually Transmitted Diseases 16: 11–14

Arya O P, Hobson D, Hart C A, Bartzokas C, Pratt B C 1986 Evaluation of ciprofloxacin 500mg twice daily for one week in treating uncomplicated gonococcal, chlamydial, and non-specific urethritis in men. Genitourinary Medicine 62: 170–174

Attenburrow A A, Barker C M 1985 Chlamydial pneumonia in the low birthweight neonate. Archives of Disease in Childhood 60: 1169–1172

Barnes R C 1989 Laboratory diagnosis of human chlamydial infections. Clinical Microbiology Reviews 2: 119–136

Barnes R C, Suchland R J, Wang S-P, Kuo C-C, Stamm W E 1985 Detection of multiple serovars of Chlamydia trachomatis in genital infections. Journal of Infectious Diseases 152: 985–989

Barnes R C, Roddy R E, Stamm W E 1986 Serovars of Chlamydia trachomatis causing repeated genital infection. In: Oriel D et al (eds) Chlamydial infections. Cambridge University Press, Cambridge. pp 503–506

Baron A L (ed) 1988 Microbiology of Chlamydia. CRC Press Inc, Florida

Barton S E, Thomas B J, Taylor-Robinson D, Goldmeier D 1985 Detection of Chlamydia trachomatis in the vaginal vault of women who have had hysterectomies. British Medical Journal 291: 250

Batteiger B E, Newhall W J, Jones R B 1985 Differences in outer membrane proteins of the lymphogranuloma venereum and trachoma biovars of Chlamydia trachomatis. Infection and Immunity 50: 488–494

Batteiger B E, Fraiz J, Newhall W J, Katz B P, Jones R B 1989 Association of recurrent chlamydial infection with gonorrhea. Journal of Infectious Diseases 159: 661–669

Bell T A 1988 Chlamydia trachomatis infection in dizygotic twins delivered by caesarean section. Genitourinary Medicine 64: 347–348

Bell T A, Sandström I, Gravett M G et al 1987 Comparison of ophthalmic silver nitrate solution and erythromycin ointment for prevention of natally acquired Chlamydia trachomatis. Sexually Transmitted Diseases 14: 195–200

Benes S, McCormack W M 1985 Inhibition of growth of Chlamydia trachomatis by nonoxynol-9 in vitro. Antimicrobial Agents and Chemotherapy 27: 724–726

Bentsi C, Klufio C A, Perine P L et al 1985 Genital infections with Chlamydia trachomatis and Neisseria gonorrhoeae in Ghanaian women. Genitourinary Medicine 61: 48–50

Berger R E, Alexander E R, Monda G D, Ansell J, McCormick G, Holmes K K 1978 Chlamydia trachomatis as a cause of acute 'idiopathic' epididymitis. New England Journal of Medicine 298: 301–304

Berger R E, Krieger J N, Kessler D et al 1989 Case control study of men with suspected chronic idiopathic prostatitis. Journal of Urology 141: 328–331

Berman S M, Harrison H R, Boyce W T, Haffner W J J, Lewis M, Arthur J B 1987 Low birth weight, prematurity, and postpartum endometritis. Association with prenatal cervical Mycoplasma hominis and Chlamydia trachomatis infections. Journal of the American Medical Association 257: 1189–1194

Bianchi A, Scieux C, Saleron C M, Casin I, Perol Y 1988 Rapid determination of MICs of 15 antichlamydial agents by using an enzyme immunoassay (Chlamydiazyme). Antimicrobial Agents and Chemotherapy 32: 1350–1353

Bischoff W 1986 Ofloxacin: therapeutic results in Chlamydia trachomatis urethritis. Infection 14 (Suppl), 316–317

Boslego J W, Hicks C B, Greenup R et al 1988 A prospective randomized trial of ofloxacin vs. doxycycline in the treatment of uncomplicated male urethritis. Sexually Transmitted Diseases 15: 186–191

Bowie W R, Yu J S, Jones H D 1986 Partial efficacy of clindamycin against Chlamydia trachomatis in men with nongonococcal urethritis. Sexually Transmitted Diseases 13: 76–80

Bowie W R, Shaw C E, Chan D G W, Black W A 1987 In vitro activity of Ro 15-8074, Ro 19-5247, A-56268, and roxithromycin (RU 28965) against Neisseria gonorrhoeae and Chlamydia trachomatis. Antimicrobial Agents and Chemotherapy 31: 470–472

Bradley M G, Hobson D, Lee N, Tait I A, Rees E 1985 Chlamydial infections of the urethra in women. Genitourinary Medicine 61: 371–375

British Co-operative Clinical Group 1987 Survey of diagnostic facilities for Chlamydia trachomatis and herpes simplex virus, 1984. Genitourinary Medicine 63: 26–27

Brunham R C, Maclean I W, Binns B, Peeling R W 1985 Chlamydia trachomatis: its role in tubal infertility. Journal of Infectious Diseases 152: 1275–1282

Brunham R C, Binns B, McDowell J, Paraskevas M 1986 Chlamydia trachomatis infection in women with ectopic pregnancy. Obstetrics and Gynecology 67: 722–726

Brunham R C, Maclean I, McDowell J, Peeling R, Persson K, Osser S 1986a Chlamydia trachomatis antigen specific serum antibodies among women who did and did not develop acute salpingitis following therapeutic abortion. In: Oriel D et al (eds) Chlamydial infections. Cambridge University Press, Cambridge pp221–224

Brunham R C, Peeling R, Maclean I, McDowell J, Persson K, Osser S 1986b Postabortal

Chlamydia trachomatis salpingitis: correlating risk with antigen-specific serological responses and with neutralization. Journal of Infectious Diseases 155: 749–755

Brunham R C, Binns B, Guijon F, Danforth D, Kosseim M L, Rand F, McDowell J, Rayner E 1988 Etiology and outcome of acute pelvic inflammatory disease. Journal of Infectious Diseases 158: 510–517

Bump R C, Copeland W E 1985 Urethral isolation of the genital mycoplasmas and Chlamydia trachomatis in women with chronic urologic complaints. American Journal of Obstetrics and Gynecology 152: 38–41

Buxton D 1986 Potential danger to pregnant women of Chlamydia psittaci from sheep. Veterinary Record 118: 510–511

Bygdeman S, Lidbrink P, Ahlin A, Teichert C, Ahmed H J 1988 Comparison between two different commercial test kits for detection of Chlamydia trachomatis antigen with EIA technique (IDEIA and Chlamydiazyme) and culture in urogenital specimens. In: Oriel J D, Waugh M (eds) Anglo-Scandinavian Conference on Sexually Transmitted Diseases, Royal Society of Medicine Services Limited p 67.

Campbell L A, Kuo C-C, Grayston J T 1987 Characterization of the new Chlamydia agent, TWAR, as a unique organism by restriction endonuclease analysis and DNA-DNA hybridization. Journal of Clinical Microbiology 25: 1911–1916

Campbell L A, Kuo C-C, Thissen R W, Grayston J T 1989 Isolation of a gene encoding a Chlamydia sp. strain TWAR protein that is recognized during infection of humans. Infection and Immunity 57: 71–75

Caul E O, Paul I D 1985 Monoclonal antibody based ELISA for detecting Chlamydia trachomatis. Lancet i: 279

Caul E O, Paul I D, Milne J D, Crowley T 1988 Non-invasive sampling method for detecting Chlamydia trachomatis. Lancet ii: 1246–1247

Cevenini R, Rumpianesi F, Sambri V, La Placa M 1986a Antigenic specificity of serological response in Chlamydia trachomatis urethritis detected by immunoblotting. Journal of Clinical Pathology 39: 325–327

Cevenini R, Rumpianesi F, Donati M, Moroni A, Sambri V La Placa M 1986b Class specific immunoglobulin response in individual polypeptides of Chlamydia trachomatis, elementary bodies, and reticulate bodies in patients with chlamydial infection. Journal of Clinical Pathology 39: 1313–1316

Cevenini R, Donati M, Sambri V, Rumpianesi F, La Placa M 1987 Enzyme-linked immunosorbent assay for the in-vitro detection of sensitivity of Chlamydia trachomatis to antimicrobial drugs. Journal of Antimicrobial Chemotherapy 20: 677–684

Chaudhuri P, Sng E H, Yuen W S 1986 Chlamydia trachomatis infection in unmarried women seeking abortions. Genitourinary Medicine 62: 17–18

Chernesky M A, Mahony J B, Castricianos et al 1986 Detection of Chlamydia trachomatis antigens by enzyme immunoassay and immunofluorescence in genital specimens from symptomatic and asymptomatic men and women. Journal of Infectious Diseases 154: 141–148

Chi E Y, Kuo C-C, Grayston J T 1987 Unique ultrastructure in the elementary body of Chlamydia sp. strain TWAR. Journal of Bacteriology 169: 3757–3763

Chisholm S M, Matheson B A, Ho-Yen D 1988 Limitations of Chlamydiazyme in general hospital laboratories. Journal of Clinical Pathology 41: 357

Chow A W, Jewesson P 1985 Pharmacokinetics and safety of antimicrobial agents during pregnancy. Reviews of Infectious Diseases 7: 287–313

Ciotti R A, Sondheimer S J, Nachamkin I 1988 Detecting Chlamydia trachomatis by direct immunofluorescence using a Cytobrush sampling technique. Genitourinary Medicine 64: 245–246

Clarke I N, Ward M E, Lambden P R 1988 Molecular cloning and sequence analysis of a developmentally regulated cysteine-rich outer membrane protein from Chlamydia trachomatis. Gene 71: 307–314

Cleary R W, Jones R B 1985 Recovery of Chlamydia trachomatis from the endometrium in infertile women with serum antichlamydial antibodies. Fertility and Sterility 44: 233–235

Cles L D, Bruch K, Stamm W E 1988 Staining characteristics of six commercially available monoclonal immunofluorescence reagents for direct diagnosis of Chlamydia trachomatis infections. Journal of Clinical Microbiology 26: 1735–1737

Close C E, Wang S P, Roberts P L, Berger R E 1987 The relationship of infection with

Chlamydia trachomatis to the parameters of male fertility and sperm autoimmunity. Fertility and Sterility 48: 880–883

Cohen I, Tenenbaum E, Fejgin M, Altaras M, Ben-Aderet N, Sarov I 1988 Serum-specific antibodies for Chlamydia trachomatis in premature contractions. Americal Journal of Obstetrics and Gynecology 158: 579–582

Conlan J W, Clarke I N, Ward M E 1988 Epitope mapping with solid-phase peptides: identification of type-, subspecies-, species-, and genus-reactive antibody binding domains on the major outer membrane protein of Chlamydia trachomatis. Molecular Microbiology 2: 673–679

Conlan J W, Kajbaf M, Clarke I et al 1989 The major outer membrane protein of Chlamydia trachomatis: critical binding site and conformation determine the specificity of antibody binding to viable chlamydiae. Molecular Microbiology 3: 311–318

Cox R L, Kuo C-C, Grayston J T, Campbell L A 1988 Deoxyribonucleic acid relatedness of Chlamydia sp. strain TWAR to Chlamydia trachomatis and Chlamydia psittaci. International Journal of Systematic Bacteriology 38: 265–268

Cramers M, Kaspersen P, From E, Møller B R 1988 Pivampicillin compared with erythromycin for treating women with genital Chlamydia trachomatis infection. Genitourinary Medicine 64: 247–248

Cromer B A, Heald F P 1987 Pelvic inflammatory disease associated with Neisseria gonorrhoeae and Chlamydia trachomatis: clinical correlates. Sexually Transmitted Diseases 14: 125–129

Csángó P A, Gundersen T, Martinsen I-M 1985 Effect of amoxicillin on simultaneous Chlamydia trachomatis infection in men with gonococcal urethritis: comparison of three dosage regimens. Sexually Transmitted Diseases 12: 93–96

Csángó P A, Sarov B, Schiøtz H, Sarov I 1988 Comparison between cell culture and serology for detecting Chlamydia trachomatis in women seeking abortion. Journal of Clinical Pathology 41: 89–92

Dean D, Palmer L, Pant C R, Courtright P, Falkow S, O'Hanley P 1989 Use of a Chlamydia trachomatis DNA probe for detection of ocular chlamydiae. Journal of Clinical Microbiology 27: 1062–1067

De Jong Z, Pontonnier F, Plante P et al 1988 The frequency of Chlamydia trachomatis in acute epididymitis. British Journal of Urology 62: 76–78

Doble A, Taylor-Robinson D, Thomas B J, Jalil N, Harris J R W, Witherow R O'N 1989a Acute epididymitis: a microbiological and ultrasonographic study. British Journal of Urology 63: 90–94

Doble A, Thomas B J, Walker M M, Harris J R W, Witherow R O'N, Taylor-Robinson D 1989b The role of Chlamydia trachomatis in chronic abacterial prostatitis: a study utilising ultrasound guided biopsy. Journal of Urology 141: 332-333

Duffy S, Cawdell G, Fieldman N 1985 Unusual presentation of chlamydial peritonitis: case report. Genitourinary Medicine 61: 202–203

Dunlop E M C, Goh B T, Darougar S, Woodland R 1985 Triple-culture tests for diagnosis of chlamydial infection of the female genital tract. Sexually Transmitted Diseases 12: 68–71

Dunlop E M C, Garner A, Darougar S, Treharne J D, Woodland R M 1989 Colposcopy, biopsy, and cytology results in women with chlamydial cervicitis. Genitourinary Medicine 65: 22–31

Dutilh B, Bebear C, Taylor-Robinson D, Grimont P A D 1988 Detection of Chlamydia trachomatis by in situ hybridization with sulphonated total DNA. Annales di l'Institut Pasteur (Microbiologie) 139: 115–127

Dutilh B, Bebear C, Rodriguez P, Vekris A, Bonnet J, Garret M 1989 Specific amplification of a DNA sequence common to all Chlamydia trachomatis serovars using the polymerase chain reaction. Research in Microbiology 140: 7–16

Edelman D A 1988 The use of intrauterine contraceptive devices, pelvic inflammatory disease, and Chlamydia trachomatis infection. American Journal of Obstetrics and Gynecology 158: 956–959

Ehret J M, Judson F N 1988a Activity of nonoxynol-9 against Chlamydia trachomatis. Sexually Transmitted Diseases 15: 156–157

Ehret J M, Judson F N 1988b Susceptibility testing of Chlamydia trachomatis: from eggs to monoclonal antibodies. Antimicrobial Agents and Chemotherapy 32: 1295–1299

Elder H A, Santamarina B A G, Smith S, Kass E H 1971 The natural history of asymptomatic bacteriuria during pregnancy: the effect of tetracycline on the clinical course and the outcome of pregnancy. American Journal of Obstetrics and Gynecology 111: 441–442

Estany A, Todd M, Vasquez M, McLaren R 1989 Early detection of genital chlamydial infection in women: an economic evaluation. Sexually Transmitted Diseases 16: 21–27

Fehler H G, Ballard R C, Dangory et al 1989 Sexually acquired acute epididymitis. Southern African Journal of Epidemiology and Infection 4: 23–24

Fish A N, Fairweather D V, Oriel J D, Ridgway G L 1988 Isolation of Chlamydia trachomatis from endometriums of women with and without symptoms. Genitourinary Medicine 64: 75–77

Forbes B A, Bartholoma N, McMillan J, Roefaro M, Weiner L, Welych L 1986 Evaluation of a monoclonal antibody test to detect chlamydia in cervical and urethral specimens. Journal of Clinical Microbiology 23: 1136–1137

Ford D K, Reid G D, Magge S, Schumacher H R 1988 Synovial lymphocyte response to chlamydial stimulation associated with intrasynovial chlamydial antigen in a patient with 'rheumatoid arthritis'. Arthritis and Rheumatism 31: 914–917

Forslin L, Danielsson D, Kjellander J, Falk V 1982 Antibiotic treatment of acute salpingitis. A study of plasma concentrations of two tetracyclines (doxycycline and lymecycline) Acta Obstetrica Gynecol Scandinavica 61: 59–64

Forster G E, Cookey I, Munday P E et al 1985 Investigation into the value of Papanicolaou stained cervical smears for the diagnosis of chlamydial cervical infection. Journal of Clinical Pathology 38: 399–402

Foulkes S J, Deighton R, Feeney A R B, Mohanty K C, Freeman C W J 1985 Comparison of direct immunofluorescence and cell culture for detecting Chlamydia trachomatis. Genitourinary Medicine 61: 255–257

Foulon W, Naessens A, Cammu H, Guossens A, Lauwers S 1986 Epidemiology and pathogenesis of Ureaplasma urealyticum and spontaneous abortion and early preterm labor. Pediatric Infectious Disease 5 (Suppl): 353

Fox A S, Saxon E M, Doveikis S, Beem M O 1989 Chlamydia trachomatis and parainfluenza 2 virus: a shared antigenic determinant? Journal of Clinical Microbiology 27: 1407–1408

Fransen L, Nsanze H, D'Costa L J, Brunham R C, Piot P 1985 Parents of infants with ophthalmia neonatorum: a high-risk group for sexually transmitted diseases. Sexually Transmitted Diseases 12: 150–154

Fransen L, Avonts D, Piot P 1986a Treatment of genital chlamydial infection with ofloxacin. Infection 14 (Suppl): 318–320

Fransen L, Nsanze H, Klauss V, van der Stuyft P, D'Costa L, Brunham R C, Piot P 1986b Ophthalmia neonatorum in Nairobi, Kenya: the roles of Neisseria gonorrhoeae and Chlamydia trachomatis. Journal of Infectious Diseases 153: 862–869

Frost E, Collet M, Reniers J, Leclerc A, Ivanoff B, Meheus A 1987 Importance of chlamydial antibodies in acute salpingitis in central Africa. Genitourinary Medicine 63: 176–178

Ghirardini C, Boselli F, Messi P, Rivasi F, Trentini G P 1989 Chlamydia trachomatis infections in asymptomatic women. Results of a study employing different staining techniques. Acta Cytologica 33: 115–119

Gibbs R S, Schachter J 1987 Chlamydial serology in patients with intra-amniotic infection and controls. Sexually Transmitted Diseases 14: 213–215

Gønnaess H, Dalaker K, Urnes A et al 1982 Treatment of pelvic inflammatory disease. Effects of lymecycline and clindamycin. Current Therapeutic Research 29: 885–892

Glenney K F, Glassman D M, Cox S W, Brown H P 1988 The prevalence of positive test results for Chlamydia trachomatis by direct smear for fluorescent antibodies in a south Texas family planning population. Journal of Reproductive Medicine 33: 457–462

Goh B T, Dunlop E M C, Darougar S, Woodland R 1985 Three sequential methods of collecting material from the urethra of men for culture for Chlamydia trachomatis. Sexually Transmitted Diseases 12: 173–176

Goudswaard J, Sabbe L, van Belzen C 1989 Interference by Gram-negative bacteria in the enzyme immunoassay for detecting Chlamydia trachomatis. Journal of Infection 18: 94–96

Grant J B F, Costello C B, Sequeira P J L, Blacklock N J 1987 The role of Chlamydia trachomatis in epididymitis. British Journal of Urology 60: 355–359

Grayston J T, Kuo C-C, Campbell L A, Wang S-P 1988 Proposal to create the Chlamydia pneumoniae sp. nov. for Chlamydia strain TWAR. International Journal of Systematic

Bacteriology 39: 88–90

Grayston J T, Wang S P, Kuo C C 1989 Current knowledge of Chlamydia TWAR, an important cause of pneumonia and other acute respiratory diseases. European Journal of Clinical Microbiology and Infectious Disease 8:191–202

Greenberg S B, Harris D, Giles P, Martin R R, Wallace R J 1985 Inhibition of Chlamydia trachomatis growth in McCoy, HeLa, and human prostate cells by zinc. Antimicrobial Agents and Chemotherapy 27: 953–957

Greenblatt R M, Handsfield H H, Sayers M H, Holmes K K 1986 Screening therapeutic insemination donors for sexually transmitted diseases: overview and recommendations. Fertility and Sterility 46: 351–364

Grillner L, Beckman S, Hammer H 1986 Comparison of two enzyme immunoassays and an immunofluourescence test for detection of Chlamydia trachomatis. European Journal of Clinical Microbiology 5: 559–562

Guaschino S, Stola E, Spinillo A 1988 Chlamydia trachomatis and cervical intraepithelial neoplasia. Clinical and Experimental Obstetrics and Gynecology 15: 98–101

Gump D W, Gibson M 1985 Antibodies to Chlamydia trachomatis in cervical secretions and serum: effect of blood in such secretions. Fertility and Sterility 43: 814–815

Hackstadt T 1986 Identification and properties of chlamydial polypeptides that bind eucaryotic cell surface components. Journal of Bacteriology 165: 13–20

Hagay Z J, Sarov B, Sachs J, Shaked O, Sarov I 1989 Detecting Chlamydia trachomatis in men with urethritis: serology v isolation in cell culture. Genitourinary Medicine 65: 166–170

Hammerschlag M R, Roblin P M, Cummings C, Williams T H, Worku M, Howard L V 1987 Comparison of enzyme immunoassay and culture for diagnosis of chlamydial conjunctivitis and respiratory infections in infants. Journal of Clinical Microbiology 25: 2306–2308

Hammerschlag M R, Cummings C, Roblin P M, Williams T H, Delke I 1989 Efficacy of neonatal ocular prophylaxis for the prevention of chlamydial and gonococcal conjunctivitis. New England Journal of Medicine 320: 769–772

Handsfield H H 1986 Problems in the treatment of bacterial sexually transmitted diseases. Sexually Transmitted Diseases 13 (Suppl): 179–184

Handsfield H H, Jasman L L, Roberts P L, Hanson V W, Kothenbeutel R L, Stamm W E 1986 Criteria for selective screening for Chlamydia trachomatis infection in women attending family planning clinics. Journal of the American Medical Association 255: 1730–1734

Hanuka N, Glasner M, Sarov I 1988 Detection of IgG and IgA antibodies to Chlamydia trachomatis in sera of patients with chlamydial infections: use of immunoblotting and immunoperoxidase assays. Sexually Transmitted Diseases 15: 93–99

Hardy P H, Hardy J B, Nell E E, Graham D A, Spence M R, Rosenbaum R C 1984 Prevalence of six sexually transmitted disease agents among pregnant inner-city adolescents, and pregnancy outcome. Lancet i: 333–337

Harper I, Shearman M, Dalgety F, Cole D 1985 Fluorescein-conjugated monoclonal antibodies to detect Chlamydia trachomatis in smears. Lancet ii: 509

Harrison H R 1986 Chlamydial infection in neonates and children. In: Oriel D et al (eds) Chlamydial infections. Cambridge University Press, Cambridge. pp283–292

Harrison H R, Riggins R M, Alexander E R, Weinstein L 1984 In vitro activity of clindamycin against strains of Chlamydia trachomatis, Mycoplasma hominis and Ureaplasma urealyticum isolated from pregnant women. American Journal of Obstetrics and Gynecology 149: 447–480

Harrison H R, Costin M, Meder J B et al 1985 Cervical Chlamydia trachomatis infection in university women: relationship to history, contraception, ectopy and cervicitis. American Journal of Obstetrics and Gynecology 153: 244–251

Hartford S L, Silva P D, diZerega G S, Yonekura M L 1987 Serologic evidence of prior chlamydial infection in patients with tubal ectopic pregnancy and contralateral tubal disease. Fertility and Sterility 47: 118–121

Hartmann A A, Elsner P, Wecker I 1986 Isolation of Chlamydia trachomatis from a gonad biopsy specimen of a man with sterile pyospermia. Journal of Infectious Diseases 154: 731–733

Hawkins D A, Wilson R S, Thomas B J, Evans R T 1985 Rapid, reliable diagnosis of chlamydial ophthalmia by means of monoclonal antibodies. British Journal of

Ophthalmology 69: 640–644

Hawkins D A, Taylor-Robinson D, Thomas B J, Harris J R W 1986 Microbiological survey of acute epididymitis. Genitourinary Medicine 62: 342–344

Heinonen P K, Teisala K, Punnonen R et al 1986 Treating pelvic inflammatory disease with doxycycline and metronidazole or penicillin and metronidazole. Genitourinary Medicine 62: 235–239

Heisterberg L, Møller B R, Manthorpe T, Sørensen S S, Petersen K, Nielsen N C 1985 Prophylaxis with lymecycline in induced first-trimester abortion: a clinical, controlled trial assessing the role of Chlamydia trachomatis and Mycoplasma hominis. Sexually Transmitted Diseases 12: 72–75

Hellstrom W J G, Schachter J, Sweet R L, McClure R D 1987 Is there a role for Chlamydia trachomatis and genital mycoplasma in male infertility? Fertility and Sterility 48: 337–339

Heppleston C, Richmond S, Bailey J 1985 Antichlamydial activity of quinolone carboxylic acids. Journal of Antimicrobial Chemotherapy 15: 645–647

Hillier S L, Krohn M J, Kiviat N, Martius J, Eschenbach D A 1986 The association of Ureaplasma urealyticum with preterm birth, chorionamnionitis, postpartum fever, intrapartum fever and bacterial vaginosis. Pediatric Infectious Disease 5 (Suppl): 349

Hipp S S, Han Y, Murphy D 1987 Assessment of enzyme immunoassay and immunofluorescence tests for detection of Chlamydia trachomatis. Journal of Clinical Microbiology 25: 1938–1943

Hobson D, Lee N, Bushell A A, Withana N 1982 The activity of beta-lactam antibiotics against Chlamydia trachomatis in McCoy cell cultures. In: Mårdh P-A et al (eds) Chlamydial infections. Elsevier Biomedical Press, Amsterdam. pp 249–252

Horn J E, Hammer M L, Falkow S, Quinn T C 1986 Detection of Chlamydia trachomatis in tissue culture and cervical scrapings by in situ DNA hybridization. Journal of Infectious Diseases 153: 1155–1159

Horn J E, Kappus E W, Falkow S, Quinn T C 1988 Diagnosis of Chlamydia trachomatis in biopsied tissue specimens by using in situ DNA hybridization. Journal of Infectious Diseases 157: 1249–1253

Hough A J, Rank R G 1989 Pathogenesis of acute arthritis due to viable Chlamydia trachomatis (mouse pneumonitis agent) in C57Bl/6 mice. American Journal of Pathology 134: 903–912

How S J, Hobson D, Hart C A, Webster R E 1985 An in vitro investigation of synergy and antagonism between antimicrobials against Chlamydia trachomatis. Journal of Antimicrobial Chemotherapy 15: 533–538

Howard L V, Coleman P F, England B J, Herrman J E 1986 Evaluation of Chlamydiazyme for the detection of genital infections caused by Chlamydia trachomatis. Journal of Clinical Microbiology 23: 329–332

Hughes E G, Mowatt J, Spence J E 1989 Endocervical Chlamydia trachomatis infection in Canadian adolescents. Canadian Medical Association Journal 140: 297–301

Hyypiä T, Jalava A, Larsen S H, Terho P, Hukkanen V 1985 Detection of Chlamydia trachomatis in clinical specimens by nucleic acid spot hybridization. Journal of General Microbiology 131: 975–978

Ibsen H H W, Møller B R, Halkier-Sørensen L, From E 1989 Treatment of nongonococcal urethritis: comparison of ofloxacin and erythromycin. Sexually Transmitted Diseases 16: 32–35

Ishikawa H, Ohno O, Yamasaki K, Ikuta S, Hirohata K 1986 Arthritis presumably caused by Chlamydia in Reiter syndrome. Case report with electron microscopic studies. Journal of Bone and Joint Surgery 68: 777–779

Jensen B L, Hoff G, Weismann K 1988 A comparison of an enzyme immunoassay and cell culture for detection of Chlamydia trachomatis in genito-urinary specimens. Sexually Transmitted Diseases 15: 123–126

Jones R B, Batteiger B E 1986 Human immune response to Chlamydia trachomatis infections. In: Oriel D et al (eds) Chlamydial infections. Cambridge University Press, Cambridge. pp423–432

Jones R B, Rabinovitch R A, Katz B P et al 1985 Chlamydia trachomatis in the pharynx and rectum of heterosexual patients at risk for genital infection. Annals of Internal Medicine 102: 757–762

Jones R B, Katz B P, van der Pol B, Caine V A, Batteiger B E, Newhall W J 1986a Effect of blind passage and multiple sampling on recovery of Chlamydia trachomatis from urogenital specimens. Journal of Clinical Microbiology 24: 1029–1033

Jones R B, Mammel J B, Shepard M K, Fisher R R 1986b Recovery of Chlamydia trachomatis from the endometrium of women at risk for chlamydial infection. American Journal of Obstetrics and Gynecology 155: 35–39

Jones R B, van der Pol B, Katz B P 1989 Effect of differences in specimen processing and passage technique on recovery of Chlamydia trachomatis. Journal of Clinical Microbiology 27: 894–898

Judson B A, Lambert P P 1988 Improved Syva MicroTrak Chlamydia trachomatis direct test method. Journal of Clinical Microbiology 26: 2657–2658

Judson F N, Tavelli B G 1986 Comparison of clinical and epidemiological characteristics of pelvic inflammatory disease classified by endocervical cultures of Neisseria gonorrhoeae and Chlamydia trachomatis. Genitourinary Medicine 62: 230–234

Kaneti J, Sarov B, Sarov I 1988 IgA and IgG antibodies specific for Chlamydia trachomatis in acute epididymitis. European Urology 14: 323–327

Kappus EW, Quinn TC 1986 The spermicide nonoxynol-9 does not inhibit Chlamydia trachomatis in vitro. Sexually Transmitted Diseases 13: 134–137

Karam G H, Martin D H, Flotte T R et al 1986 Asymptomatic Chlamydia trachomatis infections among sexually active men. Journal of Infectious Diseases 154: 900–903

Katz B P, Batteiger B E, Jones R B 1987 Effect of prior sexually transmitted disease on the isolation of Chlamydia trachomatis. Sexually Transmitted Diseases 14: 160–164

Katz B P, Danos C S, Quinn T S, Caine V, Jones R B 1988 Efficiency and cost-effectiveness of field follow-up for patients with Chlamydia trachomatis infection in a sexually transmitted diseases clinic. Sexually Transmitted Diseases 15: 11–16

Katzman D K, Friedman I M, McDonald C A, Litt I F 1988 Chlamydia trachomatis Fitz-Hugh-Curtis syndrome without salpingitis in female adolescents. American Journal of Diseases of Children 142: 996–998

Kaul R, Roy K L, Wenman W M 1987 Cloning, expression, and primary structure of a Chlamydia trachomatis binding protein. Journal of Bacteriology 169: 5152–5156

Keat A, Thomas B J, Taylor-Robinson D 1983 Chlamydial infection in the aetiology of arthritis. British Medical Bulletin 39: 168–174

Keat A, Thomas B, Dixey J, Osborn M, Sonnex C, Taylor-Robinson D 1987 Chlamydia trachomatis and reactive arthritis: the missing link. Lancet i: 72–74

Kellogg J A, Seiple J W, Levisky J S 1989 Efficacy of duplicate genital specimens and repeated testing for confirming positive results for Chlamydiazyme detection of Chlamydia trachomatis antigen. Journal of Clinical Microbiology 27: 1218–1221

Kent G P, Harrison H R, Berman S M, Keenlyside R A 1988 Screening for Chlamydia trachomatis infection in a sexually transmitted disease clinic: comparison of diagnostic tests with clinical and historical risk factors. Sexually Transmitted Diseases 15: 51–57

Kinghorn G R, Duerden B I, Hafiz S 1986 Clinical and microbiological investigation of women with acute salpingitis and their consorts. British Journal of Obstetrics and Gynaecology 93: 869–880

Kirshon B, Faro S, Phillips L E, Pruett K 1988 Correlation of ultrasonography and bacteriology of the endocervix and posterior cul-de-sac of patients with severe pelvic inflammatory disease. Sexually Transmitted Diseases 15: 103–107

Kiviat N B, Paavonen J A, Brockway J et al 1985a Cytologic manifestations of cervical and vaginal infections. I. Epithelial and inflammatory cellular changes. Journal of the American Medical Association 253: 989–996

Kiviat N B, Peterson M, Kinney-Thomas E, Tam M, Stamm W E, Holmes K K 1985b Cytologic manifestations of cervical and vaginal infections. II. Confirmation of Chlamydia trachomatis infection by direct immunofluorescence using monoclonal antibodies. Journal of the American Medical Association 253: 997–1000

Kiviat N B, Wølner-Hanssen P, Petersen M et al 1986 Localization of Chlamydia trachomatis infection by direct immunofluorescence and culture in pelvic inflammatory disease. American Journal of Obstetrics and Gynecology 154: 865–873

Klingebiel T, Pickert A, Dopfer R, Ranke M B, Siedner R 1989 Unusual course of a Chlamydia pneumonia in an infant with IgG2/IgG4-deficiency. European Journal of Pediatrics 148: 431–434

Knight S T, Lee S H, Davis C H, Moorman D R, Hodinka R L, Wyrick P B 1987 In vitro activity of nonoxynol-9 on McCoy cells infected with Chlamydia trachomatis. Sexually Transmitted Diseases 14: 165–173

Kojima H, Wang S P, Kuo C C, Grayston J T 1988 Local antibody in semen for rapid diagnosis of Chlamydia trachomatis epididymitis. Journal of Urology 140: 528–531

Krech T, Gerhard-Fsadni D, Hofmann N, Miller S M 1985 Interference of Staphylococcus aureus in the detection of Chlamydia trachomatis by monoclonal antibodies. Lancet i: 1161–1162

Kristensen G B, Bollerup A C, Lind K et al 1985 Infections with Neisseria gonorrhoeae and Chlamydia trachomatis in women with acute salpingitis. Genitourinary Medicine 61: 179–184

Kroon F P, van't Wout J W, Weiland H T, van Furth R 1989 Chlamydia trachomatis pneumonia in an HIV-seropositive patient. New England Journal of Medicine 320: 806–807

Kuo C-C, Chen H-H, Wang S-P, Grayston J T 1986 Identification of a new group of Chlamydia psittaci strains called TWAR. Journal of Clinical Microbiology 24: 1034–1037

Laga M, Plummer F A, Nzanze H et al 1986 Epidemiology of ophthalmia neonatorum in Kenya. Lancet ii: 1145–1149

Lamont R F, Taylor-Robinson D, Wigglesworth J S, Furr P M, Evans R T, Elder M G 1987 The role of mycoplasmas, ureaplasmas and chlamydiae in the genital tract of women presenting in spontaneous early preterm labour. Journal of Medical Microbiology 24: 253–257

Larsen J H, Wulf H C, Friis-Møller A 1986 Comparison of a fluorescent monoclonal antibody assay and a tissue culture assay for routine detection of infections caused by Chlamydia trachomatis. European Journal of Clinical Microbiology 5: 554–558

LeBar W, Herschman B, Jemal C, Pierzchala J 1989 Comparison of DNA probe, monoclonal antibody enzyme immunoassay, and cell culture for the detection of Chlamydia trachomatis. Journal of Clinical Microbiology 27: 826–828

Leclerc A, Frost E, Collet M, Goeman J, Bedjabaga L 1988 Urogenital Chlamydia trachomatis in Gabon: an unrecognised epidemic. Genitourinary Medicine 64: 308–311

Lee C T, Lim K B, Thirumoorthy T, Nadarajah M 1989 Bacampicillin to treat non-gonococcal urethritis in men: pilot study. Genitourinary Medicine 65: 32–34

Lefebvre J, Laperrière H, Rousseau H, Massé R 1988 Comparison of three techniques for detection of Chlamydia trachomatis in endocervical specimens from asymptomatic women. Journal of Clinical Microbiology 26: 726–731

Lefèvre J C, Averous S, Bauriaud R, Blanc C, Bertrand M A, Lareng M B 1988 Lower genital tract infections in women: comparison of clinical and epidemiologic findings with microbiology. Sexually Transmitted Diseases 15: 110–113

Levy R A, Warford A L 1986 Evaluation of the modified Chlamydiazyme immunoassay for the detection of chlamydial antigen. American Journal of Clinical Pathology 86: 330–335

Liebowitz L D, Saunders J, Fehler G, Ballard R C, Koornhof H J 1986 In vitro activity of A-56619 (difloxacin), A-56620, and other new quinolone antimicrobial agents against genital pathogens. Antimicrobial Agents and Chemotherapy 30: 948–950

Lindner L E, Geerling S, Nettum J A, Miller S L, Altman K H 1988 Clinical characteristics of women with chlamydial cervicitis. Journal of Reproductive Medicine 33: 684–690

Linnemann C C, Heaton C L, Ritchey M 1987 Treatment of Chlamydia trachomatis infections: comparison of 1- and 2-g doses of erythromycin daily for seven days. Sexually Transmitted Diseases 14: 102–106

Lipkin E S, Moncada J V, Shafer M-A, Wilson T E, Schachter J 1986 Comparison of monoclonal antibody staining and culture in diagnosing cervical chlamydial infection. Journal of Clinical Microbiology 23: 114–117

Livengood C H, Schmitt J W, Addison W A, Wrenn J W, Magruder-Habib K 1988 Direct fluorescent antibody testing for endocervical Chlamydia trachomatis: factors affecting accuracy. Obstetrics and Gynecology 72: 803–809

Longhurst H J, Flower N, Thomas B J et al 1987 Journal of the Royal College of General Practitioners 37: 255–256

Louv W C, Austin H, Alexander W J, Stagno S, Cheeks J 1988 A clinical trial of nonoxynol-9 for preventing gonococcal and chlamydial infections. Journal of Infectious Diseases 158: 518–523

Louv W C, Austin H, Perlamn J, Alexander W J 1989 Oral contraceptive use and the risk of chlamydial and gonococcal infections. American Journal of Obstetrics and Gynecology 160: 396–402

Mabey D C W, Booth-Mason S 1986 The detection of Chlamydia trachomatis by direct immunofluorescence in conjunctival smears from patients with trachoma and patients with ophthalmia neonatorum using a conjugated monoclonal antibody. Journal of Hygiene 96: 83–87

Mabey D C W, Forsey T, Treharne J D 1987 Serotypes of Chlamydia trachomatis in the Gambia. Lancet ii: 452

Maeda H, Fujii A, Nakata K, Arakouva S, Kamidono S 1988 In vitro activities of T-3262, NY-198, fleroxacin (AM-833; RO23-6240), and other new quinolone agents against clinically isolated Chlamydia trachomatis strains. Antimicrobial Agents and Chemotherapy 32: 1080–1081

Magder L S, Harrison H R, Ehret J M, Anderson T S, Judson F N 1988 Factors related to genital Chlamydia trachomatis and its diagnosis by culture in a sexually transmitted disease clinic. American Journal of Epidemiology 128: 298–308

Mahony J B, Chernesky M A 1985 Effect of swab type and storage temperature on the isolation of Chlamydia trachomatis from clinical specimens. Journal of Clinical Microbiology 22: 865–867

Mahony J B, Chernesky M A, Bromberg K, Schachter J 1986 Accuracy of immunoglobulin M immunoassay for diagnosis of chlamydial infections in infants and adults. Journal of Clinical Microbiology 24: 731–735

Mantell J, Goh B T 1987 Occult chlamydial ophthalmia in men with non-gonococcal urethritis. British Medical Journal 294: 707

Mantell J, Goh BT, Woodland R M, Walpita P 1988 Dual infection of the conjunctiva with herpes simplex virus and Chlamydia trachomatis. Sexually Transmitted Diseases 15: 167–168

Manuel A R G, Veeravahu M, Matthews R S, Clay J C 1987 Pooled specimens for Chlamydia trachomatis: new approach to increase yield and cost efficiency. Genitourinary Medicine 63: 172–175

Mårdh P-A 1986 Ascending chlamydial infection in the female genital tract. In: Oriel D et al (eds) Chlamydial infections. Cambridge University Press, Cambridge. pp173–184

Mårdh P-A, Paavonen J, Puolakkainen M 1989 Chlamydia. Plenum Medical, London.

Martin D H, Pastorek J G, Faro S 1986 In-vitro and in-vivo activity of parenterally administered β-lactam antibiotics against Chlamydia trachomatis. Sexually Transmitted Diseases 13: 81–87

Martius J, Krohn M, Hillier S, Stamm W E, Holmes K K, Eschenbach D A 1988 Relationships of vaginal Lactobacillus species, cervical Chlamydia trachomatis, and bacterial vaginosis to preterm birth. Obstetrics and Gynecology 71: 89–95

Maslow A S, Davis C H, Choong J, Wyrick P B 1988 Estrogen enhances attachment of , Chlamydia trachomatis to human endometrial epithelial cells in vitro. American Journal of Obstetrics and Gynecology 159: 1006–1014

Matthews R S, Wise R 1989 Non-invasive sampling method for detecting Chlamydia trachomatis. Lancet i: 96

Mearns G, Richmond S J, Storey C C 1988 Sensitive immune dot blot test for diagnosis of Chlamydia trachomatis infection. Journal of Clinical Microbiology 26: 1810–1813

Mecsei R, Haugen O A, Halvorsen L E, Dalen A 1989 Genital Chlamydia trachomatis infections in patients with abnormal cervical smears: effect of tetracycline treatment on cell changes. Obstetrics and Gynecology 73: 317–321

Meddens M J M, Quint W G V, van der Willigen H, Wagenvoort J T H, v. Dijk W C, Lindeman J, Herbrink P 1988 Detection of Chlamydia trachomatis in culture and urogenital smears by in situ DNA hybridization using a biotinylated DNA probe. Mollecular and Cellular Probes 2: 261–268

Medici A, Sollecito D, Rossi D, Midulla M 1988 Family outbreak of Chlamydia trachomatis. Lancet ii: 682

Meijer C J L M, Calame J J, de Windt E J G et al 1989 Prevalence of Chlamydia trachomatis infection in a population of asymptomatic women in a screening program for cervical cancer. European Journal of Clinical Microbiology and Infectious Diseases 8: 127–130

Melekos M D, Asbach H W 1988 The role of chlamydiae in epididymitis. International Urology and Nephrology 20: 293–297

Mentis A F, Tzouvelekis L S, Mavrommati L 1989 Susceptibility of fifteen Chlamydia trachomatis strains isolated in Greece. Journal of Antimicrobial Chemotherapy 24: 1989

Meyer M P, Amortegui 1987 Evaluation of single whole inclusion serum test for IgG antibody to Chlamydia trachomatis in asymptomatic women. Genitourinary Medicine 63: 22–25

Midulla M, Sollecito D, Feleppa F, Assensio A M, Ilari S 1987 Infection by airborne Chlamydia trachomatis in a dentist cured with rifampicin after failures with tetracycline and doxycycline. British Medical Journal 294: 742

Miettinen A, Saikku P, Jansson E, Paavonen J 1986 Epidemiologic and clinical characteristics of pelvic inflammatory disease associated with Mycoplasma hominis, Chlamydia trachomatis, and Neisseria gonorrhoeae. Sexually Transmitted Diseases 13: 24–28

Mohammed N R S, Hilary I B 1985 Improved method for isolation and growth of Chlamydia trachomatis in McCoy cells treated with cycloheximide using polyethylene glycol. Journal of Clinical Pathology 38: 1052–1054

Mohanty K C, O'Neill J J, Hambling M H 1986 Comparison of enzyme immunoassays and cell culture for detecting Chlamydia trachomatis. Genitourinary Medicine 62: 175–176

Moi H, Danielsson D 1986 Diagnosis of genital Chlamydia trachomatis infection in males by cell culture and antigen detection test. European Journal of Clinical Microbiology 5: 563–568

Møller B R, Cramers M, From E 1985 Pivampicillin in treating genital infection with Chlamydia trachomatis. Genitourinary Medicine 61: 264–265

Møller B R, Kaspersen P, Kristiansen F V, Mårdh P-A 1986 Chlamydia trachomatis in the upper female genital tract with negative cervical culture. Lancet ii: 390

Moncada J V, Schachter J, Wolfsy C 1986 Prevalence of Chlamydia trachomatis lung infection in patients with acquired immune deficiency syndrome. Journal of Clinical Microbiology 23: 986

Moncada J V, Schachter J, Golbus M S 1987 Chlamydia trachomatis infection among patients undergoing chorionic villus sampling. American Journal of Obstetrics and Gynecology 156: 915–916

Moncada J, Schachter J, Shipp M, Bolan G, Wilber J 1989 Cytobrush in collection of cervical specimens for detection of Chlamydia trachomatis. Journal of Clinical Microbiology 27: 1863–1866

Monteiro E F, Bradbury J A, O'Donnell M, Rennie I G, Kinghorn G R 1987 Occult chlamydial ophthalmia in men with non-gonococcal urethritis. British Medical Journal 294: 394

Morgan-Capner P, Hudson P, Cansfield J A, Saeed A 1986 Detection of Chlamydia trachomatis by enzyme immunoassay, immunofluorescence, and cell culture. Journal of Clinical Pathology 39: 232

Moss T R, Hawkswell J 1987 Clinical and microbiological investigation of women with acute salpingitis and their consorts. British Journal of Obstetrics and Gynaecology 94: 187–188

Moss T R, Steptoe P C 1984 Chlamydia trachomatis: importance in in vitro fertilization? Journal of the Royal Society of Medicine 77: 70–72

Moss T R, Nicholls A, Viercant P, Gregson S, Hawkswell J 1986 Chlamydia trachomatis and infertility. Lancet ii: 281–282

Mulcahy F M, Lacey C J N 1987 Sexually transmitted infections in adolescent girls. Genitourinary Medicine 63: 119–121

Mulcahy F M, Bignell C J, Rajakumar R et al 1987 Prevalence of chlamydial infection in acute epididymo-orchitis. Genitourinary Medicine 63: 16–18

Mumtaz G, Mellars B J, Ridgway G L, Oriel J D 1985 Enzyme immunoassay for the detection of Chlamydia trachomatis antigen in urethral and endocervical swabs. Journal of Clinical Pathology 38: 740–742

Mumtaz G, Nayagam A, Ridgway G L, Oriel J D 1988a Comparison of novel EIA (Pharmacia) with cell culture and immunofluorescence for the diagnosis of genital chlamydial infection. In: Oriel J D, Waugh M (eds) Anglo-Scandinavian Conference on Sexually Transmitted Diseases. Royal Society of Medicine Services, London. p68

Mumtaz G, Ridgway G L, Felmingham D 1988b In vitro activity of sulphamethoxazole/trimethoprim and sulfadoxine/pyrimethamine against Chlamydia trachomatis SA$_2$f in McCoy cell culture. European Journal of Clinical Microbiology and Infectious Diseases 7: 415–417

Munday P E, Stacey C M, Ison C A, Thomas B J, Taylor-Robinson D 1987 Clinical and microbiological investigation of women with acute salpingitis and their consorts. British Journal of Obstetrics and Gynaecology 94: 281–282

Nachamkin I, Sawyer K, Skalina D, Crooks G W, Ciotti R, Sondheimer S J 1987

Test-of-cure analysis by direct immunofluorescence for Chlamydia trachomatis after antimicrobial therapy. Journal of Clinical Microbiology 25: 1774–1775

Nagashima T 1987 A high prevalence of chlamydial cervicitis in postmenopausal women. American Journal of Obstetrics and Gynecology 156: 31–32

Nagayama A, Nakao T, Taen H 1988 In vitro activities of ofloxacin and four other new quinolone-carboxylic acids against Chlamydia trachomatis. Antimicrobial Agents and Chemotherapy 32: 1735–1737

Nägel T C, Tagatz G E, Campbell B F 1986 Transmission of Chlamydia trachomatis by artificial insemination. Fertility and Sterility 46: 959–960

Näher H, Petzoldt D 1986 Evaluation of an enzyme immunoassay (Chlamydiazyme) and a direct immunofluorescence technique (MicroTrak) for the detection of Chlamydia trachomatis antigen in urogenital specimens. European Journal of Sexually Transmitted Diseases 3: 217–222

Näher H, Petzoldt D, Sethi K K 1988 Evaluation of non-radioactive in situ hybridisation method to detect Chlamydia trachomatis in cell culture. Genitourinary Medicine 64: 162–164

Nayagam A T, Ridgway G L, Oriel J D 1988 Efficacy of ofloxacin in the treatment of non-gonococcal urethritis in men and genital infections caused by Chlamydia trachomatis in men and women. Journal of Antimicrobial Chemotherapy 22 (Suppl): 155–160

Nettleman M D, Jones R B 1988 Cost-effectiveness of screening women at moderate risk for genital infections caused by Chlamydia trachomatis. Journal of the American Medical Association 260: 207–213

Nettleman M D, Jones R B, Roberts S D et al 1986 Cost-effectiveness of culturing for Chlamydia trachomatis. A study in a clinic for sexually transmitted diseases. Annals of Internal Medicine 105: 189–196

Newhall W J 1987 Biosynthesis and disulfide cross-linking of outer membrane components during the growth cycle of Chlamydia trachomatis. Infection and Immunity 55: 162–168

Newhall W J, Basinski M B 1986 Purification and structural characterization of chlamydial outer membrane proteins. In: Oriel et al (eds) Chlamydial infections. Cambridge University Press, Cambridge. pp93–96

Newhall W J, Batteiger B, Jones R B 1982 Analysis of the human serological response to proteins of Chlamydia trachomatis. Infection and Immunity 38: 1181–1189

Newhall W J, Terho P, Wilde C E, Batteiger B E, Jones R B 1986 Serovar determination of Chlamydia trachomatis isolates by using type-specific monoclonal antibodies. Journal of Clinical Microbiology 23: 333–338

Nielsen P B, Christensen J D, Frentz G 1984 A comparison of oxytetracycline and trimethoprim, in the treatment of Chlamydia trachomatis urethritis. Infection 12: 274–275

Numazaki K, Chiba S, Moroboshi T, Kudoh T, Yamanaka T, Nakao T 1985 Comparison of enzyme linked immunosorbent assay and enzyme linked fluorescence immunoassay for detection of antibodies against Chlamydia trachomatis. Journal of Clinical Pathology 38: 345–350

Numazaki K, Chiba S, Kogawa K, Umetsu M, Motoya H, Nakayo T 1986 Chronic respiratory disease in premature infants caused by Chlamydia trachomatis. Journal of Clinical Pathology 39: 84–88

Ogawa H, Yamazaki Y, Hashiguchi K 1988 Chlamydia trachomatis: a currently recognized pathogen of tonsillitis. Acta Oto-Laryngologica 454 (Suppl): 197–201

Oriel J D, Waugh M (eds) 1988 Anglo-Scandinavian Conference on Sexually Transmitted Diseases. Royal Society of Medicine Services, London.

Oriel D, Ridgway G, Schachter J, Taylor-Robinson D, Ward M (eds) 1986 Chlamydial infections. Cambridge University Press, Cambridge

Orfila J, Haider F, Thomas D 1988 Activity of spiramycin against chlamydia, in vitro and in vivo. Journal of Antimicrobial Chemotherapy 22 Suppl B: 73–76

Paavonen J, Aine R, Teisala K et al 1985a Chlamydial endometritis. Journal of Clinical Pathology 38: 726–732

Paavonen J, Kiviat N, Brunham R C et al 1985b Prevalence and manifestations of endometritis among women with cervicitis. American Journal of Obstetrics and Gynecology 152: 280–286

Paavonen J, Critchlow C W, DeRouen T et al 1986 Etiology of cervical inflammation. American Journal of Obstetrics and Gynecology 154: 556–564

Palva A, Korpela K, Lassus A, Ranki M 1987 Detection of Chlamydia trachomatis from genito-urinary specimens by improved nucleic acid sandwich hybridization. FEMS Microbiology Letters 40: 211–217

Pao C C, Lin S-S, Yang T-E, Soong Y-K, Lee P-S, Lin J-Y 1987 Deoxyribonucleic acid hybridization analysis for the detection of urogenital chlamydia trachomatis infections in women. American Journal of Obstetrics and Gynecology 156: 195–199

Pastorek J G, Mroczkowski T F, Martin D H 1988 Fine-tuning the fluorescent antibody test for chlamydial infections in pregnancy. Obstetrics and Gynecology 72: 957–960

Patton D L, Halbert S A, Kuo C-C, Wang S-P, Holmes K K 1983 Host response to primary Chlamydia trachomatis infection of the fallopian tube in pig-tailed monkeys. Fertility and Sterility 40: 829–840

Patton D L, Kuo C-C, Wang S-P, Halbert S A 1987 Distal tubal obstruction induced by repeated Chlamydia trachomatis salpingeal infections in pig-tailed macaques. Journal of Infectious Diseases 155: 1292–1299

Perea E J, Aznar J, Herrera A, Mazuecos J, Rodriguez-Pichardo A 1989 Clinical efficacy of new quinolones for therapy of nongonococcal urethritis. Sexually Transmitted Diseases 16: 7–10

Peterson E M, Oda R, Tse P, Gastaldi C, Stone S C, de la Maza L M 1989 Comparison of a single-antigen microimmunofluorescence assay and inclusion fluorescent-antibody assay for detecting chlamydial antibodies and correlation of the results with neutralizing ability. Journal of Clinical Microbiology 27: 350–352

Phillips L E, Faro S, Smith P B, Martens M G, Riddle G D, Goodrich K H 1988 Premarket evaluation of Monofluor reagent for detecting Chlamydia trachomatis in adolescent outpatients. Genitourinary Medicine 64: 165–168

Phillips R S, Aronson M D, Taylor W C, Safran C 1987a Should tests for Chlamydia trachomatis cervical infection be done during routine gynecologic visits? An analysis of the costs of alternative strategies. Annals of Internal Medicine 107: 188–194

Phillips R S, Hanff P A, Klauffman R S, Aronson M D 1987b Use of a direct fluorescent antibody test for detecting Chlamydia trachomatis cervical infection in women seeking routine gynecologic care. Journal of Infectious Diseases 156: 575–581

Poletti F, Medici M C, Alinovi A et al 1985 Isolation of Chlamydia trachomatis from the prostatic cells in patients affected by nonacute abacterial prostatitis. Journal of Urology 134: 691–693

Pothier P, Kazmierczak A 1986 Comparison of cell culture with two direct chlamydia tests using immunofluorescence or enzyme — linked immunosorbent assay. European Journal of Clinical Microbiology 5: 569–572

Pouletty P, Martin J, Catalan F et al 1988 Optimization of a rapid test by using fluorescein-conjugated monoclonal antibodies for detection of Chlamydia trachomatis in clinical specimens. Journal of Clinical Microbiology 26: 267–270

Preece P M, Anderson J M, Thompson R G 1989 Chlamydia trachomatis infection in infants. Archives of Disease in Childhood 64: 525–529

Proceedings (1988) The European Society for Chlamydia Research. 1st Meeting, Bologna, Italy (May 30-June 1, 1988)

Pugh S F, Slack R C B, Caul E O, Paul I D, Appleton P N, Gatley S 1985 Enzyme amplified immunoassay: a novel technique applied to direct detection of Chlamydia trachomatis in clinical specimens. Journal of Clinical Pathology 38: 1139–1141

Puolakkainen M, Saikku P, Leinonen M, Nurminen M, Väänänen P, Mäketä P H 1985 Comparative sensitivity of different serological tests for detecting chlamydial antibodies in perihepatitis. Journal of Clinical Pathology 38: 929–932

Puolakkainen M, Vesterinen E, Purola E, Saikku P, Paavonen J 1986 Persistence of chlamydial antibodies after pelvic inflammatory disease. Journal of Clinical Microbiology 23: 924–928

Puolakkainen M, Kousa M, Saikku P 1987 Clinical conditions associated with positive complement fixation serology for Chlamydiae. Epidemiology and Infection 98: 101–108

Pust R A, Ackenheil-Köppe H R, Weidner W, Meier-Ewert H 1988 Clinical efficacy and tolerance of fleroxacin in patients with urethritis caused by Chlamydia trachomatis. Journal of Antimicrobial Chemotherapy 22 (Suppl): 227–230

Quinn T C, Warfield P, Kappus E, Barbacci M, Spence M 1985 Screening for Chlamydia trachomatis infection in an inner-city population: a comparison of diagnostic methods. Journal of Infectious Diseases 152: 419–423

Quinn P A, Petric M, Barkin M et al 1987 Prevalence of antibody to Chlamydia trachomatis in spontaneous abortion and infertility. American Journal of Obstetrics and Gynecology 156: 291–296

Rahm V A, Gnarpe H, Oldlind V 1988 Chlamydia trachomatis among sexually active teenage girls. Lack of correlation between chlamydial infection, history of the patient and clinical signs of infection. British Journal of Obstetrics and Gynaecology 95: 916–919

Rank R G, Batteiger B E 1989 Protective role of serum antibody in immunity to chlamydial genital infection. Infection and Immunity 57: 299–301

Rank R G, Ramsey K H, Hough A J 1988 Antibody-mediated modulation of arthritis induced by Chlamydia. American Journal of Pathology 132: 372–381

Rapoza P A, Quinn T C, Kiessling L A, Green W R, Taylor H R 1986 Assessment of neonatal conjunctivitis with a direct immunofluorescent monoclonal antibody stain for Chlamydia. Journal of the American Medical Association 255: 3369–3373

Reed B D, Huck W 1987 Differences in the prevalence of Chlamydia trachomatis reported by two laboratories using the direct immunofluorescence test. Journal of the American Medical Association 257: 2593

Reid R 1985 Genital chlamydial infection and cervical cancer. American Journal of Obstetrics and Gynecology 152: 364

Rettig P J, Rollerson W J, Macks M I 1986 In vitro activity of six fluoroquinolones against Chlamydia trachomatis. In: Oriel D et al (eds) Chlamydial infections, Cambridge University Press, Cambridge. pp 528–531

Richmond S J, Bhattacharyya M N, Maiti H, Chowdhury F H, Stirland R M, Tooth J A 1988 The efficacy of ofloxacin against infection caused by Neisseria gonorrhoeae and Chlamydia trachomatis. Journal of Antimicrobial Chemotherapy 22 (Suppl):149–153

Ridgway G L 1986 Antimicrobial Chemotherapy of chlamydial infection: where next? European Journal of Clinical Microbiology 5: 550–553

Riordan T, Ellis D A, Matthews P I, Ratcliffe S F 1986 False positive results with an ELISA for detection of chlamydia antigen. Journal of Clinical Pathology 39: 1276–1277

Robertson J N, Ward M E, Conway D, Caul E O 1987 Chlamydial and gonococcal antibodies in sera of infertile women with tubal obstruction. Journal of Clinical Pathology 40: 377–383

Robertson J N, Hogston P, Ward M E 1988 Gonococcal and chlamydial antibodies in ectopic and intrauterine pregnancy. British Journal of Obstetrics and Gynaecology 95: 711–716

Rompalo A M, Price C B, Roberts P L, Stamm W E 1986 Potential value of rectal-screening cultures for Chlamydia trachomatis in homosexual men. Journal of Infectious Diseases 153: 888–892

Rompalo A M, Suchland R J, Price C B, Stamm W E 1987 Rapid diagnosis of Chlamydia trachomatis rectal infection by direct immunofluorescence staining. Journal of Infectious Diseases 155: 1075–1076

Rosenberg M J, Feldblum P J, Rojanapithayakorn W, Sawasdivorn W 1987 The contraceptive sponge's protection against Chlamydia trachomatis and Neisseria gonorrhoeae. Sexually Transmitted Diseases 14: 147–152

Ross J M, Furr P M, Taylor-Robinson D, Altman D G, Coid C R 1981 The effect of genital mycoplasmas on human fetal growth. British Journal of Obstetrics and Gynaecology 88: 749–755

Rothburn M M, Mallinson H, Mutton K J 1986 False-positive ELISA for Chlamydia trachomatis recognised by atypical morphology in fluorescent staining. Lancet ii: 982–983

Rowland G F, Forsey T, Moss T R, Steptoe P C, Hewitt J, Darougar S 1985 Failure of in vitro fertilization and embryo replacement following infection with Chlamydia trachomatis. Journal of in vitro Fertilization and Embryo Transfer 2: 151–155

Royal College of Physicians Committee on Genitourinary Medicine 1987 Chlamydial diagnostic services in the United Kingdom and Eire: current facilities and perceived needs. Genitourinary Medicine 63: 371–374

Ruijs G J, Kauer F M, van Gijssel P M, Schirm J, Schroder F P 1988 Direct immunofluorescence for Chlamydia trachomatis on urogenital smears for epidemiological purposes. European Journal of Obstetrics, Gynaecology and Reproductive Biology 27: 289-297

Saikku P, Puolakkainen M, Leionen M, Nurminen M, Nissinen A 1986 Cross reactivity between Chlamydiazyme and acinetobacter strains. New England Journal of Medicine 314: 922–923

Sanders L L, Harrison H R, Washington A E 1986 Treatment of sexually transmitted chlamydial infections. Journal of the American Medical Association 255: 1750–1756

San Joaquin V H, Rettig P J 1986 Role of Chlamydia trachomatis in upper-respiratory-tract infections in children. Journal of Infectious Diseases 154: 193

Sanyal D, Oates S 1987 Chlamydia trachomatis in antenatal clinics. Lancet ii: 855

Sarov I, Sarov B, Hanuka N, Glasner M, Kaneti J 1986 The significance of serum specific IgA antibodies in diagnosis of active Chlamydia trachomatis infections. In: Oriel D et al (eds) Chlamydial infections. Cambridge University Press, Cambridge. pp 566–569

Saul H M, Grossman M B 1988 The role of Chlamydia trachomatis in Bartholin's gland abscess. American Journal of Obstetrics and Gynecology 158: 576–577

Schachter J 1967 Isolation of Bedsoniae from human arthritis and abortion tissues. American Journal of Ophthalmology 63: 1082–1086

Schachter J 1986a Chlamydia trachomatis infections: epidemiology and disease spectrum. In: Oriel J D, Harris J R W (eds) Recent advances in sexually transmitted diseases, Churchill Livingstone, Edinburgh, pp 39–58

Schachter J 1986b Human Chlamydia psittaci infection. In: Oriel D et al (eds) Chlamydial infections. Cambridge University Press. Cambridge. pp 311–320

Schachter J 1989 Why we need a program for the control of Chlamydia trachomatis. New England Journal of Medicine 320: 802–804

Schachter J, Martin D H 1987 Failure of multiple passages to increase chlamydial recovery. Journal of Clinical Microbiology 25: 1851–1853

Schachter J, Grossman M, Sweet R L, Holt J, Jordan C, Bishop E 1986a Prospective study of perinatal transmission of Chlamydia trachomatis. Journal of the American Medical Association 255: 3374–3377

Schachter J, Sweet R L, Grossman M, Landers D, Robbie M, Bishop E 1986b Experience with the routine dose of erythromycin for chlamydial infections in pregnancy. New England Journal of Medicine 314: 276–279

Schumacher H R, Magge S, Cherian P V et al 1988 Light and electron microscopic studies on the synovial membrane in Reiter's syndrome. Immunocytochemical identification of chlamydial antigen in patients with early disease. Arthritis and Rheumatism 31:937–946

Scott BD, Fortenberry JD 1986 Postgonococcal conjunctivitis due to Chlamydia trachomatis. Sexually Transmitted Diseases 13: 172–173

Segreti J, Kessler H A, Kapell K S, Trenholme G M 1989 In vitro activities of temafloxacin (A-62254) and four other antibiotics against Chlamydia trachomatis. Antimicrobial Agents and Chemotherapy 33: 118–119

Sekhri A, Le Faou A E, Tardieu J C, Antz M, Fabre M 1988 What can be expected from the cytologic examination of cervicovaginal smears for the diagnosis of Chlamydia trachomatis infections? Acta Ctyologica 32: 805–810

Sellors J W, Mahony J B, Chernesky M A, Rath D J 1988 Tubal factor infertility: an association with prior chlamydial infection and asymptomatic salpingitis. Fertility and Sterility 49: 451–457

Shafer M-A, Chew K L, Kromhout L K et al 1985 Chlamydial endocervical infections and cytologic findings in sexually active female adolescents. American Journal of Obstetrics and Gynecology 151: 765–771

Shafer M-A, Prager V, Shalwitz J et al 1987 Prevalence of urethral Chlamydia trachomatis and Neisseria gonorrhoeae among asymptomatic, sexually active adolescent boys. Journal of Infectious Diseases 156: 223–224

Shanahan D, Lord P H, Grogono J, Wastell C 1988 Clinical acute cholecystitis and the Curtis-Fitz-Hugh syndrome. Annals of the Royal College of Surgeons of England 70: 44–46

Sherman J K, Jordan G W 1985 Cryosurvival of Chlamydia trachomatis during cryopreservation of human spermatozoa. Fertility and Sterility 43: 664–666

Singal S S, Reichman R C, Graman P S, Greisberger C, Trupei M A, Menegus M A 1986 Isolation of Chlamydia trachomatis from men with urethritis: relative value of one vs. two swabs and influence of concomitant gonococcal infection. Sexually Transmitted Diseases 13: 50–52

Slaney L, Plummer F, Ronald R R, Degagne P, Hoban D, Brunham R C 1987 In vitro activity of azithromycin (AZM) against Neisseria gonorrhoeae (gc), Haemophilus ducreyi (Hd), Chlamydia trachomatis and Chlamydia psittaci. In Abstracts of the 1987 ICAAC, Abstract No. 728, p 1224

Smeltzer M P, Marchiarullo A G, Dorian K J 1985 Establishing Chlamydia trachomatis isolation capability in a local laboratory. Sexually Transmitted Diseases 12: 44–48

Smith J W, Rogers R E, Katz B P 1987 Diagnosis of Chlamydial infection in women attending antenatal and gynecologic clinics. Journal of Clinical Microbiology 25: 868–872

Soren K, Willis E 1989 Chlamydia and the adolescent girl. The enzyme immunoassay as a screening tool. American Journal of Diseases of Children 143: 51–54

Stamm W E 1988 Diagnosis of Chlamydia trachomatis genitourinary infections. Annals of Internal Medicine 108: 710–717

Stamm WE, Cole B 1986 Asymptomatic Chlamydia trachomatis urethritis in men. Sexually Transmitted Diseases 13: 163–165

Stamm W E, Suchland R 1986 Antimicrobial activity of U–70138F (paldimycin), roxithromycin (RU965), and ofloxacin (ORF18489) against Chlamydia trachomatis in cell culture. Antimicrobial Agents and Chemotherapy 30: 806–807

Stamm W E, Koutsky L A, Benedetti J K, Jourden J L, Brunham R C, Holmes K K 1984 Chlamydia trachomatis urethral infections in men. Annals of Internal Medicine 100: 47–51

Stary A, Kopp W, Gebhart W, Söltz-Szöts J 1985 Culture versus direct specimen test: comparative study of infections with Chlamydia trachomatis in Viennese prostitutes. Genitourinary Medicine 61: 258–260

Stenberg K, Mårdh P-A 1986 Persistent neonatal chlamydial infection in a 6-year-old girl. Lancet ii: 1278–1279

Stephens R S, Inouye C J, Wagar E A 1986 A species-specific major outer membrane domain. In: Oriel D et al (eds) Chlamydial infections. Cambridge University Press, Cambridge pp 110–113

Stephens R S, Sanchez-Pescador R, Wagar E A, Inouye C, Urdea M S 1987 Diversity of Chlamydia trachomatis major outer membrane protein genes. Journal of Bacteriology 169: 3879–3885

Stephens R S, Wagar E A, Schoolnik G K 1988 High-resolution mapping of serovar-specific and common antigenic determinants of the major outer membrane protein of Chlamydia trachomatis. Journal of Experimental Medicine 167: 817–831

Storey C C, Mearns G, Richmond S J 1987 Immune dot blot technique for diagnosing infection with Chlamydia trachomatis. Genitourinary Medicine 63: 375–379

Su H, Zhang Y-X, Barrera O et al 1988 Differential effect of trypsin on infectivity of Chlamydia trachomatis: loss of infectivity requires cleavage of major outer membrane protein variable domains II and IV. Infection and Immunity 56: 2094

Sulaiman M Z C, Foster J, Pugh S F 1987 Prevalence of Chlamydia trachomatis infection in homosexual men. Genitourinary Medicine 63: 179–181

Svensson L, Mårdh P-A, Ahlgren M, Nordenskjöld F 1985 Ectopic pregnancy and antibodies to Chlamydia trachomatis. Fertility and Sterility 44: 313–317

Sweet R L 1986 Pelvic inflammatory disease. Sexually Transmitted Diseases 13 (Suppl): 192–198

Sweet R L, Blankfort-Doyle M, Robbie M O, Schachter J 1986 The occurrence of chlamydial and gonococcal salpingitis during the menstrual cycle. Journal of the American Medical Association 255: 2062–2064

Sweet R L, Landers D V, Walker C, Schachter J 1987 Chlamydia trachomatis infection and pregnancy outcome. American Journal of Obstetrics and Gynecology 156: 824–833

Swenson C E, Sung M L, Schachter J 1986 The effect of tetracycline treatment on chlamydial salpingitis and subsequent fertility in the mouse. Sexually Transmitted Diseases 13: 40–44

Swinker M L, Young S A, Cleavenger R L, Neely J L, Palmer J E 1988 Prevalence of Chlamydia trachomatis cervical infection in a college gynecology clinic: relationship to other infections and clinical features. Sexually Transmitted Diseases 15: 133–136

Syrjänen K, Mäntyjärvi R, Väyrynen M et al 1986 Coexistent chlamydial infections related to natural history of human papillomavirus lesions in uterine cervix. Genitourinary Medicine 62: 345–351

Taylor-Robinson D 1986 The role of animal models in chlamydial research. In: Oriel D et al (eds) Chlamydial infections. Cambridge University Press, Cambridge. pp 355–366

Taylor-Robinson D 1987a Occult chlamydial ophthalmia in men with non-gonococcal urethritis. British Medical Journal 294: 706–707

Taylor-Robinson D 1987b Infection by airborne Chlamydia trachomatis in a dentist cured with rifampicin after failures with tetracycline and doxycycline. British Medical Journal 294: 1161–1162

Taylor-Robinson D 1989 Detecting Chlamydia trachomatis by direct immunofluorescence using a Cytobrush sampling technique. Genitourinary Medicine 65: 130

Taylor-Robinson D, Thomas B J 1980 The role of Chlamydia trachomatis in genital-tract and associated diseases. Journal of Clinical Pathology 33: 205–233

Taylor-Robinson D, Tuffrey M 1987 Comparison of detection procedures for Chlamydia trachomatis, including enzyme immunoassays, in a mouse model of genital infection. Journal of Medical Microbiology 24: 169–173

Taylor-Robinson D, Ward M E 1989 Immunity to chlamydial infections and the outlook for vaccination. In : Meheus A Spier RE (eds) Vaccines for sexually transmitted diseases. Butterworths, London pp 67–85

Taylor-Robinson D, Thomas B J, Osborn M F 1987 Evaluation of enzyme immunoassay (Chlamydiazyme) for detecting Chlamydia trachomatis in genital tract specimens. Journal of Clinical Pathology 40: 194–199

Taylor-Robinson D, Thomas B J, Dixey J, Osborn M F, Furr P M, Keat A C 1988 Evidence that Chlamydia trachomatis causes seronegative arthritis in women. Annals of Rheumatic Diseases 47: 295–299

Temmerman M, Laga M, Ndynia-Achola J O et al 1988 Microbial aetiology and diagnostic criteria of postpartum endometritis in Nairobi, Kenya. Genitourinary Medicine 64: 172–175

Thomas G D H 1986 Lymphoid reaction in chlamydial endometritis. Journal of Clinical Pathology 39: 464

Thomas B J, Taylor-Robinson D 1988 Limitations of Chlamydiazyme in general hospital laboratories. Journal of Clinical Pathology 41: 357–358

Thomas B J, Evans R T, Hawkins D A, Taylor-Robinson D 1984 Sensitivity of detecting Chlamydia trachomatis elementary bodies in smears by use of a fluorrescein labelled monoclonal antibody: comparison with conventional chlamydial isolation. Journal of Clinical Pathology 37: 812–816

Thomas B J, Osborn M F, Gilchrist C, Taylor-Robinson D 1989 Improved sensitivity of an enzyme immunoassay IDEIA for detecting Chlamydia trachomatis. Journal of Clinical Pathology 42: 759–762

Tilton R C, Judson F N, Barnes R C, Gruninger R P, Ryan R W, Steingrimsson O 1988 Multicenter comparative evaluation of two rapid microscopic methods and culture for detection of Chlamydia trachomatis in patient specimens. Journal of Clinical Microbiology 26: 167–170

Tjiam K H, Zeilmaker G H, Alberda A T et al 1985 Prevalence of antibodies to Chlamydia trachomatis, Neisseria gonorrhoeae, and Mycoplasma hominis in infertile women. Genitourinary Medicine 61: 175–178

Tjiam K H, van Heijst B Y M, van Zuuren A et al 1986 Evaluation of an enzyme immunoassay for the diagnosis of chlamydial infection in urogenital specimens. Journal of Clinical Microbiology 23: 752–754

Tjiam K H, van Heijst B Y M, Polak-Vogelzang A A et al 1987 Sexually communicable micro-organisms in human semen samples to be used for artificial insemination by donor. Genitourinary Medicine 63: 116–118

Todd W J, Caldwell H D 1985 The interaction of Chlamydia trachomatis with host cells: ultrastructural studies of the mechanism of release of a biovar II from HeLa 229 cells. Journal of Infectious Diseases 151: 1037–1044

Tomioka E S, Anzai R Y, Kwang W N et al 1987 Endometrial damage in acute salpingitis. Sexually Transmitted Diseases 14: 63–68

Torode H W, Wheeler P A, Saunders D M, Petrie R A, Medcalf S C, Ackerman V A 1987 The role of chlamydial antibodies in an in vitro fertilization program. Fertility and Sterility 48: 987–990

Trachtenberg A I, Washington A E, Halldorson S 1988 A cost-based decision analysis for Chlamydia screening in California family planning clinics. Obstetrics and Gynecology 71: 101–108

Tuffrey M 1988 The contribution of animal models to chlamydial research. In: Proceedings of the European Society for Chlamydial Research, 1st meeting, Bologna. pp 117–120

Tuffrey M, Falder P, Gale J, Quinn R, Taylor-Robinson D 1986 Infertility in mice infected genitally with a human strain of Chlamydia trachomatis. Journal of Reproduction and Fertility 78: 251–260

Tuffrey M, Alexander F, Taylor-Robinson D 1990 Severity of salpingitis in mice after primary and repeated inoculation with a human strain of Chlamydia trachomatis. Journal of Experimental Pathology 71: 403–410

Tullo A B, Richmond S J, Easty D L 1981 The presentation and incidence of paratrachoma in adults. Journal of Hygiene 87: 63–69

Van der Willigen A H, Polak-Vogelzang A A, Habbema L, Wagenvoort J H 1988 Clinical efficacy of ciprofloxacin versus doxycycline in the treatment of non-gonococcal urethritis in males. European Journal of Clinical Microbiology and Infectious Diseases 7: 658–661

Viswalingam M, Goh B T, Mantell J, Treharne J D 1987 Infection by airborne Chlamydia trachomatis. British Medical Journal 295: 119

Wagenvoort J H, Suchland R J, Stamm W E 1988 Serovar distribution of urogenital Chlamydia trachomatis strains in The Netherlands. Genitourinary Medicine 64: 159–161

Walsh M, Kappus E W, Quinn T C 1987 In vitro evaluation of CP-62,993, erythromycin, clindamycin, and tetracycline against Chlamydia trachomatis. Antimicrobial Agents and Chemotherapy 31: 811–812

Walters M D, Eddy C A, Gibbs R S, Schachter J, Holden A E, Pauerstein C J 1988 Antibodies to Chlamydia trachomatis and risk for tubal pregnancy. American Journal of Obstetrics and Gynecology 159: 942–946

Wang S-P, Kuo C-C, Barnes R C, Stephens R S, Grayston J T 1985 Immunotyping of Chlamydia trachomatis with monoclonal antibodies. Journal of Infectious Diseases 152: 791–800

Ward M E 1983 Chlamydial classification, development and structure. British Medical Bulletin 39: 109–115

Ward M E 1986 Outstanding problems in chlamydial cell biology. In: Oriel J D et al (eds) Chlamydial infections. Cambridge University Press, Cambridge. pp 3–14

Ward M E 1988 The chlamydial development cycle. In: Barron A L (ed) Microbiology of Chlamydia, CRC Press, Baton Rouge, Florida. pp 71–95

Washington A E, Johnson R E, Sanders L L 1987 Chlamydia trachomatis infections in the United States. What are they costing us? Journal of the American Medical Association 257: 2070–2072

Wasserheit J N, Bell T A, Kiviat N B et al 1986 Microbial causes of proven pelvic inflammatory disease and efficacy of clindamycin and tobramycin. Annals of Internal Medicine 104: 187–193

Watkins N G, Caldwell H D 1986 Delayed hypersensitivity as a pathogenic mechanism in chlamydial disease. In: Oriel D et al (eds) Chlamydial infections. Cambridge University Press, Cambridge. pp 408–411

Weidner W, Schiefer H G, Krauss H 1988 Role of Chlamydia trachomatis and mycoplasmas in chronic prostatitis. A review. Urologia Internationalis 43: 167–173

Weiland T L, Noller K L, Smith T F, Ory S J 1988 Comparison of Dacron-tipped applicator and cytobrush for detection of chlamydial infections. Journal of Clinical Microbiology 26: 2437–2438

Weismeier E, Bruckner D A, Malotte C K, Manduke L 1988 Enzyme-linked immunosorbent assays in the detection of Chlamydia trachomatis: how valid are they? Diagnostic Microbiology and Infectious Disease 9: 219–223

Wenman W M, Meuser R U 1986 Chlamydia trachomatis elementary bodies possess proteins which bind to eucaryotic cell membranes. Journal of Bacteriology 165: 602–607

Weström L, Mårdh P-A 1983 Chlamydial salpingitis. British Medical Bulletin 39: 145–150

Whittum-Hudson J A, Prendergast R A, Taylor H R 1986 Effects of oral preimmunization on chlamydial eye infection. In: Oriel D et al (eds) Chlamydial infections. Cambridge University Press, Cambridge. pp 469–472

Williams T, Maniar A C, Brunham R C, Hammond G W 1985 Identification of Chlamydia trachomatis by direct immunofluorescence applied in specimens originating in remote areas. Journal of Clinical Microbiology 22: 1053–1054

Wise R, Ashby J P, Andrews J M 1988 In vitro activity of PD 127,391, an enhanced-spectrum quinolone. Antimicrobial Agents and Chemotherapy 32: 1251–1256

Wølner-Hanssen P, Patton D L, Stamm W E, Holmes K K 1986 Severe salpingitis in pig-tailed macaques after repeated cervical infections followed by a single tubal inoculation with Chlamydia trachomatis. In: Oriel D et al (eds) Chlamydial infections. Cambridge University Press, Cambridge. pp 371–374

Wølner-Hanssen P, Paavonen J, Kiviat N et al 1988 Ambulatory treatment of suspected pelvic inflammatory disease with Augmentin, with or without doxycycline. American Journal of

Obstetrics and Gynecology 158: 577–579

Woodland R M, Kirton R P, Darougar S 1987 Sensitivity of mitomycin C treated McCoy cells for isolation of Chlamydia trachomatis from genital specimens. European Journal of Clinical Microbiology and Infectious Diseases 6: 653–656

Worm A-M, Petersen C A 1987 Transmission of chlamydial infections to sexual partners. Genitourinary Medicine 63: 19–21

Worm A-M, Hoff G, Kroon S, Petersen C S, Christensen J J 1989 Roxithromycin compared with erythromycin against genitourinary chlamydial infections. Genitourinary Medicine 65: 35–38

Wreghitt T G, Robinson V J, Caul E O, Paul I D, Gatley S 1988 The development and evaluation of a μ-capture ELISA detecting chlamydia-specific IgM. Epidemiology and Infection 101: 387–395

Yearsley P J, Treharne J D, Ballard R C 1988 Emergence of resistance to rifampicin and rifabutin in C. trachomatis. In: Proceedings of the European Society for Chlamydial Research, 1st Meeting, Bologna. p 284

Yong D C T, Paul N R 1986 Micro direct inoculation method for the isolation and identification of Chlamydia trachomatis. Journal of Clinical Microbiology 23: 536–538

Yuan Y, Zhang Y-X, Watkins N G, Caldwell H D 1989 Nucleotide and deduced amino acid sequences for the four variable domains of the major outer membrane proteins of the 15 Chlamydia trachomatis serovars. Infection and Immunity 57: 1040–1049

Zdrodowska-Stefanow B, Manikowska-Lesinska W 1988 Epidemiologic and clinical studies of Chlamydia trachomatis infection in Northeastern Poland. Sexually Transmitted Diseases 15: 137–140

Zhang Y-X, Stewart S, Joseph T, Taylor H R, Caldwell H D 1987a Protective monoclonal antibodies recognize epitopes located on the major outer membrane protein of Chlamydia trachomatis. Journal of Immunology 138: 575–581

Zhang Y-X, Watkins N G, Stewart S, Caldwell H D 1987b The low-molecular-mass, cysteine-rich outer membrane protein of Chlamydia trachomatis possesses both biovar- and species-specific epitopes. Infection and Immunity 55: 2570–2573

Zhong G M, Peterson E M, Czarniecki C W, Schreiber R D, de la Maza L M 1989 Role of endogenous gamma interferon in host defence against Chlamydia trachomatis infections. Infection and Immunity 57: 152–157

Zurenko G E, Yagi B H, Vavra J J, Wentworth B B 1988 In vitro antibacterial activity of trospectomycin (U-63366F), a novel spectinomycin analog. Antimicrobial Agents and Chemotherapy 32: 216–223

Zvillich M, Sarov I 1989 The persistence of Chlamydia trachomatis elementary body cell walls in human polymorphonuclear leucocytes and induction of a chemiluminescent response. Journal of General Microbiology 135: 95–104

# Index

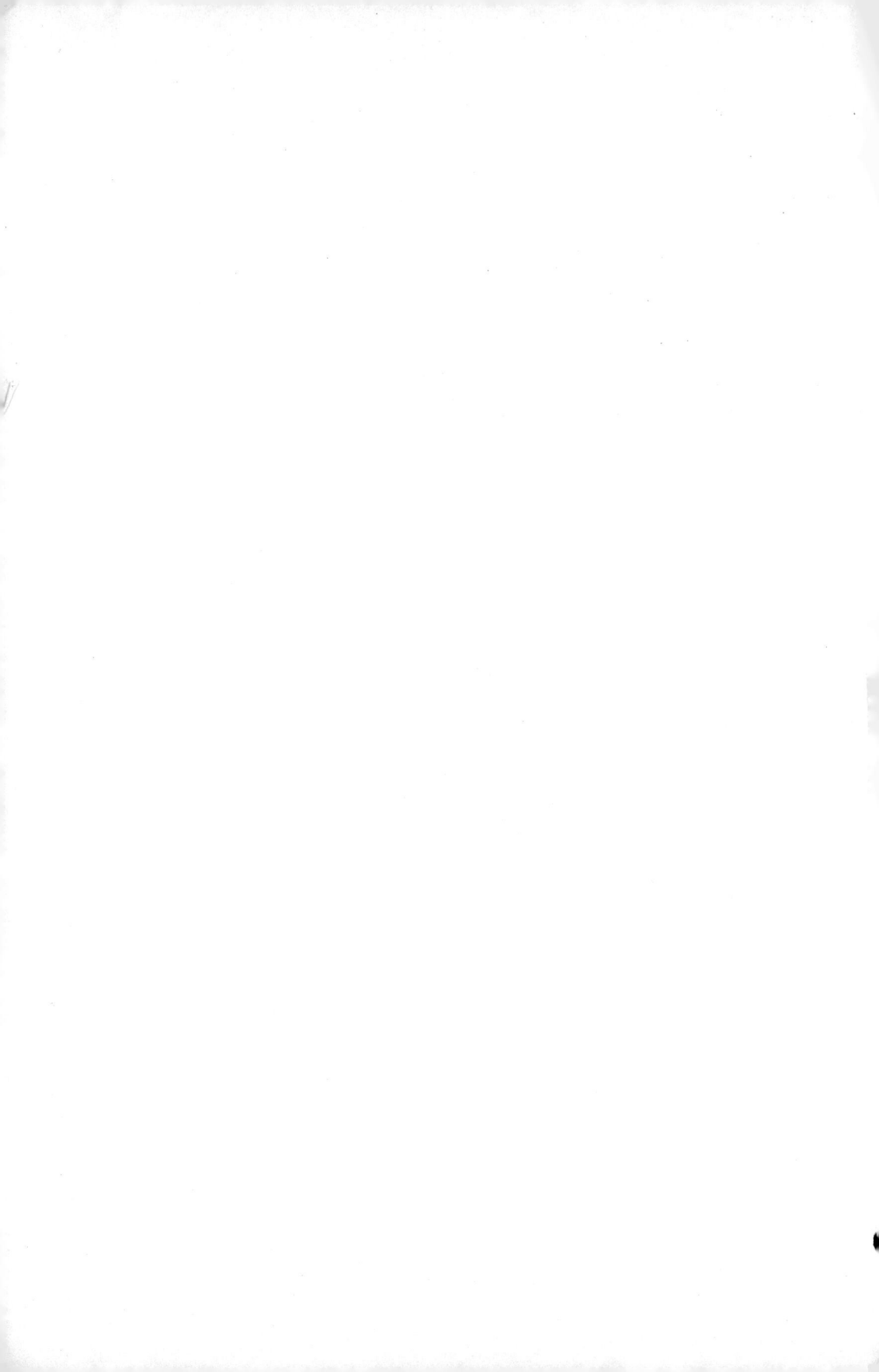